Contents

Acknowledgements

We wish to express our thanks to our husbands and children, Ken, David and Michael Ward, and David, Edward and Annabel Cartwright, and our families and friends for their patience, support and encouragement whilst researching and writing this book.

Special thanks go to Zaf Ansari (Profile Aesthetics), Judy Naake (Beauty Source) and Kim Dainty (Warwickshire College) for work used in this book. Thanks also go to: Rod Fabes, Angela Barbagelata Fabes and Christophe Barbagelata (Carlton Professional); Laurence Green (Ellisons); Sean Harrington (Steiners); Christina Jenkins and Bernadette Fava (Matis); Simon Grogan (Cosmetronic); Jayne Lewis-Orr and Moira Paulusz (Health & Beauty Salon); Kate Jenkins (Beauty Express); Gerri Moore (VTCT); Vanessa Puttick (The Hairdressing & Beauty Equipment Centre); Mark Maloney (Professional Beauty); Thomas Scholz (Balnea); Eve Taylor (Institute of Clinical Aromatherapy); John Birtwistle (Silhoutte); Deborah Hale (Forest Mere Health Farm); Richard Warden (Helionova); Sharon Curtis (The International Dermal Institute); Hilary Allison, Andrea Freeman, Joanne Latham and Pam Snape (Warwickshire College); and to Delvis Bona, Pam Baddersley, Val Cooke, Chris Elliot, Sheila Godfrey, Pedro Lopes, Heather Lulham-Robinson, Rita Roberts, Gaye Wensley and Jean Worth for their technical assistance.

Acknowledgements and thanks are due to Lyn Goldberg, author of *Massage and Aromatherapy*, for work reproduced in Chapter 1 of this book.

We are grateful to our colleagues in the beauty industry, in particular the companies that have kindly allowed us to reproduce photographs:

AIM International School, Bangkok, Thailand p.218 (bottom)
Balnea p.162
BelleSante (UK) Ltd p.109
CACI p.107
Caplin Naake Associates pp.249, 292
Carlton Professional pp.30, 112, 113, 116, 117, 121. 144, 163, 187, 188, 191, 192, 383
Chiva Som International Health Resort, Thailand pp.171, 177
Chubb Fire p.306
Clynol p.243
Cosmetronic (UK) Ltd pp.5, 142, 147, 193
Elemis UK Ltd p.289
Endolite UK p.190
Forest Mere Health Farm pp.167, 173
Helionova Ltd p.218 (top)
Martin Sookias pp.11, 40, 44, 45, 48, 49, 307
Matis p.253
Pat Shirreff-Thomas, Ovation Productions, London p.303
Photodisc 75 (NT) p.241
Profile UK pp.221, 222, 230
Rita Roberts p.236
Silhouette International p.146
Steiners Training Ltd pp.284, 303
St Tropez pp.198, 199, 200, 203, 206, 210, 292
The Hairdressing and Beauty Equipment Centre pp.126, 195, 248
Ultratone Bodyshapters p.132
Vibrosaun p.157.

3rd edition

Health and Beauty Therapy

A Practical Approach for NVQ Level 3

Dawn Mernagh-Ward

Jennifer Cartwright

Published in 2004 by:
Nelson Thornes Ltd
Delta Place
27 Bath Road
CHELTENHAM
GL53 7TH
United Kingdom

04 05 06 07 08 / 10 9 8 7 6 5 4 3 2 1

A catalogue record for this book is available from the British Library

ISBN 0 7487 9035 7

Illustrations by Angela Lumley
Page make-up by Florence Production Ltd, Stoodleigh, Devon

Printed in Croatia by Zrinski

Introduction

A career in therapies has never been more exciting as public awareness and interest in the health and beauty sector has grown phenomenally over the past few years. There appears to be no slowing down in the fastest growing industry sector. It is now far more acceptable to acknowledge 'me time', which has generated a huge demand in stress-related services and treatments. The traditional beauty salon has changed to the 'day spa' to meet the changing market, and the range and breadth of treatments includes holistic approaches, manual and electrotherapy treatments for skin and body improvement, and a vast array of water-based and specialist treatments. Hotels have identified this growing trend in leisure time and have introduced spa facilities to maximise their business potential. Clients are travelling worldwide and wanting to recapture eastern techniques and treatments back home. Training today has to reflect these worldwide treatments and standards; we have to continue to learn from each other to afford our clients the best possible service and advice. It is, however, a very challenging profession due to the fact that by its nature it is a caring industry, requiring a great deal of sympathy, empathy and understanding from the therapist. The range and breadth of the skills and knowledge covered are vast and it is essential that the therapist remembers that they will continue to learn new skills and further enhance existing ones throughout their career. Opportunities for the therapist expand every year, particularly as advancements in technology and travel have made the world a much smaller place.

Health and Beauty Therapy: A Practical Approach for NVQ Level 3, 3rd edition, is intended as a guide for learners studying any of the paths in the NVQ level 3 or internationally-recognised Beauty Therapy qualifications. The integration of the essential key skills – communication, application of numbers and working with others – needed to work within the health and beauty sector are covered within this book and *Good Practice in Salon Management*. They are linked to the beauty therapy curriculum through reception, stock control, dispensing products, costing treatments, working with others and liaising with clients and visitors. Lecturers can map the three main key skills – communication, application of numbers and information technology (IT) – to these areas by setting assignments. The lecturer must ensure that the appropriate level of key skill is matched and that IT can be used to display graphs and charts of measurement and study produced by the individual student. For example, the findings from a stock control, the day's client profiles, or monies taken on treatment and retail services could all be displayed in pie charts. It must be remembered that there is a requirement for uniqueness of portfolios, therefore assignment work must reflect this, perhaps by setting one research assignment in purchasing, equipping and planning the opening of a new salon. This would give a great deal of scope for individualism as well as matching the majority of key skill requirements.

This book is also a useful reference book for beauty therapy examinations offered by CIBTAC, CIDESCO, C&G, Edexcel, ITEC, NOCN, NCFE, OCR and VTCT.

It will also assist in updating qualified therapists, especially those who work on their own.

We have had fantastic, exciting and worthwhile careers in beauty therapy and we hope that you will find this book a useful vehicle whilst studying and working in the best profession in the world.

Wishing you success and happiness in your future careers

Dawn Mernagh-Ward

Jennifer Cartwright

Dedication

This third edition is dedicated to our parents, John and Mary Mernagh, Valerie Peake, and to the memory of Roy Peake, for their love, support and guidance throughout our lives. They inspired us to be confident and believe that we would be successful and fulfil our dreams and ambitions.

We would also like to recognise the inspirational figures who have influenced and shaped our careers. These include: Wallace Sharpes, Heather Mole and Gerri Moore (VTCT); Jean Worth, Eve Taylor and Elisabeth Peet (BABTAC, part Chairpersons); Jo Wackett (CIDESCO/Steiners); Ritta Salmi (CIDESCO, past President); William Arnould-Taylor (ITEC, founder); Rod Fabes (Carlton Professional); Lynnette Wright, Pam Linforth, Margaret Philpott, Lesley Parkes, Penny Turvey and Helena Bielecka-McElroy (tutors/lecturers); Mike Bates (Birmingham College of Food, former Head of Department); Eddie McIntyre (BCFTCS, Principal); Ioan Morgan (Warwickshire College, Principal); Doc Slattery (uncle and mentor).

Mapping grid

Unit number	Chapter
G1 Ensure your own actions reduce risks to health and safety	5 Facial and body electrotherapy treatments 9 Reception, stock control and health and safety 10 The business environment and related salon administration 11 Related business legislation
G6 Promote additional products or services to clients	9 Reception, stock control and health and safety 10 The business environment and related salon administration
G11 Contribute to the financial effectiveness of the business	9 Reception, stock control and health and safety 10 The business environment and related salon administration
BT16 Epilate the hair follicle using diathermy, galvanic and blend techniques	4 Electro-epilation 9 Reception, stock control and health and safety 11 Related business legislation 12 Anatomy and physiology 13 Elementary science
BT17 Provide head and body massage treatments	1 Head and body massage 5 Facial and body electrotherapy treatments 9 Reception, stock control and health and safety 11 Related business legislation 12 Anatomy and physiology 14 Elementary diet and exercise
BT18 Improve body condition using electro-therapy	5 Facial and body electrotherapy treatments 9 Reception, stock control and health and safety 11 Related business legislation 12 Anatomy and physiology 13 Elementary science 14 Elementary diet and exercise
BT19 Improve face and skin condition using electro-therapy	5 Facial and body electrotherapy treatments 9 Reception, stock control and health and safety 11 Related business legislation 12 Anatomy and physiology 13 Elementary science 14 Elementary diet and exercise
BT20 Provide Indian Head Massage treatment	2 Indian head massage 9 Reception, stock control and health and safety 11 Related business legislation 12 Anatomy and physiology
BT21 Provide massage using pre-blended aromatherapy oils	3 Aromatherapy 9 Reception, stock control and health and safety 11 Related business legislation 12 Anatomy and physiology 14 Elementary diet and exercise

BT26 Enhance appearance using cosmetic camouflage	8 Make-up 9 Reception, stock control and health and safety 11 Related business legislation 12 Anatomy and physiology
BT27 Design and create images for fashion and photographic make-up	8 Make-up 9 Reception, stock control and health and safety 11 Related business legislation 12 Anatomy and physiology
BT28 Set up, monitor and shut down water, temperature and spa facilities	6 Spa and specialised treatments 9 Reception, stock control and health and safety 11 Related business legislation 13 Elementary science
BT29 Provide specialist spa treatments	6 Spa and specialised treatments 9 Reception, stock control and health and safety 11 Related business legislation 12 Anatomy and physiology 13 Elementary science
BT30 Provide UV tanning treatments	7 Tanning and light treatments 9 Reception, stock control and health and safety 11 Related business legislation 13 Elementary science
BT31 Provide self tanning treatments	7 Tanning and light treatments 9 Reception, stock control and health and safety 11 Related business legislation
BT36 Improve the appearance of the skin using micro-dermabrasion	5 Facial and body electrotherapy treatments 9 Reception, stock control and health and safety 11 Related business legislation 12 Anatomy and physiology 13 Elementary science
G12 Check how successful your business idea will be	10 The business environment and related salon administration 11 Related business legislation
G13 Check what law and other regulations will affect your business	10 The business environment and related salon administration 11 Related business legislation

This book does not include the following specialist optional units

BT23 Maintain, repair and enhance artificial nail structures

BT24 Plan, design and provide nail art services to clients

BT25 Design and create images incorporating nail art techniques

BT32 Prepare to change the performer's appearance

BT33 Assist with the continuity of the performer's appearance

BT34 Apply make-up to change the performer's appearance

BT35 Apply special effects

Chapter 1

Head and body massage

After working through this chapter you will be able to:

- explain the equipment required for massage
- describe how a welcoming environment can be created for a client having a body massage
- list the contraindications to massage
- name the main massage movements and their effects on the body
- describe the effects of massage
- perform an effective massage treatment for a range of clients including: male, female, apprehensive, for stress and relaxation, muscular aches and pains, weight loss, poor muscle tone and for a variety of times, e.g. 1 hour, 30 minutes
- identify different types of massage.

Introduction

Massage is much more than just manipulation of soft body tissue; it has deep psychological implications. Records show that ancient civilisations practised massage in varying forms before medicine was developed.

Our earliest childhood memories of when we were injured are of adults insisting on 'rubbing' it better. Hippocrates, who is regarded as the father of modern medicine, made reference to the benefit of physicians being able to rub and knead.

So it can be seen that massage has firmly established itself as a therapeutic treatment and one which enjoys rediscovered popularity in our stress-laden times.

Over the last decade, massage therapy has expanded greatly. It is widely practised as a specialist field but is also offered by beauty therapists in salons, health spas, leisure centres, etc. One of the main benefits the therapist can offer the client is relaxation to release the stress that can lead to aches and pains, postural problems, and physical and emotional illness.

Every client from the high-powered executive to the busy houseperson will suffer with stress at some time, if not for a large part of their life, whether through day-to-day problems encountered at work, in their social life or through a particular crisis. Stress can cause physical and emotional illness and therefore it is paramount that the therapist truly considers each client as an individual and views information gathered in the consultation to establish a full picture of that individual client.

A professional massage can be extremely exhausting both physically and emotionally for the therapist as they are not just laying on hands but giving of themselves. The majority of massage therapists ensure that they have booked sufficient time between each client to gather themselves and focus on the next person.

The consultation period spent with each client is highly important, it gives the therapist and client an opportunity to establish a professional bond and it enables the therapist to assess the individual clients' needs. On average the therapist would allow approximately 10 minutes at the first appointment and thereafter a minimum of 5 minutes should be taken prior to the massage to assess the client's reaction to the previous treatment and to establish their individual needs for this treatment.

Throughout the world, trainee therapists may learn different European massage routines depending on their individual tutor. When a trainee commences a massage programme, the instructor will design an introductory massage routine lasting 1 hour, which will encompass the classical massage movements to cover the whole of a female body. This form of massage predominantly affects the muscular and circulatory systems and is seen as a starting point to introduce the trainee to massage and develop their:

- manual dexterity and postural stance
- understanding of rate, rhythm, pressure and contact
- understanding of the classical massage movements and their benefits
- communication, organisation and management skills
- ability to analyse the individual's needs.

From the commencement of their training until the day they decide to stop practising and learning, the therapist will broaden their knowledge and technical skills by:

- observing various techniques by different instructors
- observing technical representatives from product companies
- observing fellow therapists in the industry
- watching demonstrations at beauty exhibitions
- receiving treatment from other therapists
- reading textbooks on massage.

Once a trainee has learnt an introductory massage routine, mastering the correct posture, stance, rhythm, rate, pressure and client care, they will be encouraged to adapt their massage by drawing on their instructors' and other trainees' knowledge to suit the individual client's needs, e.g. male client massage is generally much firmer; clients suffering from stress in the upper back may prefer the time they have booked to be spent concentrating on this area.

Classification of massage movements and their effects on the body

Massage movements are generally divided into five main categories: effleurage, petrissage, tapotement, frictions and vibrations.

Effleurage

Effleurage can be defined as a stroking movement in the direction of venous return involving the passage of the hand or part of the hand over the skin. The hand should be moulded to the area being treated and the fingers and thumbs should be kept together. It is important that the pressure is constant and even throughout the movement. The pressure will vary depending on the area being treated; therefore effleurage movements can be subdivided into two forms.

Superficial stroking

As the name suggests, superficial stroking is performed using very light pressure. The hand should be flexible and under perfect control so that the entire palmar surface is in contact with the area being massaged.

Deep stroking

Deep stroking refers to the depth of pressure on the tissues rather than the use of force. Again the movement is performed using the entire palmar surface of the hand, but a greater depth of pressure is applied. The return stroke should be of a superficial nature, otherwise it may reverse some of the effects achieved, e.g. return of venous circulation and lymph.

The beneficial effects of effleurage

- Aids venous circulation and return to the heart by the mechanical effect on the tissues.
- Aids lymphatic circulation by the mechanical effects on the tissues.
- Speeds the absorption of waste materials.
- Promotes relaxation by the reflex effect on the tissues.
- Enables the client to become accustomed to the therapist's hands.

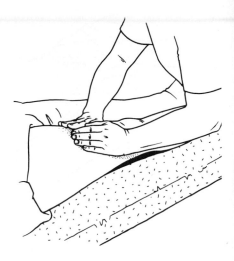

Deep effleurage

Petrissage

Petrissage can be defined as pressure and/or relaxing of pressure. The movements consist of repeatedly grasping and releasing the tissues with one or both hands in a lifting, rolling or pressing fashion. Petrissage movements are often named according to the part of the hand used and include palmar kneading, palmar lifting, wringing, thumb kneading, finger kneading, skin rolling and picking up.

Although the pressure is intermittent, care must be taken to avoid pinching the skin. This is prevented by gently relaxing the pressure as the bulk of the tissues diminishes.

The beneficial effects of petrissage

- Aids venous circulation.
- Increases lymphatic flow.
- Improves absorption of substances within the tissues.
- Loosens adherent tissues.
- Moves the tissues over bone.

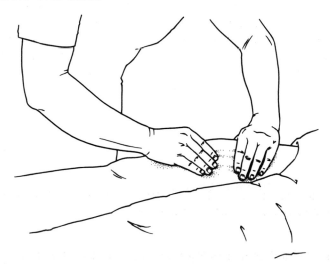

Petrissage

Tapotement

Tapotement movements are sometimes defined as percussion-type movements which can be light tapping to beating movements applied in a brisk fashion. The whole hand or part of the hand can be used depending on the type of tapotement movement being given.

Tapotement movements include:

- Tapping – using the fingertips only.
- Hacking – using the ulnar border of the hands.
- Cupping – using the fingers and palms of the hands in a concave position.
- Pounding – using the ulnar border of a lightly clenched fist.
- Beating – using lightly clenched fists palms down.

The beneficial effects of tapotement

- Very stimulating – causes erythema.
- Produces localised heat.
- Stimulates muscle fibres.
- Increases cellular activity.

Frictions

Frictions are normally performed with either the palms, the fingers or the thumbs. The superficial tissues are moved over the underlying structures keeping the hand in firm contact whilst performing small circular movements in a restricted area before gliding on to the next part. The movement is applied in a direction which produces tension on the tissues and has a loosening effect. Pressure should not be too firm otherwise bruising may occur.

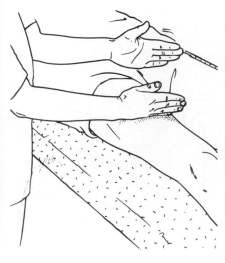

Hacking

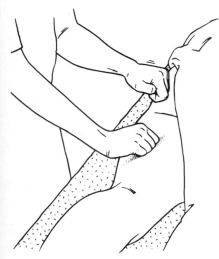

Beating

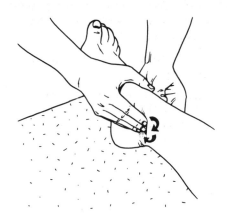

Frictions

The beneficial effects of frictions

- Loosen adherent tissues.
- Greatly increase localised circulation.
- Speed cellular activity.

Vibrations

Vibrations are defined as rapid muscular contractions of the therapist's arms being transmitted through the fingers or palms to produce a highly stimulating, shaking-type movement. Vibrations are normally applied on areas overlying muscular motor points.

The beneficial effects of vibrations

- Increase blood circulation.
- Stimulate localised nerve endings.

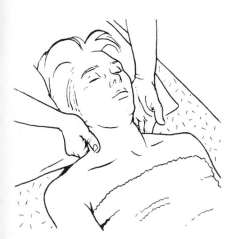

Light vibrations

Preparation for massage

Treatment area

Massage treatment areas vary in appearance depending on the environment in which they are found. Some salons have individual rooms for therapists to work in, designed to allow complete privacy for the client. Others screen the salon into a number of cubicles by using rails and curtains, like those you see in hospitals.

Equipment required for massage
Beauty couches
In order for the massage to be performed, a sturdy, comfortable treatment couch of the correct height for the individual therapist is needed. There are a wide variety of couches available for the therapist or salon owner to choose from.

A general purpose massage or treatment couch with an adjustable back support is available in standard heights. They can be purchased with a 'breathe hole' (which can be removed when performing back and neck massage) to allow the client to breathe easily. A face cushion can also be purchased and used where the couch does not have a breathe hole or when the therapist or client feels the need to use one to aid comfort during the treatment.

A multi-purpose couch/chair is available in standard heights. It enables the therapist to convert the couch from a massage plinth to a couch suitable for facial treatments by lifting and lowering the client's legs for comfort and raising the back support.

Adjustable-height couches have been developed over recent years to enhance the working life of the therapist as they can be adjusted to suit the height of the individual and/or the particular treatment they are performing.

There is a wide selection of adjustable-height couches/chairs and they are very useful. Their versatility is an important factor when different height therapists work from the same room, as for example in massaging or waxing, and where a treatment room is multi-functional and used for body and face treatments. The height-adjustable chair/couch is especially recommended for body wrapping treatments when client mobility is restricted and lower bed height is advantageous.

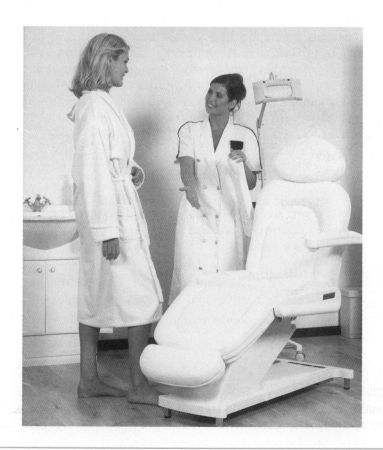

Electrically-operated beauty couch

The heavy-duty hydraulic height-adjustable bed or chair/couch will have a central hydraulic pump, operated by the foot to adjust plinth height – the usual range being about 18–20 cm. On some models the head and leg sections are raised and lowered with either a gas strut-assisted mechanism or a foot-operated hydraulic system.

The heavy-duty electrically-operated hydraulic bed or chair/couch is considered to be the present top-of-the range choice. It has all the advantages of the standard hydraulic operation but can also have the additional advantages of a greater height range (up to 50 cm), often leg and head sections that are operated electronically, and for a chair/couch model it is also possible to have an electronic tilt to the mid-section for greater client comfort. Wheels and brakes to the base frame are often standard and are advantageous as they afford easy positioning around a room and cleaning of the floor area.

It is important to note that hydraulic couches:

- Protect therapists and employees from possible postural problems due to the use of couches of incorrect height and thus enable the therapist to perform a treatment more accurately.
- Enable a variety of therapists of differing heights to perform different treatments in the same treatment area.

Prior to the client's arrival the therapist or their assistant should ensure the couch is covered with clean linen, towels and/or blankets depending upon the salon policy or the client's preference. The couch may be covered with paper towels to maintain hygienic conditions, protect the linen and reduce laundry bills. Pillows or rolled towels should be available for client comfort throughout the treatment.

Couch steps

Couch steps are available to assist clients who are particularly small or who for medical reasons have difficulty getting onto the general purpose non-hydraulic couch. They should be used with care and always with the therapist in attendance.

Beauty chairs (stools)

As part of some massage treatments, the therapist may need to sit to ensure they are able to apply the appropriate pressure and at the same time protect their own posture. Therefore an operator's chair or stool should be in the treatment area. Two important things to note with this piece of furniture are that it should have well-oiled castors to allow the therapist to manoeuvre into different positions smoothly and prevent any unnecessary noise and that it should be adjusted correctly to suit the height of the therapist.

It is important to observe general safety in the treatment area by ensuring the chair or stool is safely stored to prevent any accidents.

Beauty trolleys

Most therapists use a sturdy trolley with easy-moving castors to hold the products and materials needed to perform a massage. Some holistic therapists may use a convenient surface such as a table rather than a traditional trolley to lessen the clinical aspect of massage.

Whatever surface is being used it is essential that it is cleaned and prepared with the necessary items before the client arrives and is suited for the purpose.

First impressions count, so it is essential that the therapist and treatment area are well prepared for each client.

ACTIVITY

Research the variety of massage equipment available. Draw up a chart detailing cost, durability and features of each piece of equipment.

The therapist

To establish a professional ethos, the therapist should take great care of his or her appearance and personal hygiene, particularly for massage treatments where they will be working in close contact with their clients.

They should always note the following:

- A high standard of personal hygiene should be observed at all times.
- Professional dress should be worn in the salon environment. It should be non-restrictive, clean and pressed.
- Items required to ensure personal hygiene can be maintained throughout the day should be kept in the therapist's locker, e.g. soap, towel, deodorant, a change of clothes, toothbrush and toothpaste.
- Hair should be clean and well groomed. Long hair should be styled to prevent it from falling into the client's or therapist's face.
- Comfortable, supportive, low-heeled, closed-in shoes should be worn to prevent poor posture and subsequent back problems.
- Nails should be short, so that they do not disturb the flow of the massage or cause discomfort to the client, and should be unvarnished for hygienic practice and in case of client allergy.
- Jewellery should be removed from the wrists and hands, along with dangling earrings or chains, again to ensure the flow of the massage and so as not to disturb the client's relaxation.
- A calm, relaxed, reassuring therapist is essential for a massage treatment.

Items required for massage

Essential items:

- Massage medium (lubricant).
- Tissues.
- Cotton wool.
- Protection for the client's hair.
- Waste receptacle.

Optional items:

- Eau de cologne (for refreshing client's feet and/or removing oil/cream).
- Hot, damp towels (for removing excess oil/cream).
- Hot, dry towels (for therapeutic purposes).
- Footspray (for refreshing client's feet).

Massage mediums

Traditionally a variety of massage mediums have been used.

Oils

Oil still tends to be the most popular lubricant for body massage as it gives the therapist more 'slip'. The oils selected by today's therapists generally have a base of vegetable or plant oils and may have other active ingredients added to create a particular effect on the body, e.g. lemon (stimulating). Aromatherapy is a specialised massage treatment using essential oils for therapeutic purposes. This can be studied in depth by attending specialised training courses. (See Chapter 3.)

Modern therapists tend not to use mixtures high in mineral oil as these are generally considered to be comedogenic.

Creams

Cream is not a particularly popular medium for a full body massage, though it has been used in the past for spot areas of massage or because of a client's preference. Today you are far more likely to find creams being used as part of a particular manual body treatment for skin improvement, i.e. cellulite or stretch mark treatments.

Talcum powder

Talcum powder tends to be used as a lubricant when an electrotherapy treatment is carried out in conjunction with massage and the client or therapist does not want to use an oil or cream, e.g. during high frequency treatments. Talcum powder is popular with reflexologists as it gives 'slip' to the therapist's hands. It is often believed that greater depth can be achieved by using talcum powder as the massage medium.

In recent years product manufacturers have greatly developed products available for salon massage treatments as well as for complementary home care use. It is more popular to find a salon using one or two product companies' ranges rather than the old-fashioned bulk products of the late twentieth century. One of the main reasons for this has been the huge technological advances of the new millennium, and a great increase in the general public's product knowledge combined with their thirst for improved appearance and health. Therapists have also realised the professional and financial rewards that can be gained from retailing products such as body scrubs and lotions.

ACTIVITY

Research the different professional massage mediums available. Compare their ingredients and costs.

Creating a welcoming environment

As one of the main benefits of massage is relaxation, it is extremely important to create the right environment to enhance the massage treatment. This can be done in a number of ways.

Heating

As the client will be undressed during the massage, it is important to ensure they are kept comfortable.

The room or treatment area may be heated to a higher than normal working temperature prior to the client's arrival and the temperature reduced as necessary throughout the treatment.

Blankets can be used to wrap the client up snugly.

Towels can be warmed over a radiator or in a tumble drier and placed on the couch for the client or over the area that has just been worked on, particularly on cold, damp, winter days.

Electronically heated under- and over-blankets are now available which offer safe, professional and controllable heating ranges. These add great client comfort-value and gentle sedation is very beneficial for many of the new spa-type salon treatments involving envelopment/cocoon protocols.

Ventilation

A well-ventilated treatment area is essential to prevent cross-infection of communicable diseases. It also ensures that stagnant air, saturated with carbon dioxide due to exhalation from clients and therapists, is removed. A build-up of stale air, containing heat, odours and carbon dioxide, can make the treatment room uninviting and the therapist lethargic, which can affect their work.

Aroma

The treatment area needs to be inviting to the client and one of the ways the therapist can enhance this is by introducing aroma essence into the area. Qualified

information point

- Consideration should be given to the climate, e.g. in hot, humid countries the majority of clients like therapists to work in cool, air-conditioned rooms and to use cold (iced) towels on the areas that have been treated.
- Consideration should be given to the client's needs. Some people feel the cold more than others, e.g. in warm weather one client may not want to be wrapped up snugly in blankets and warm towels whereas another may prefer it.

aromatherapists use essential oils for treatment and this obviously can create a pleasant smell in the treatment area. As no two clients are alike, the therapist must ensure that they know their client's likes and dislikes in smells. The introduction of a smell the client dislikes will automatically prevent the client from relaxing and returning for further treatment.

Recently, a number of manufacturers have developed a small piece of equipment, a diffuser, which is used to introduce aromas into the atmosphere. Aromatherapy burners may also be used to further enhance the environment.

Aroma diffuser

Colour

When planning a treatment area of a salon, the therapist should spend a great deal of time considering the decor (wall and floor coverings, towels, etc.) to ensure they create the right sort of environment for their clients. Generally therapists select warm colours, e.g. pinks, oranges and yellows, or relaxing colours, e.g. greens. The type of client plays a large role in selection of colour schemes, e.g. sports therapists may select white as a clinical colour and a beauty salon with mixed gender clients would generally avoid what are considered by some people to be feminine colours, e.g. pinks.

Colour used in a superficial form, such as in decor, towels and lighting, can contribute to a client's relaxation and should therefore be considered by the therapist when preparing the treatment area.

In recent years colour therapists have undertaken a great deal of research not only into the therapeutic effects of colour but into the use of light to heal (chromatherapy).

Lighting

Ideally the lighting of the treatment area for massage should be soft to induce relaxation. The use of strong bright lights can be very distracting to clients.

Chromatic light therapy (using the pure colours of the visible light spectrum, see page 212) is used to help improve problem skin conditions and promote good body equilibrium.

Sound

The therapist can perform the massage in a tranquil area and/or they may wish to complement the treatment (with the client's agreement) with therapeutic music to aid relaxation. Some therapists retail taped music to clients who need to unwind and relax between treatments.

Health, safety, legislation and local bye-laws

Health and safety is of paramount importance and should be foremost in the therapist's mind. Therefore the therapist must be aware of certain legislative requirements in order to practise massage therapy. These are:

- The Health and Safety at Work Act 1974.
- The Office, Shops and Railway Premises Act 1963.
- Local government bye-laws relating to massage, e.g. Birmingham City Council Act 1990.
- Public Liability insurance.
- Employers Liability insurance.

(For further information of these legislative requirements and principles of good practice, see Chapter 12.)

information point

Colours are thought to have the following effects:
- Red – motivation and circulation are increased.
- Orange – boosts energy levels.
- Yellow – stimulates mental activity and movement.
- Green – helps to balance nerves and is calming and sedatory.
- Blue – reduces anxiety and tension.
- Violet – deeply relaxing.

ACTIVITY

Through work experience, discuss with your colleagues how different salons have created a welcoming environment.

Massage consultation and assessment

The introduction to massage given in the earlier part of this chapter along with the section in Chapter 9 on consultation highlight the importance of performing a thorough consultation prior to the massage treatment to establish the individual client's needs, their views and preconceived ideas and to develop a professional relationship.

When training in massage therapy, it is important to use a detailed consultation card which acts as a reminder to the trainee therapist to ensure they use all sources of information in order to establish a clear picture of each client. Once qualified, the therapist can purchase professional record cards or design their own for recording consultations and treatment depending upon their environment, e.g. salons offering a variety of treatments may use a multi-purpose record card whereas health centres specialising in alternative therapies may use a specialised record card.

In order to perform an effective consultation the therapist must know what the general effects of massage are, along with the conditions that may prevent the client from having treatment.

The general effects of massage

- Improves blood circulation, therefore hastening the interchange of oxygen, nutrients, carbon dioxide and waste.
- Relieves muscular tension due to removal of waste.
- Increases lymphatic circulation, again hastening the removal of toxins.
- Causes hyperaemia which temporarily increases heat in the area of treatment.
- Helps to soften fatty tissue deposits depending on the movements used.
- Softens and nourishes the skin, depending on the medium chosen.
- Causes slight desquamation, thus improving the skin's texture.
- Skin tone and elasticity are improved.
- Stimulates or soothes the sensory nerve endings, depending on the massage movements used.
- Deeply relaxing – it gives the client a feeling of wellbeing.
- Helps to prevent stress-related disorders.

CONTRAINDICATIONS

to massage
- Skin diseases.
- Infectious skin disorders.
- Vascular conditions – history of thrombosis, severe varicose veins.
- Heart disorders, high/low blood pressure (medical approval should be obtained before giving treatment in these cases).
- Unidentified swellings or lumps.
- Oedema.
- Raised body temperature.
- Burns/sunburn.
- Later stages of pregnancy (avoid abdominal massage once pregnancy is known).

GOOD PRACTICE

- If in doubt about the client's medical condition, refer the client tactfully to their medical practitioner without causing the client concern.
- Do not attempt to diagnose a medical condition.
- Some conditions do not prevent entire treatment, only treatment to specific areas or the omission of certain movements.

Points to note in performing a consultation

On greeting the client, the therapist takes them through to the treatment area to carry out the consultation.

Details taken in the consultation should include:

- General details, e.g. the client's name, address and contact telephone number.
- Medical history details.
- General physical health details.
- Lifestyle details.
- Posture/figure analysis.
- Further salon treatments.
- Retail and home-care advice.

(For further information on the reception of clients and client consultation, see Chapter 10.)

Principles of good massage practice

- Perform a detailed consultation in order to devise the most appropriate form of massage to be given. The consultation is the basis to establish how best to treat the client's needs, i.e. type, duration and frequency of massage. The consultation is also needed to rule out contraindications.
- Maintain good posture throughout massage. The therapist needs to ensure that throughout the massage routine he/she maintains correct postural stance for the movements and area of the body being treated to provide a beneficial treatment for the client and to prevent fatigue of the therapist. When working on the body in a longitudinal direction use walk-standing and when working in a transverse direction use stride-standing.

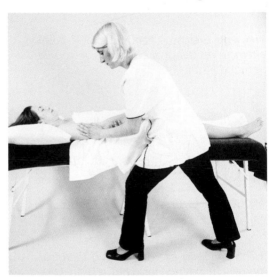

Walk-standing – keeping the back straight, commence effleurage on client's arm, then glide up the arm rocking the body weight forward from heel to toe

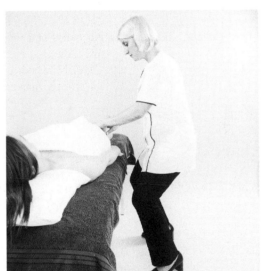

Stride-standing – knees bent, back straight

- Maintain an even rate and rhythm. Massage movements should be gentle, slow and rhythmical – with the exception of tapotement. The acceptable rate of coverage is 18 cm (7 inches) per second and this should remain consistent throughout the massage to give the most beneficial effects.
- Ensure hand flexibility. Manual massage treatment involves the use of the hands for manipulation of body tissues. It is therefore essential that the therapist has complete control of his/her hands in order to mould them to the area being

treated and provide the optimum treatment. When commencing training you should practise simple hand and wrist exercises to increase mobility and flexibility and use these exercises prior to a massage if the hands and arms are not suitably relaxed.

- Adapt pressure according to the area being treated and the individual client's needs. The secret of a successful massage is to vary the pressure for maximum benefit to the client, but without being too heavy as to be uncomfortable or to cause pain or bruising. Pressure should be increased or decreased gradually.
- Always maintain contact with the client during the massage. When changing movements always keep a reassuring hand on the area to avoid breaking continuity of the sequence.

Preparation for treatment

- Ensure the treatment room creates a welcoming environment.
- Ensure the couch is protected appropriately.
- The therapist should present him/herself professionally and ensure their hands are relaxed, ready for treatment.

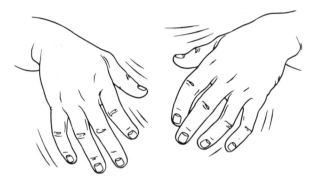

Hand and wrist exercise – loosely shaking hands and wrists

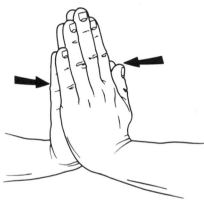

Hand and wrist exercise – hands in prayer position, using alternate resistance push from side to side

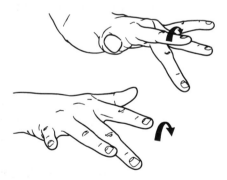

Hand and wrist exercise – rotate each finger and thumb individually in a circular fashion clockwise and anticlockwise

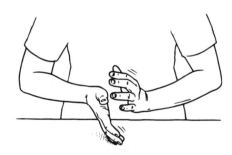

Hand and wrist exercise – using the ulnar borders of both hands, with relaxed fingers and wrists alternately flick the hands lightly onto a hard surface

Massage treatment

1 The client is greeted at reception and taken to the changing area.
2 The consultation is carried out to check for contraindications, to establish the client's needs and to explain the benefits of the treatment.
3 The client or therapist may have selected a heat treatment to relax the muscles ready for massage and this treatment is carried out first.
4 The client relaxes on the couch, and using the selected massage medium the therapist performs a massage routine to benefit the individual client.

5 The client is allowed time to relax and then offered a drink of mineral water. If the client wishes, the oil can be removed, either by the therapist or by showering. (Aromatherapy oil is generally left on the skin.)

SELF-CHECKS

1 State the equipment needed to perform a body massage.

2 List six factors that will contribute towards a welcoming environment.

3 Give six contraindications to massage treatment and explain why each is a contraindication.

4 List the five classical types of massage movement and describe two benefits of each type.

5 State five specific effects of massage.

Introductory massage routine (for a female client)

The client should first be prepared by being asked to undress and put on a clean towelling robe. If possible, it is better to offer a heat treatment before commencing massage to relax the client and warm the body tissues. The heat treatment could be a steam bath, sauna, jacuzzi or even just a warm shower.

In the prepared treatment area, ask the client to remove their gown and get on to the couch lying face upwards (supine), assisting the client and providing couch steps where needed. Then cover the client in clean, warm towels.

Front of leg massage

Preparation

a Remove the towel from the front of the leg area, keeping other parts of the body well covered for warmth.

b Apply the selected massage medium to the area by first warming it on your own hands and then applying it to the client's leg from foot to thigh following the effleurage pattern.

c Ensure your posture is good with a straight back.

Massage sequence

1 **Effleurage to the whole leg**
Place the entire palmar surface of both hands on the dorsal surface of the foot. With one hand leading, keep fingers and thumbs together and glide hands along the entire leg to the top of the thigh. Glide hands apart laterally, lightly returning to ankle.

(Main muscles affected: tibialis anterior, soleus, quadriceps, abductors, adductors.)

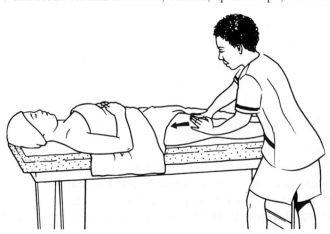

Effleurage to the whole leg

> **information point**
>
> The movements in the introductory massage routine (for a female client) are repeated a number of times to suit an individual client's needs.

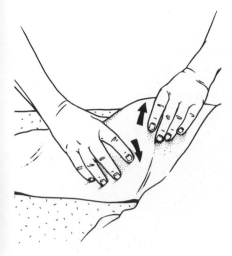

Wringing to the quadriceps

2 **Deep wringing of the quadriceps**

   a Slide hands to the interior aspect of the thigh and then with hands parallel, pick and lift the tissues and squeeze gently in a wringing action. Work the entire quadriceps area.

     (Main muscles affected: quadriceps, abductors, adductors.)

   b Effleurage to the quadriceps area.

3 **Alternate palmar lifting of the quadriceps**

   a Starting with hands on either side at the top of the thigh, use the entire palmar surface of both hands to gently compress the tissues against each other and lift from side to side. Keep repeating until the knee is reached and then slide the hands back up the leg.

     (Main muscles affected: quadriceps, abductors, adductors.)

   b Effleurage to the quadriceps area.

4 **Hacking to the quadriceps**

   a Using the ulnar border of both hands, briskly but lightly hack the quadriceps area in a rhythmical pattern.

     (Main muscles affected: quadriceps, abductors, adductors.)

   b Effleurage to the quadriceps area.

5 **Cupping to the quadriceps**

   a Holding the fingers and palms of the hands in a concave position, briskly but lightly cup the quadriceps area.

     (Main muscles affected: quadriceps, abductors, adductors.)

   b Effleurage to the quadriceps area.

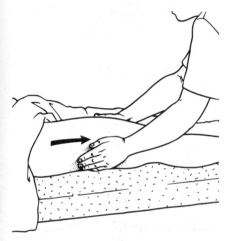

Effleurage to the quadriceps area

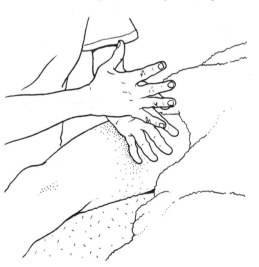

Hacking to the quadriceps

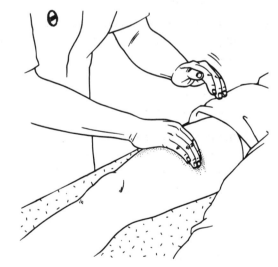

Cupping to the quadriceps

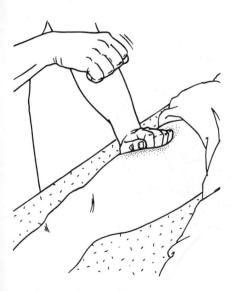

Beating to the quadriceps

6 **Beating to the quadriceps area**

   a Using lightly clenched fists, palms down, lightly beat the quadriceps area.

     (Main muscles affected: quadriceps, abductors, adductors.)

   b Effleurage to the quadriceps.

7 **Thumb friction circles around the patella**

   a Using the thumb digits, gently perform friction circles around the patella.

     (Main muscles affected: tibialis anterior, coleus, quadriceps, abductors, adductors.)

   b Effleurage the whole leg.

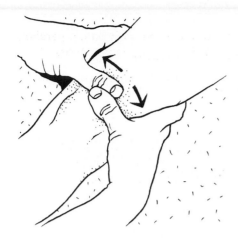

Thumb friction circles around the patella

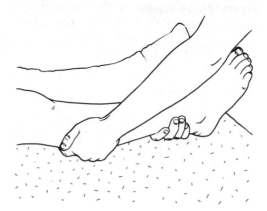

Palmar kneading to the soleus

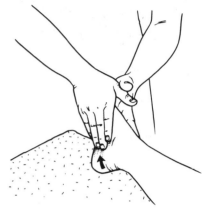

Deep stroking around the ankle malleolus

8 **Palmar kneading to the soleus**
   Using the thenar eminence of the hand (see p. 369) push upwards along the soleus muscle towards the knee. Continue using the thenar eminence of the hand to apply friction circles in a clockwise movement, slowly working down towards the ankle.

   (Main muscle affected: soleus.)

9 **Deep stroking around the ankle malleolus**
   Using the digits of both hands gently stroke around the ankle malleolus.

10 **Friction circles between the metatarsal bones**
   Using the thumbs of both hands apply friction circles between the metatarsal bones.

11 **Toe circles**
   Support the toe joints with one hand underneath the foot and the other on top. Circle hands in a clockwise then anticlockwise direction a number of times.

12 **Scissor friction on the sole of the foot**
   a Using the thumbs of both hands, friction in a scissor pattern down the sole of the foot returning with a deep push back.
   b Effleurage to the whole leg to finish.

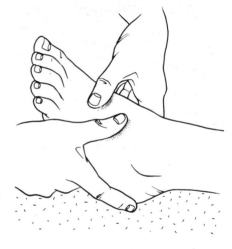

Friction circles between the metatarsals

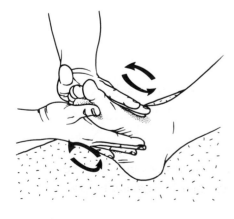

Toe circling

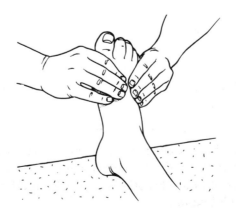

Scissor friction on the sole of the foot

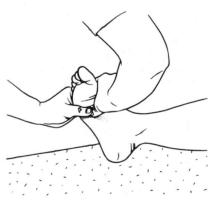

Arm massage

Preparation

a   Ask the client to gently lift her arm out of the towel covering.

b   Apply the selected massage medium to the area using effleurage movements.

Massage sequence

1   **Effleurage to the whole arm**

    Place the entire palmar surface of one hand on the client's wrist and support with the other hand. Glide up the arm, around the deltoid, then lightly return.

    (Main muscles affected: biceps, triceps, brachialis, deltoid.)

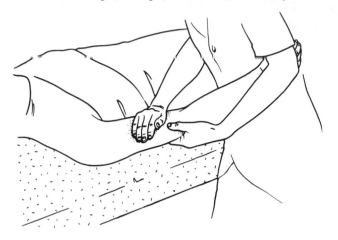

Effleurage to the whole arm

2   **Deep stroking to the deltoids**

    Using the palmar surface of both hands, alternately effleurage around the deltoid area.

    (Main muscle affected: deltoid.)

3   **Wringing and hacking to the biceps and triceps**

    a   Slide hands to the biceps area and with both parallel, pick and lift the tissues and gently squeeze in a wringing action.

    b   Effleurage the area.

    c   Using the ulnar border of both hands, briskly but lightly hack the area in a rhythmical pattern.

    d   Effleurage the area.

    e   Gently rest the client's arm in a crooked position at the side of her head (a towel support may be used under the wrist) and repeat wringing, effleurage and hacking movements to the triceps area.

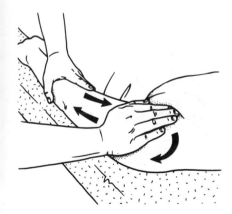

Deep stroking to the deltoids

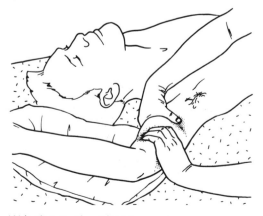

Wringing to the triceps

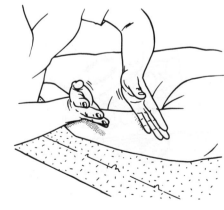

Hacking to the biceps

HEALTH AND BEAUTY THERAPY: A PRACTICAL APPROACH

1 Return the client's arm to its previous position and effleurage the top of the arm.

(Main muscles affected: biceps, triceps.)

4 **Effleurage to lower arm**
Using the entire palmar surface of the hand, stroke the lower arm from wrist to elbow in an alternate fashion.

(Main muscle affected: brachialis.)

5 **Friction circles**
  a Friction circle from the wrist to the elbow with a deep push back.

  (Main muscle affected: brachialis.)

  b Friction circle around the wrist joint using both thumbs simultaneously.

  c Friction circle between each metacarpal bone with a deep push back and continue this action down each finger to the tip.

  d Effleurage the hand and then turn over so the palm is uppermost.

6 **Friction circles to the hand**
Friction circles across the palm of the hands.

7 **Passive exercise**
Turn the client's hand back to a proline position and grasp the hand in your own, supporting the client's wrist with your other hand, then perform gentle, passive exercises clockwise, anticlockwise, forwards and backwards.

8 **Effleurage the whole arm to finish**
(Main muscles affected: biceps, triceps, brachialis, deltoid.)

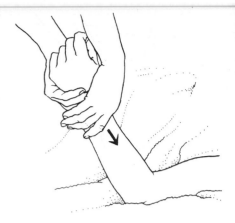

Effleurage to the lower arm

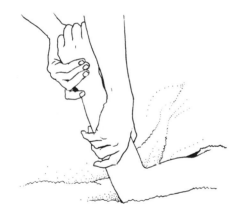

Friction circles from the wrist to the elbow

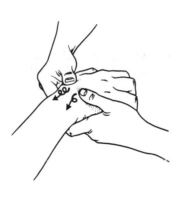

Friction circles around the wrist

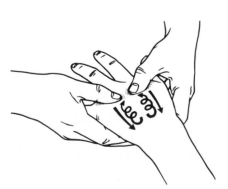

Friction circles between the metacarpals

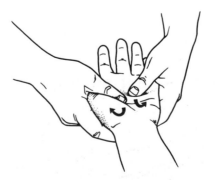

Friction circles to the palm

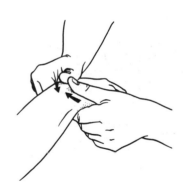

information point

When performing the passive hand and wrist mobility exercises, it is very important not to force the joint beyond its natural range.

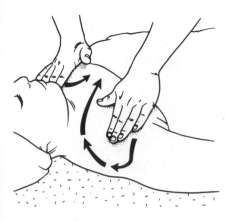

Chest massage

Preparation

a   Gently lower the towel in the area to expose the upper chest area.

b   Ensure the client's arms are tucked into the towel unless otherwise requested.

c   Apply massage medium to the selected area using effleurage strokes.

Massage sequence

1   **Effleurage to the chest**

Place the entire palmar surface of both hands in the middle of the chest area, then gently work each hand outwards separately, sweeping around the deltoids, over the trapezius, and back over to the starting area.

(Main muscles affected: pectoralis major, deltoid, trapezius.)

Effleurage to the chest

2   **Knuckling of the pectorals**

Clench fists lightly and then knuckle across the front of the pectoral area.

(Main muscles affected: pectoralis major.)

3   **Friction circles to the top of the shoulder**

Friction circle a number of times using both thumbs simultaneously in the bicipital groove of the humerus and shoulder area.

4   **Stroking of the deltoids**

a   Using the entire palmar surface of both hands, simultaneously stroke around the deltoid area in a clockwise direction and then in an anticlockwise direction.

(Main muscle affected: deltoid.)

b   Effleurage the chest area.

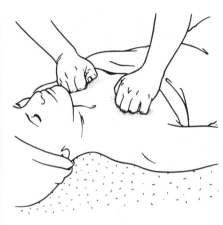

Knuckling of the pectorals

5   **Reinforced ironing**

Using double hand pressure, effleurage across the pectoral area in a figure of eight.

(Main muscles affected: pectoralis major, deltoid, trapezius.)

6   **Effleurage to the chest area to finish**

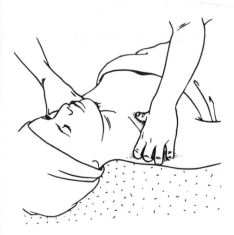

Friction circles to the shoulders

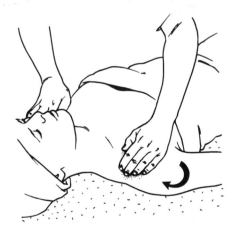

Stroking of the deltoids

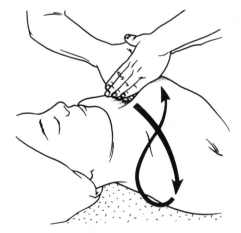

Reinforced ironing

Abdominal massage

CONTRAINDICATIONS

to abdominal massage
- Pregnancy.
- Diarrhoea.
- Within one hour of a heavy meal.

HEALTH AND BEAUTY THERAPY: A PRACTICAL APPROACH

Preparation

a   Place a rolled towel or small pillow under the client's knees to relax the abdominal wall. Remove the towel in the abdominal area keeping other parts of the body well covered for warmth.

b   Apply the selected massage medium to the area by first warming it on your own hands and then applying it to the client's abdomen following the effleurage pattern.

c   Ensure that your posture is good, with a straight back and stand with your right thigh towards the couch but facing forwards as in walk-standing position.

Massage sequence

1   **Effleurage to the abdomen**

Place the entire palmar surface of both hands on the abdomen and keeping fingers together, glide hands down towards the symphysis pubis, then glide under to the upper lumber spine where hands should meet and then glide lightly back on to the front of the abdomen.

(Main muscles affected: rectus abdominis, external obliques, internal obliques.)

GOOD PRACTICE

- Avoid abdominal massage if the client has just eaten a heavy meal.
- Abdominal massage needs to be lighter than massage on other parts of the body.
- Advise the client the abdominal massage may stimulate bowel and/or bladder action.
- Clients who are menstruating may prefer this area to be left out of the sequence.

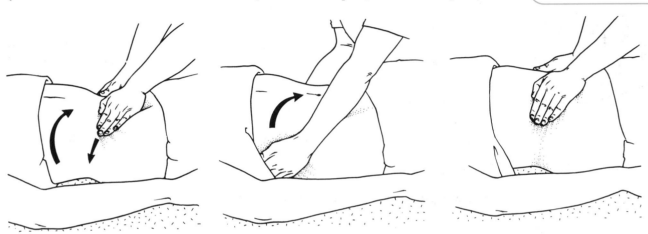

Effleurage to the abdomen

2   **Deep stroking of the abdomen**

Place the palmar surface of both hands on the middle of the abdomen and then stroke in a circular motion following the direction of the colon.

(Main muscle affected: rectus abdominis.)

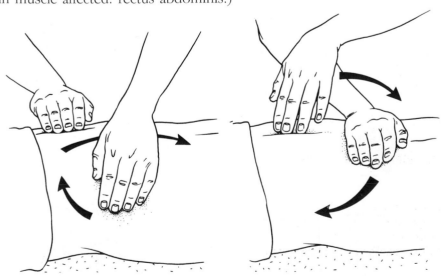

Deep stroking to the abdomen

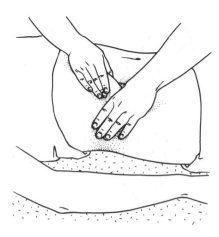

Wringing to the external obliques

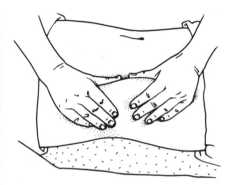

Skin rolling to the external obliques

3 **Wringing of the external obliques**
   a Still standing adjacent to the couch with the hands parallel, pick and lift the tissues and squeeze gently in a wringing action.
   b Glide both hands across the abdomen and repeat to the other side.
     (Main muscles affected: external obliques.)

4 **Skin rolling to the external obliques**
   a Still standing in the same position with hands parallel, slide down the obliques and then feed the tissues through your fingers and thumbs in a rolling motion.
   b Glide both hands across the abdomen and repeat to the other side.
     (Main muscles affected: external obliques.)

5 **Effleurage to the abdomen to finish**
   (Main muscles affected: rectus abdominis, external obliques, internal obliques.)

REMEMBER

The number of massage repetitions should be appropriate to the individual client's needs.

At this point in the massage routine you are now ready to ask the client to turn over so that she is lying prone on the couch. This needs to be done as quickly and discreetly as possible with the least disruption to the client. Lift the towels slightly and ask the client to gently turn over. Re-arrange the towels neatly.

Back of the leg and buttock massage
Preparation
a Remove the towel from the back leg area exposing the leg and gluteal area, but keeping other parts of the body well covered for warmth.

b Place a small rolled towel under the client's ankle for support.

c Apply the selected massage medium to the area by first warming it on your own hands and then applying it to the client's leg from ankle to buttocks using effleurage movements.

d Ensure your posture is good with a straight back.

Massage sequence
1 **Effleurage to the back of the leg and buttock**
   Place the entire palmar surface of both hands on the Achilles tendon area of the ankle. With one hand leading, keep fingers and thumbs together and glide the

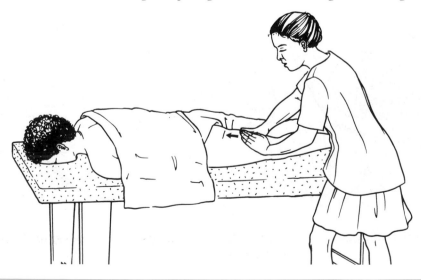

Effleurage to back of the leg and buttock

hands along the entire leg to the gluteal area, glide hands around the gluteal, lightly returning down to the ankle.

(Main muscles affected: soleus, gastrocnemius, hamstrings, gluteals, adductors, abductors.)

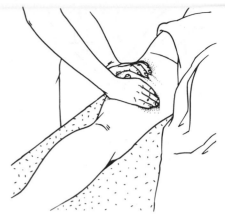

2 **Deep wringing to the hamstrings and gluteals**
   a Slide the hands to the interior aspect of the thigh and then with hands parallel, pick and lift the tissues and squeeze gently in a wringing action. Work the entire hamstring and gluteal areas.
   b Effleurage the hamstrings and gluteals.

   (Main muscles affected: hamstrings, gluteals, adductors, abductors.)

Deep wringing of the hamstrings and gluteals

3 **Alternate palmar lifting of the hamstrings**
   a Starting with hands on either side at the top of the thigh, use the entire palmar surface of both hands to gently compress the tissues against each other, lifting from side to side. Keep repeating until the back of the knee is reached and then slide back to repeat the sequence.
   b Effleurage the hamstrings area.

   (Main muscles affected: hamstrings, adductors, abductors.)

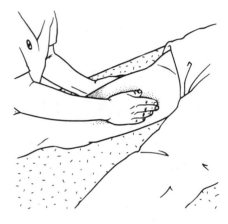

4 **Hacking to the hamstrings and gluteals**
   a Using the ulnar border of both hands, briskly but lightly hack the hamstring and gluteal areas in a rhythmical pattern.
   b Effleurage the hamstring and gluteal areas.

   (Main muscles affected: hamstrings, gluteals, adductors, abductors.)

5 **Cupping to the hamstrings and gluteals**
   a Holding the fingers and palms of the hands in a concave position, briskly but lightly cup the hamstrings area.
   b Effleurage the hamstrings and gluteals.

   (Main muscles affected: hamstrings, gluteals, adductors, abductors.)

Alternate palmar lifting of the hamstrings

6 **Beating to the hamstrings and gluteals**
   a Using lightly clenched fists, palms down, lightly beat the hamstrings and gluteals.
   b Effleurage the hamstrings and gluteals.

   (Main muscles affected: hamstrings, gluteals, adductors, abductors.)

7 **Pounding to the gluteals**
   a Using the ulnar border of lightly clenched fists, gently pound the gluteal area.

   (Main muscles affected: gluteals.)

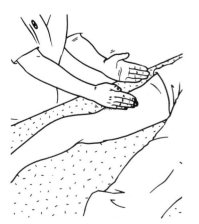

Hacking to the hamstrings and gluteals

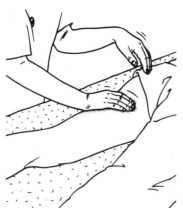

Cupping to the hamstrings and gluteals

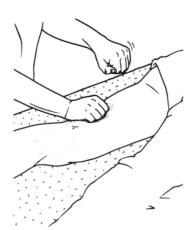

Beating to the hamstrings and gluteals

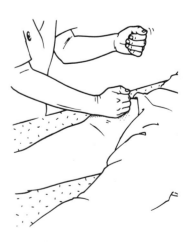

Pounding to the gluteals

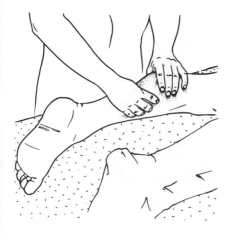

Deep wringing to the gastrocnemius/soleus

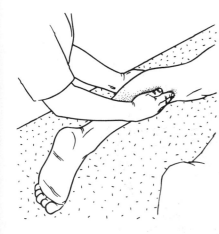

Alternate palmar lifting to the gastrocnemius/soleus

information point

On the lower leg area do not perform the beating movement as the muscles are more superficial.

   b Effleurage the gluteal area.

   c Effleurage the entire leg.

8 **Deep wringing to the gastrocnemius and soleus**

   a Slide the hands to the interior aspect of the calf, and then with hands parallel, pick and lift the tissues and squeeze gently in a wringing action.

   b Effleurage the gastrocnemius and soleus.

   (Main muscles affected: gastrocnemius, coleus.)

9 **Alternate palmar lifting to the gastrocnemius and soleus**

   a Starting with the hands on either side at the top of the lower leg, use the entire palmar surface of both hands to gently compress the tissues against each other and lift from side to side. Keep repeating until reaching the ankle, then slide back to repeat the sequence.

   b Effleurage the gastrocnemius and soleus.

   (Main muscles affected: gastrocnemius, soleus.)

10 **Light hacking to the gastrocnemius and soleus**

   a Using the ulnar border of both hands, briskly but lightly hack the gastrocnemius and soleus areas in a rhythmical pattern.

   b Effleurage the gastrocnemius and soleus.

   (Main muscles affected: gastrocnemius, soleus.)

11 **Light cupping to the gastrocnemius and soleus**

   a Holding the fingers and palms of the hands in a concave position, briskly, but lightly and gently, cup the gastrocnemius and soleus areas.

   b Effleurage the gastrocnemius and soleus.

   (Main muscles affected: gastrocnemius, soleus.)

12 **Digital stroking to the calcaneal (Achilles) tendon**

   Using all the digits of one hand, gently stoke the area. (The other hand can be placed on the calf for support.)

13 **Effleurage the entire leg to finish**

   (Main muscles affected: soleus, gastrocnemius, hamstrings, gluteals, adductors, abductors.)

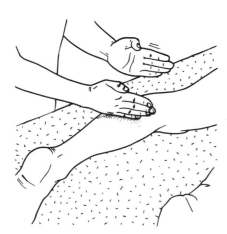

Light hacking to the gastrocnemius/soleus

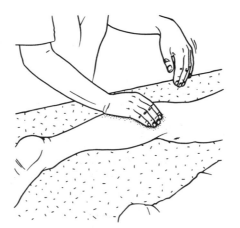

Light cupping to the gastrocnemius/soleus

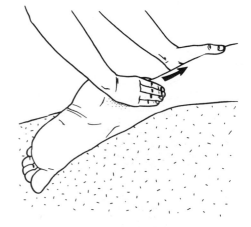

Digital stroking to the calcaneal tendon

Back massage

Preparation

a   Unless the couch has a breathe hole facility, place a support cushion, rolled towel or similar under the client's forehead to ensure that the neck is straight.

b   Remove towel from the back area keeping other parts of the body well covered for warmth.

c   Apply the selected massage medium to the area by first warming it on your own hands and then applying it to the client's back area.

d   Ensure that your posture is good with a straight back and stand with your right thigh towards the couch but facing forwards.

Massage sequence

1   **Effleurage to the back area**
    Place the entire palmar surface of both hands either side of the spine in the lower lumbar region. Glide up the back area and over the deltoids firmly, then return back to the lumbar area with a light stroke.

    (Main muscles affected: trapezius, deltoids, obliques, latissimus dorsi, serratus anterior.)

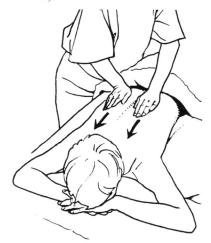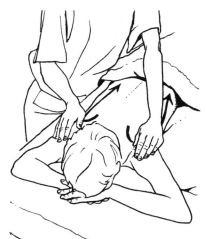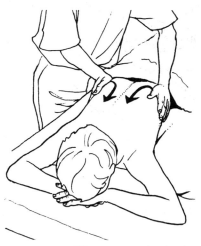

Effleurage to the back

2   **Wringing of the upper trapezius and deltoid**
    a   Slide both hands to the right side of the client's back in the external oblique area. Then with both hands parallel pick and lift the tissues and gently squeeze in a wringing action. The pressure can be increased over the upper trapezius and deltoid area to suit the client.

    b   Effleurage the back.

    (Main muscles affected: trapezius, deltoids, obliques, latissimus dorsi, serratus anterior.)

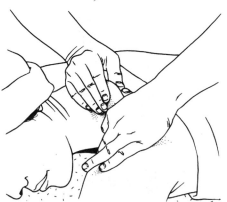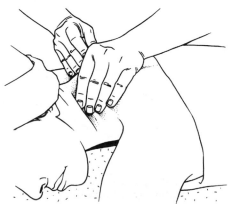

Wringing to the upper trapezius/deltoid

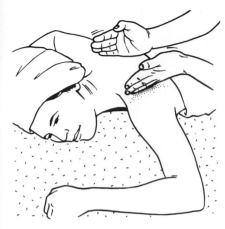

Light hacking of the trapezius and deltoids

information point

- Do not apply any tapotement movements over the spine.
- Tapotement movements are often omitted from the back massage routine.

3 **Light hacking of the trapezius and deltoids**
  a Using the ulnar border of both hands, briskly but lightly hack the trapezius and deltoids in rhythmical pattern.

   (Main muscles affected: trapezius, deltoids, obliques, latissius dorsi, serratus anterior.)

  b Effleurage the back.

4 **Light cupping of the trapezius and deltoids**
  a Holding the fingers and palms of the hands in a concave position, briskly but lightly cup the trapezius and deltoids.

  b Effleurage to back.

   (Main muscles affected: trapezius, deltoids, obliques, latissimus dorsi, serratus anterior.)

5 **Friction circles along the erector spinae muscles**
  a Starting at the sacrum, place both thumbs either side of the spine. Working upwards gently, perform friction circles until reaching the seventh cervical vertebrae. Gently work into the area, then return with index and middle fingers down either side of the spine.

  b Effleurage the back.

   (Main muscle affected: erector spinae.)

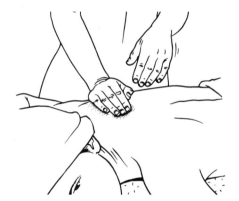

Light cupping of the trapezius and deltoids

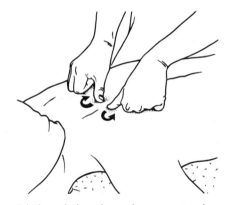

Friction circles along the erector spinae

6 **Deep wringing of the trapezius**
  a Slide the hands to the trapezius area and then with the hands parallel, pick and lift the tissues and squeeze gently in a wringing action.

  b Effleurage the back.

   (Main muscles affected: trapezius.)

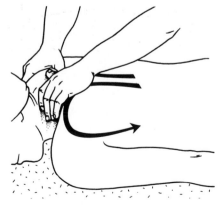
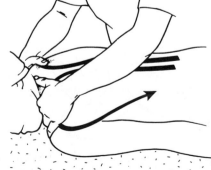
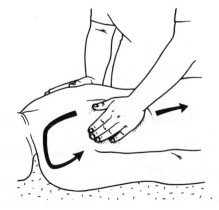

Deep wringing of the trapezius

7 Friction circles across the trapezius
Using the thumb digits, gently perform friction circles across the entire trapezius area, working on any nodules of tension.

8 Deep stroking of the trapezius

  a Place the palmar surface of both hands on either side of the neck. Firmly stroke down either side of the spine to the thoracic region, then glide out across the scapulae and up and over the deltoids to the starting position.

  b Effleurage the back.

    (Main muscles affected: trapezius, deltoids, obliques, latissimus dorsi, serratus anterior.)

9 Deep stroking of the spine to finish

  a Place the entire palmar surface of one hand in the cervical region and using alternate hands, gently stroke down towards the lumbar area.

  b Repeat the action a number of times, getting progressively lighter to finish.

    (Main muscle affected: erector spinae.)

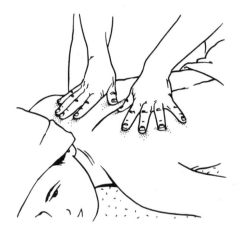
Friction circles across the trapezius

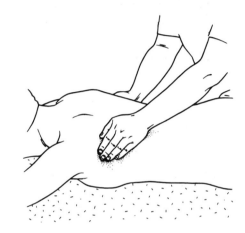
Deep stroking of the trapezius

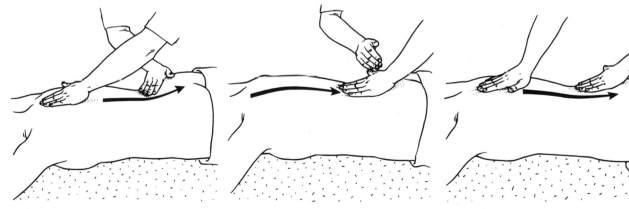
Deep stroking of the spine

This is the end of the basic massage sequence.

Face, head and scalp massage
Face massage
The client should first be prepared in the usual way and the skin needs to be cleaned and toned thoroughly to remove any traces of make-up. Apply an appropriate massage medium.

a   Starting on the shoulder area, effleurage in broad sweeping movements working upwards towards the neck.

b   Apply deep thumb frictions along the trapezius working from the outside inwards.

c   Sweep up the neck and on to the mandible and brace round returning to the chin area.

d   Perform alternate masseter lifts, sweeping around the mandible as doing so.

e   Apply frictions around the chin and mouth area and then sweep up to the forehead.

f   Apply gentle stroking movements around the eye area including some lymphatic drainage pinching across the eyebrows.

g   Apply gentle friction movements simultaneously using ring fingers, working in a small circular motion around and underneath the eye area towards the nose.

h   Gently stroke the forehead using the entire palm surface of both hands.

i   Apply scissoring movement to the forehead using the ring finger of both hands.

j   Effleurage the entire face a few times finishing at the temples with deep pressure.

Head and scalp massage

Remove the headband and or towelling protection from the client's hair and apply a small amount of massage medium to your hands before starting. This is optional and will also depend on the client's preferences.

a   Effleurage the head by placing both hands on top of the head and gently stroking alternatively down. Repeat this until the whole head has been treated.

b   Comb through the hair using the digits of both hands in a stroking movement from front to back.

c   Gently perform friction circles using the digits in a circular motion starting at the occipital bone working towards the crown and down to the frontal bone. This movement can be applied quite deeply.

d   Apply brisk friction movements working up and down the entire scalp and head area using the finger tips.

e   Using the index, middle and ring fingers, work the entire scalp area with an upwards and downwards stroking action.

f   Effleurage to finish.

SELF-CHECKS

1   Describe briefly how you would prepare a client for massage treatment.

2   Why should abdominal massage be lighter than massage on other parts of the body?

3   Carry out a massage treatment and state the key muscles affected in each area.

Adaptation of massage to suit the individual's requirements

Having mastered the basic principles of rate, rhythm and pressure for the introductory massage routine, a good therapist will develop their skills and knowledge to design a massage suitable for their client's needs.

It is extremely beneficial to take treatments from other therapists, attend short training courses, read trade journals and attend exhibitions, all of which will enable the therapist to enhance their own techniques.

There are many reasons why a client may request a massage, among some of the most popular are:

- Stress.
- Muscular aches and pains.
- Weight loss.
- Poor muscle tone.

Massage for stress and relaxation

The majority of people at some time in their lives will suffer with stress through pressure of everyday living, e.g. it is amazing how tense many drivers become particularly sitting in heavy traffic. Stress has many different physiological and psychological effects on the body: it is often responsible for causing tension in our muscles, which if left untreated will eventually affect our posture and may even affect our general state of health. As one of the main benefits of massage is relaxation, it is extremely beneficial for most people provided they are not contraindicated to the treatment.

There are many forms of massage available to clients, all of which will vary in time and price depending on the type of establishment the client visits and its location.

One-hour body massage

The therapist can use the petrissage and effleurage movements from the introductory massage routine, along with any other they have learnt from further study, demonstrations or from other therapists, to devise an individual programme for their client. This may also include lymph drainage movements if the therapist feels they are appropriate to the client's needs. They will need to carry out a consultation and ensure there are no contraindications to the massage.

Therapists may choose to alter the order of treatment depending on their own and client's preferences, e.g. many holistic massage therapists commence on the client's back, spending a great deal of time here because this is an area prone to tension. They then move on to the backs, then fronts, of the legs and quite often may effleurage both legs at the same time. The arms and chest areas are next, followed by a face and scalp massage. Note that massage of the abdomen is often omitted.

GOOD PRACTICE

- Remember that massage is a very personal, individualised treatment as no two people are alike. The therapist must ensure they prepare the treatment area and perform a massage to best enhance relaxation of the individual client.
- In European winters, therapists often use pre-heated duvets or heated under-pads to assist the relaxation of the client. Warm, dry towels may also be applied to the area that has been treated to further induce relaxation and maintain the warmth generated in the tissues.

Half-hour body massage

The majority of health spas, as part of their package, offer a half-hour massage and therefore the therapist must learn to adapt a one-hour routine without making the client feel rushed. Rate and rhythm need to remain fairly constant and pressure altered to suit the client. Some clients prefer to have the time spent on certain areas rather than the whole body, e.g. legs, arms and back. Always establish during the consultation with the client their preferences and any areas of tension. New clients will look for the therapist's professional advice or quietly accept the treatment they are offered. It is far more rewarding for the therapist to discover problem areas, which will enable them to give the client a more beneficial treatment rather than make small talk, which can often become repetitive.

Back massage

Many salons' and spas' price lists will include a half-hour back massage. This can prove to be a very popular treatment as a lot of people at some time in their life will suffer from tension in the shoulders and/or back. This can often be the first massage that clients experience. Over the years people have tended to feel inhibited about exposing their body without first knowing the salon and therapist. In many countries, whether through religion or culture, body treatments are not as popular. The therapist needs to establish a professional ethos that is reassuring to the client and embodies their culture.

During the consultation the therapist needs to establish any particular problems the client may have, e.g. tension in the lower back, along with their likes and dislikes in aromas, sound, colour, temperature and pressure. This will enable the therapist to ensure that the treatment room and product selection will assist more fully in relaxation of the client. The massage techniques selected will help relieve tension in the problem area and will include mainly effleurage and petrissage movements and in particular, deep thumb frictions to the trapezius and erector spinae muscles.

Apprehensive clients

Often clients attending for their first treatment are apprehensive and will tend to talk to overcome their fears. The therapist needs to be reassuring and encourage the client to relax to ensure maximum benefit is gained. The introduction of therapeutic music and essential oils either in the massage medium or in the aroma of the room may help.

It is important to establish the cause of the client's concern so that the therapist is conscious of their dilemma. Generally it can be assumed that the client is apprehensive as they do not understand fully what the treatment involves and/or they are nervous of exposing their body and feeling vulnerable. The therapist should bear this in mind by considering how she/he would feel semi-naked in unfamiliar surroundings with a total stranger who is fully dressed! The therapist should ensure they fully explain the treatment to the client and allow them time to get on to the couch and cover themselves before commencing.

Massage for muscular aches and pains

The therapist must first ascertain whether there are any underlying medical conditions which would contraindicate the client from treatment.

Having carried out a thorough consultation and where necessary having gained approval from the client's GP (this should be a note that the client has brought from their general practitioner) the client should be given a heat treatment, such as sauna, steam or infrared heat lamp, to relax the muscles prior to the massage. The therapist may even decide to use the infrared heat lamp during the massage to increase the heat within the tissues, thus aiding relaxation.

As muscular tension can cause aches and pains, the therapist should devote more time to particular problem areas using deep kneading and calming effleurage movements. The increase of warmth to the tissues brought about by the increase in blood and lymph circulation will assist in soothing the client's aches and pains.

REMEMBER

It is invaluable to take treatments with different therapists in different areas of your country, also when abroad, and to share these experiences with other therapists.

Massage for weight loss

It is a popular misconception that massage alone can induce weight loss. Weight loss is brought about by diet and exercise. However, if introduced as part of a planned treatment and home care programme alongside diet, exercise and electrical treatments, massage can prove to be extremely beneficial.

There are many reasons why a client may be overweight, e.g. it may be hereditary, as a result of over-eating or lack of exercise. Whatever the reason, the fact that the client has sought help indicates a determination to address the problem. Many people address the issue themselves or seek assistance through therapists or weight loss groups. The therapist must decide with the client the best plan of action to suit their individual needs and constraints such as time and finances available. They must also ensure that there are no underlying medical conditions such as hormone imbalance, e.g. an underactive thyroid gland can cause obesity.

Once a thorough consultation has been carried out and medical approval has been sought (where necessary), the therapist can use her/his knowledge and skills to devise a suitable treatment plan including diet, exercise, electrical treatments and a stimulating massage routine which should include petrissage (skin rolling, wringing and picking up) and tapotement movements (hacking, cupping, pounding and beating) on the areas of excess fat. It may prove beneficial to include manual treatments for stretch marks as often when people lose weight they tend to gain stretch marks. If the client suffers from cellulite, the therapist could also include manual treatments for cellulite in the treatment programme (see Chapter 6).

Massage for poor muscle tone

The causes of poor muscle tone are many:

- natural ageing
- lack of exercise
- after rapid weight loss which may be caused through such things as illness or stress, or may be self-induced
- after pregnancy.

To tone poor muscles the therapist would need to recommend exercises to increase the strength of the muscles. These could be supported by salon electrical treatments for muscle tone and a stimulating massage routine incorporating mainly petrissage movements to increase the client's blood and lymph circulation. Once again the therapist could also offer manual treatments and home care products for stretch marks. (See Chapter 6.)

GOOD PRACTICE

- Carry out a thorough consultation.
- Check for contraindications.
- If needed, seek medical advice.
- Ascertain the client's needs.
- As part of a treatment plan, consider the client's financial and time constraints.
- Prepare the treatment area and client to induce relaxation.
- Devise an individual routine with movements suitable for the aims of the massage.

Massage for men

Generally speaking males have more muscle bulk than females, unless of course the female client is a body builder. As the muscles are stronger and firmer, there is a

Massage therapists (male and female) may treat members of the opposite sex, particularly if they work in a health spa, and must therefore:

● respect their clients' privacy by allowing clients time to undress and cover themselves

● adapt movements and pressure accordingly.

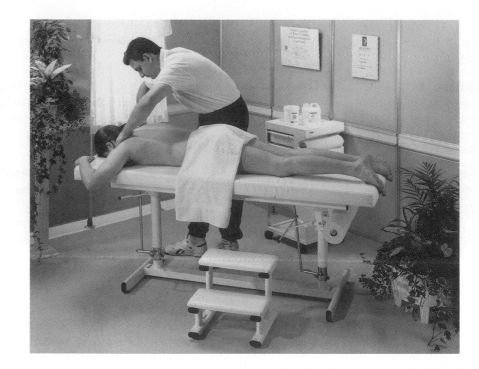

Massage treatment for men

tendency for males to have less subcutaneous (fatty) tissue. The massage movements need to be performed with a greater depth of pressure on men than on women. The type of movements used will obviously depend on the client's reason for treatment but would usually include petrissage (kneading, wringing and picking up), tapotement (hacking, cupping and pounding) and deep effleurage movements. If the massage is for relaxation then the tapotement movements would be omitted. As men usually have much more body hair than women, it is important to ensure that the massage medium selected gives enough slip for ease of movement. Generally male massage does not include working on the inner thighs, abdomen or gluteal areas.

GOOD PRACTICE

Suggestions for after/home care and further salon treatments following a massage:

● Allow a minimum of five minutes relaxation time after the massage.

● Health spas often have separate relaxation rooms with reclining chairs, therapeutic music, subdued lighting and aromatherapy burners.

● Advise the client to avoid strenuous activities for a few hours.

● Recommend the client drinks plenty of water, particularly if essential oils have been used in the massage medium.

● Having performed the massage and noted the individual client's needs, e.g. dry skin, stretch marks, cellulite, tactfully recommend a suitable treatment plan to include salon treatments and home care products considering the client's financial and time constraints.

ACTIVITY

Select a client, perform a detailed consultation, devise an appropriate massage routine and justify your choice of movements.

Types of massage

Aroma massage

Aroma massage is generally for relaxation and uses ready-blended essential oils as the massage medium. It has become increasingly popular over the last few years and is practised by many beauty therapists. The massage routine incorporates mainly effleurage and petrissage-type movements and is often enhanced by the use of therapeutic music.

The oils used in aroma massage are generally in a diluted concentration compared to those used by a qualified aromatherapist.

Aromatherapy

This type of massage is a specialist treatment which should only be offered by qualified aromatherapists. It uses plant extracts (essential oils) blended with a carrier oil to form a therapeutic treatment medium to suit the individual client's needs. The massage itself is the method used to transport the essential oils into the client's body and generally consists of effleurage movements.

The last decade has seen a great advance in the recognition of complementary treatments such as aromatherapy. Some aromatherapists work in hospitals under the direction of medical staff and a number of local health authorities have nurses trained and qualified in aromatherapy. For further information see Chapter 3.

Deep tissue massage

Deep tissue massage is considered to be a method of connective tissue massage. It involves a stroking technique which is used to stimulate the release of histamine from what are known as mast cells found within connective tissue. It increases the circulation in the surrounding area, and may produce a generalised flushed appearance and an erythema.

Lymph drainage

This type of massage involves working on the lymphatic system. True lymph drainage massage incorporates superficial effleurage and petrissage movements. Its aims are to relieve congestion within the tissues and increase the drainage of lymph to the lymph nodes. Generally clients come for treatment for specific problem areas rather than having a whole body treatment.

Multi-type massage

Multi-type massage originated in the Far East where it has been practised for many hundreds of years. It involves two therapists working in unison on the one client. It has recently become a fairly popular at a number of international spas. It involves a great deal of training to ensure the therapists are emotionally in tune and that their rate, rhythm and pressure are equal.

Oriental massage

Oriental massage has its origin in the Far East. It has been practised for centuries and is growing in popularity throughout the western world. Oriental massage is pressure massage using any surface of the body, e.g. thumbs, hands, feet, elbows, etc. It can also include gentle stretching and manipulation along with the 'laying on of hands' similar to that used in spiritual healing. The application of pressure is usually based along the meridian lines that are used in acupuncture.

Shiatsu is the Japanese name for oriental massage (*shi* meaning finger and *atsu* pressure). The majority of Far Eastern countries, such as Thailand and Malaysia, have, over the years, developed their own versions of pressure massage.

One of the main differences in oriental and European massage is that the client does not undress, though the therapist and the client need to be dressed in non-restrictive clothing. The massage is performed with the client either sitting or lying on a low bed or a mattress on the floor. It is also quite common in Far Eastern countries to see holidaymakers receiving oriental massage on the beach!

Sports massage

This type of massage has greatly increased in popularity over the last decade, particularly as more and more people are adopting various sports as part of their leisure activities. The sports person is aware of the benefits of sports massage, which include easing aches and pains, and relaxing the musculo-skeletal system or specific muscles or muscle groups. Through specialised training the massage therapist uses a variety of movements to treat the individual client problem, e.g. deep friction movements are often used to break down scar tissue and adhesions.

ACTIVITY

Perform four massage routines on a selection of clients (male and female), who display different bodily conditions and age ranges. Keep a record of the body conditions noted, age and gender of client, the choice of lubricant and the massage routine devised.

KEY TERMS

You need to know what these words and phrases mean. Go back through the chapter to find out.

Adaptation of massage

Contraindications

Creating a welcoming environment

Effleurage

Frictions

Massage consultation and assessment

Massage mediums

Petrissage

Preparation for massage

Principles of good massage practice

Tapotement

Types of massage

Vibrations

SELF-CHECKS

1   Give three reasons why massage treatment may be adapted. Explain each reason.

2   How would you deal with an apprehensive client?

3   Name and briefly describe four different forms of massage treatment.

Chapter 2 Indian head massage

After working through this chapter you will be able to:

- have an understanding of the history and origins of Indian head massage
- identify the key chakra system
- have an awareness of what an aura is and how to feel for it
- perform an effective Indian head massage treatment
- state the main benefits of Indian head massage
- expertly advise on after-care and home-care practices.

Introduction

This therapy, which is based on ancient Ayurvedic principles, has been practised in India for well over 4,000 years, often passed down from mother to child. It is a holistic treatment, which means that it works on the mind, body and soul to restore balance and harmony as well as improve health and wellbeing.

Oils can sometimes be used with the treatment – they can give additional benefits depending on the type used. Popular oils include almond, mustard seed, coconut and sometimes essential oils.

Indian head massage is a treatment that includes the scalp, face, neck, shoulders, upper back and sometimes the arms. These areas are kneaded, rubbed, squeezed and stroked in a flowing rhythmical sequence. Indian head massage is extremely relaxing but it can also be invigorating depending upon the movements used. The main benefits are that clients do not have to remove any clothing and the massage can be performed with or without oils.

Indian head massage works on what are known as chakras. Quantum physicists, devotees of vibrational medicine, believe that we are all composed of energy in the form of sub-atomic vibrating particles. Chakras are believed to be three-dimensional circling vortices that draw energy into the body and pass it through the energy network. Various therapists work on chakras to balance them and therefore improve physical and emotional health.

Ayurveda

The word Ayurveda comes from two Sanskrit words – *Ayur* meaning life, and *Veda* meaning knowledge. This traditional Indian life science is the oldest form of medicine known to man, with written texts dating back 3,500 years. Ayurveda still forms the basis of much medical practice today in India, Sri Lanka and Pakistan, where orthodox doctors work alongside Ayurvedic physicians.

Ayurvedic medicine is a complete healthcare system and involves detoxification, diet, exercise and herbs, as well as techniques to improve mental and emotional health.

The central tenet of Ayurvedic science is that each human being is unique, having a distinct individual constitution, genetic inheritance and predisposition to certain diseases. Our constitution is determined by the balance of three vital energies in the body, known as the three doshas or tridoshas. The three doshas are known by their Sanskrit names of Vata, Pitta and Kapha. Everyone's constitution is governed by the three doshas in varying degrees, but each individual is also controlled by one or possibly two dominant doshas.

Health is maintained when all three doshas are in balance. Each one has its role to play in the body. For example, Vata is the driving force: it relates mainly to the nervous system and the body's energy. Pitta is fire; it relates to metabolism, digestion, enzymes, acid and bile.

In Ayurveda good digestion is considered the key to good health. Poor digestion produces 'Ama' toxins believed to cause disease. Ama occurs when the metabolism is impaired due to an imbalance of 'agni'. Agni, when working normally, maintains all functions. Imbalance of agni is caused by irregularities in the doshas and such things as eating and drinking too much of the wrong food and repressing emotions. Agni affected by too much Kapha can slow the digestive process making you feel heavy and sluggish, while too much Vata can cause flatulence, cramps, alternating constipation and diarrhoea.

Toxins which cause illness can be produced by emotional as well as physical factors. For example, fear and anxiety relate to Vata and the large intestine. When held inside these emotions can cause bloating and intestinal pain.

Ayurvedic principles

Every living body possesses three vital energies known as Vata, Pitta and Kapha, in unique proportions. This is known as your Prakriti (the proportion you are born with).

Vata

This is the driving force within the body and its functions are similar to the functions of the nervous system. When Vata is low, it leads to accumulation of fluids, bowel infections, tiredness and poor circulation. When in excess, it can lead to dry skin, brittle hair, bone problems, flatulence, bowel disorders such as irritable bowel syndrome, worry, fear, anxiety, insomnia and depression.

Pitta

This is the metabolic force within the body. It controls appetite, thermoregulation, digestion and absorption. When balanced, people can eat and drink well without becoming over/under weight. When it is low it can cause indigestion, poor appetite, weight loss and lethargy. When in excess, stomach ulcers, inflammation, skin disorders (acne/eczema), liver, pancreatic or gall bladder disorders, burning stools and urine, anger and irritability may result.

Kapha

This constitutes water and bodily fluids. Excess Kapha leads to asthma, sinus problems, fluid retention, obesity. Low Kapha leads to weight loss, dry chest, dehydration and thirst.

The chakra system

The word 'chakra' means 'wheel' and in Indian tradition the chakras are centres of specific forces. Some people can see chakras and describe them as spinning whirlpools of energy. Actually, chakras are 'energy channels' that run throughout the body.

The Indian head massage routine includes chakra balancing work. The body has seven major chakras:

- Crown
- Brow (third eye)
- Throat
- Heart
- Solar plexus
- Hara (sacrum)
- Base (root).

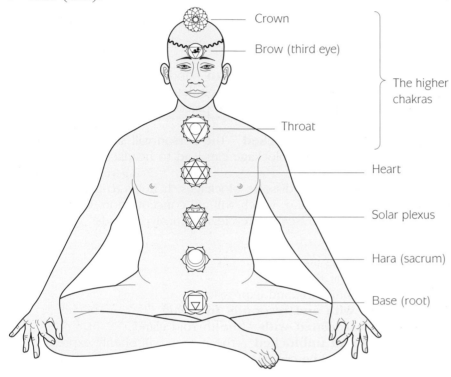

The chakras

Minor chakras are also found in the feet, on the palms of the hands and at joints. The chakras are centres of energy that are located about an inch away from the body and should ideally spin in a clockwise direction. Each chakra resembles a flower and its petals represent energy channels through which energy passes. Each chakra has a different number of petals. The energy (prana) for the chakras is supplied from the universe. Prana is an Indian word meaning 'life-force energy'. It enters the body through these energy centres. To ensure health, all the chakras need to be open, unblocked and in balance with each other.

An important part of Indian head massage is working with the higher chakras:

- the crown (sahasrara)
- third eye (ajna)
- throat (vishuddha).

Higher chakras

The crown chakra is called the master chakra and can help to open up and balance the six other chakras of the body. It is important that this chakra is not blocked, otherwise energy will not be able to run freely from all the other chakras to it. Working with this chakra will cause energy to be sent to where it is needed in the body and so promote healing. The crown chakra is the place through which the universe sends its energy into the body.

Crown chakra – seventh chakra
- **Where chakra is found** – at the top of the head
- **Concerned with** – thinking and decision-making
- **Colour it is associated with and responds to** – violet
- **Endocrine gland it is associated with** – the pineal gland in the brain
- **Effects when balanced and unblocked** – the person will be thoughtful, wise, spiritual and open-minded
- **Effects when out of balance or blocked** – the person will be apathetic and thoughtless, will have no direction in life and fear of dying
- **Essential oils** – jasmine and lavender promote spiritual growth; lavender will help to unblock this chakra

Brow chakra – sixth chakra
The brow chakra is also known as 'the third eye'.

- **Where chakra is found** – on the forehead between the eyebrows
- **Concerned with** – inner vision
- **Colour it is associated with and responds to** – indigo
- **Endocrine gland it is associated with** – the pituitary gland
- **Effects when balanced and unblocked** – the person will be intuitive, have a good memory and be perceptive
- **Effects when out of balance or blocked** – the person will suffer from poor vision, nightmares and forgetfulness; blockage can lead to headaches and nightmares
- **Essential oils** – rosemary helps to dissolve blockages. It helps to get rid of negative thoughts and clear the mind, which will aid concentration. Clary sage strengthens the inner eye to 'see' more clearly. Eucalyptus aids concentration.

Throat chakra – fifth chakra
- **Where chakra is found** – at the throat
- **Concerned with** – communication and expression
- **Colour it is associated with and responds to** – blue
- **Endocrine gland it is associated with** – the thyroid gland
- **Effects when balanced and unblocked** – the person will openly express feelings, be a good listener and be creative
- **Effects when out of balance or blocked** – the person will be shy, a poor listener and talk too much
- **Essential oils** – clary sage loosens tension in the throat chakra and helps us to energetically express what we need to say. Peppermint will aid communication and concentration. Eucalyptus helps to clear and widen the throat chakra.

Heart chakra – fourth chakra
The heart chakra is the centre of the chakra system. The energy from the heart chakra streams out strongly and if it is open it will have a healing or other positive influence on other people.

- **Where chakra is found** – the centre of the chest
- **Concerned with** – the capacity to empathise and sympathise with others
- **Colour it is associated with and responds to** – green, the colour of healing, sympathy and harmony
- **Endocrine gland it is associated with** – the thymus gland
- **Effects when balanced and unblocked** – the person will be sincere, caring, loving and warm
- **Effects when out of balance or blocked** – the person will suffer from depression and jealousy and will be cold or heartless
- **Essential oils** – rose can help to unblock the heart chakra. Bergamot can help to open this chakra and allow love to radiate from it.

Solar plexus – third chakra
- **Where chakra is found** – 5 cm above the navel
- **Concerned with** – personality, feelings and emotional strength
- **Colour it is associated with and responds to** – yellow
- **Endocrine gland it is associated with** – the pancreas
- **Effects when balanced and unblocked** – the person will be confident and responsible, with feelings of peace and inner harmony, and have high self-esteem
- **Effects when out of balance or blocked** – the person will have a low sense of self-worth and be gloomy, bad-tempered, hyperactive and stubborn
- **Essential oils** – lavender oil has a calming, relaxing and balancing effect on hyperactive third chakras. It also helps to dissolve negative bottled-up emotions. Rosemary is useful for balancing the solar plexus chakra. Juniper strengthens will power and increases self-worth. It helps to restore confidence against the fear of failure.

Hara (sacrat chakra) – second chakra
- **Where chakra is found** – 5 cm below the navel
- **Concerned with** – relationships, especially with the opposite sex
- **Colour it is associated with and responds to** – orange
- **Endocrine gland it is associated with** – reproductive organs (females: ovaries; males: testes)
- **Effects when balanced and unblocked** – the person will exhibit a zest for life and will feel sexual and attractive
- **Effects when out of balance or blocked** – the person will suffer from sexual problems, lack of self-love and mood swings
- **Essential oils** – ylang ylang is a well-known aphrodisiac. Its aroma gives feelings of safety and helps to dissolve pent-up emotions and anger. In the Far East, sandalwood oil is often used to increase sexual energy.

Base or root chakra – first chakra
- **Where chakra is found** – at the base or the spine
- **Concerned with** – connection to mother earth, health and survival
- **Colour it is associated with and responds to** – red
- **Endocrine gland it is associated with** – the adrenal glands
- **Effects when balanced and unblocked** – the person will show good health, optimism and enthusiasm for life and will feel safe and secure
- **Effects when out of balance or blocked** – fearful, disorganised and possessive
- **Essential oils** – palmarosa encourages feelings of security. Patchouli helps to unblock this chakra.

The colours of the chakras are the same as the colours of the rainbow.

Unbalanced chakras

Any type of negative stress can cause a chakra to become blocked or thrown out of balance. This can occur because of upset, shock or fear. An imbalance in one energy centre can affect the others, especially those closest to it; for example, if suffering an upsetting experience the heart chakra is affected, which may cause a bad stomach (solar plexus chakra) and difficulty in talking (throat chakra). When the chakras lose their ability to work harmoniously with each other they become unbalanced. Imbalances or blockages can be eased or corrected by contact with an energy that nourishes, or vibrates at a frequency beneficial to the chakra. To help rebalance these chakras the hands can be placed over the three higher chakras to help the energy to flow freely. Balancing means helping a chakra to achieve proper functioning so that it is not too open or closed. When in a balanced state, a person can remain calm and centred in any situation. When out of balance, people tend to withdraw, or be overwhelmed, or lose control of their emotions.

Indian head massage and chakras

Chakras act as a link between the emotional and physical body. This is why working to balance the chakras during an Indian head massage treatment can have such positive effects on the mind and body. When giving an Indian head massage treatment, imagine lavender-coloured light being brought from the universe, through the crown chakra and out through the hands. The therapist is sending healing energy to the client. If during Indian head massage treatment a client is feeling mentally tired, one hand can be placed on the crown chakra and the other on the brow chakra. This will help to re-energise the client so that they feel more mentally alert. When working on a chakra concentrate on what can be felt. Some therapists may feel heat, a tingling sensation, sometimes feelings of coldness or perhaps a magnetic force that causes their hands to be repelled.

If a client is bottling up problems and is finding it hard to talk about them, one hand can be placed on the crown and the other hand on the throat chakra. Encourage the client to breathe slowly and deeply. This causes the client to release their emotions, maybe by crying.

Auras

The energy given off by the chakras creates an aura, which is an energy field that surrounds the physical body. It is made up of levels of energy called the subtle bodies. In a healthy person the aura makes an egg shape around the whole body and for most people extends about 1 metre from the body.

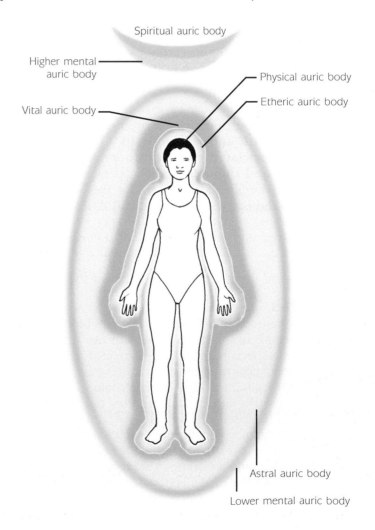

Spiritual auric body

Higher mental auric body

Physical auric body

Vital auric body

Etheric auric body

Astral auric body

Lower mental auric body

The auras

The more healthy an individual, the further the aura will extend and the more vibrant and colourful it will be. It is said that great leaders from the past had auras that extended for miles, which may explain why they had so many followers. Animals and plants have auras too. Everybody's aura is different. People with similar auras will get on well but people with dissimilar auras may well take an instant dislike to each other.

The aura is weakened by poor diet, lack of exercise, stress, lack of rest, alcohol, drugs and tobacco. The layers closest to the body are the most dense. As the aura expands it becomes less dense. The inner layers of the aura represent health matters. It is where disease begins; and disease affects the colour of the aura. The outer layers of the aura are concerned with what is going on within the mental and emotional life of a person.

The aura consists of colours. The clarity of these colours and the size and shape of the aura are all indicators of the health and emotional wellbeing of the individual. The colours and their intensity can change throughout the day.

Photographs can be taken of the aura through a process called kirlian photography. The human energy field can absorb the energies of plants, flowers, trees, animals and absorb energy from the earth too. The aura is stronger and larger when in direct contact with the earth with no shoes on. Being around nature is balancing and cleansing to the aura. Sitting under a willow tree for about 10 minutes can help to alleviate a headache. Pine trees are very cleansing to the aura as they absorb negative emotions.

The layer found directly outside the physical body is called the ethereal body. The ethereal body draws energy from the sun via the solar plexus chakra and from the earth via the base chakra. It stores these energies and feeds them in continuous streams through the chakras and into the body. The energy travels through invisible channels in the body called meridians; they are called nadis in India. These meridians connect the aura and chakras with our physical body.

The energy reaches the body's cells through the meridians and helps to maintain balance (homeostasis) in the body. When the body does not need this energy it will release it out through the chakras and through the pores of the skin. The energy that is released produces the ethereal aura. The energy sent out from the chakra points is stronger than the energy released from other areas of the body.

Negative thoughts, emotional trauma, continual stress and worry, an unhealthy lifestyle and excessive use of alcohol, nicotine and drugs may use up the ethereal energy, leading to a weakening of the energy radiating out from the aura. If this happens, holes may be seen in the aura. These enable negative vibrations and disease-causing matter such as bacteria to enter the body, as the protective effect of the aura is lessened. A weakened aura causes a person to tire more easily. Physical health problems can begin to develop.

The aura expands with positive thoughts and feelings such as joy and happiness, and contracts with negative feelings such as fear or hatred.

Feeling the aura
- Rub the palms of the hands together briskly for about 30 seconds.
- Face palms towards each other, fingers together, at about two feet apart.
- Very slowly move the hands towards each other. Bring them as close to each other without touching.
- Can you feel anything such as heat, cold, or tingling?
- Draw the hands back about 15 cm (6 inches) and bring them towards each other again.

If you do not experience anything at first, do not worry, just keep practising!

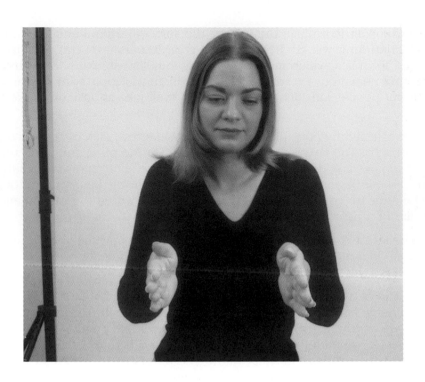

Feeling the aura

Push and pull aura exercise

The following exercise is a good way of proving there is an energy field (aura) around us that another person can affect.

- Ask a friend to stand facing away from you, preferably with their eyes closed.
- Standing about 1 metre away from your friend's back, straighten your arms out in front of you with palms facing their back.
- Gently rock your body forwards and back. Be aware of what you can feel while pushing on your partner's energy field.
- As you push and pull, it is probable that your friend's body will also be swaying forwards and backward. If there is a third person ask them to observe too.
- Now swap over with your partner and repeat the exercise.

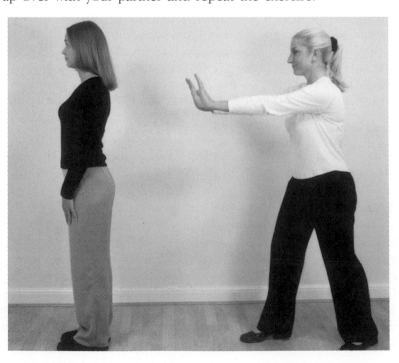

Pushing and pulling the aura

Seeing the aura

With practice, anyone can learn to see an aura. A good way to begin is to look at the energy fields of trees. Relax the gaze and look around the top of a tree and above it. Hopefully, you can start to see a slight haze or shimmer around the tree. It may appear lighter or slightly darker in colour than the sky around the tree.

During an eclipse the sun's aura can be seen; this energy field is called the corona.

Another exercise you can try is to use a piece of white card and place your hand on it. Relax your eyes and just stare at and around your hand, this exercise works better in dim light. You can also try to place your hand up near a window so that its background is the sky. Can you see any colours? Yellow is often one of the first colours that you can see; it may only slightly radiate from the hands at first.

The meaning or the colours discussed refers to bright shades. Duller, muddier shades can indicate health or emotional problems – but do not tell a client that their aura indicates health or emotional problems.

Colours of the aura

The colours of the aura frequently change. There are many different types of colour and shade within an aura. All these colours have meaning.

- Red is a sign of strong energy, passion, mind and will.
- Orange is a sign of warmth, creativity and emotion. Depending on the shade, it can also denote agitation and emotional imbalances. It may reflect worry and vanity.
- Yellow is one of the first and easiest colours to see in an aura. Pale yellow around the hairline can show optimism. It can reflect learning, wisdom and intellect. Yellow is the colour that represents the power of ideas and awakening psychic ability.
- Green is a colour of sensitivity and compassion. It can reflect a person who is reliable, friendly, dependable and open-minded. Bright greens moving towards the blue end of the spectrum indicate healing ability.
- Blue is the colour of calm and quietness. It reflects devotion, truth and seriousness. The lighter shades of blue reflect an active imagination and good intuition. A deep shade of blue can indicate loneliness. Royal blue shows honesty and good judgement.
- Violet and purple reflect independence and intuition. The lighter shades can reflect spirituality. Red purple shades indicate great passion or strength of will. They may also reflect a need for greater individual effort.

Other colours of the aura

- Pink is the colour of compassion and love. It can reflect joy and comfort.
- Gold indicates a great deal of spiritual energy. It shows great enthusiasm and inspiration.
- White is often seen in an aura before seeing any actual colours. White reflects truth and purity. It indicates that the energy of a person is cleansing and purifying itself.

The holistic approach

Massage helps to heal the body. Recent research found that massage releases chemicals which boost the immune system. The movements assist the improvement of circulation and lymphatic drainage, helping to improve nutrition to bones, muscles and skin at the area being treated. The removal of lactic acid, waste and toxins increases the efficient functioning of organs.

REMEMBER

Only a few people will be able to see chakras and auras. If you cannot see them, it does not mean that you will be an inadequate therapist. You will still be able to give an excellent treatment.

Psychological effects

Massage soothes and calms the emotional feelings of the clients, particularly if it is carried out in slow even flowing movements. Stress, depression and anxiety can eat away at a person's confidence, ability to concentrate and cope with everyday challenges. Often a problem in someone's past, e.g. accident or bereavement, can, if not correctly treated at the time, remain in their subconscious and this can develop into a severe emotional condition which the therapist would need to refer to a qualified counsellor or to a GP for referral. Minor anxieties, depression, stress and nervous tension can be treated with an Indian head massage but it may evoke strong reactions from a client, e.g. anger/crying. The release of emotions helps to ease symptoms and helps to re-establish an equal balance. Complete support, care and confidentiality are required by the therapist.

Grounding

This term is used in a lot of holistic therapies. It means making body, mind and spirit feel at one with itself. Often, stress, depression and anxiety make us feel out of control, incomplete and dysfunctional. Grounding brings back the balance. In Chinese treatments this is referred to as the yin and yang. In Indian treatments reference is made to the chakras.

Client grounding

The client should sit on a chair, both feet resting on the floor and concentrate on breathing. The client needs to imagine her feet rolling into the earth and relax. This will help to re-energise and balance the client.

Therapist grounding

Before beginning the client's treatment, the therapist should also feel at one with themselves. They must feel calm and think of peace and tranquility. When dealing with different clients they must try to turn off between each client. Grounding is necessary in order not to be drained by the client.

Introduction to the routine

The spine supports the head which incorporates the shoulder bones and muscles. Most of the weight of the head after the spine is taken by the shoulders. Tension and stress build up in this area. So it is important that this area is worked on first, in order to help the neck and head. When working on neck muscles, these must be worked on slowly to enable more when the muscles are warmed up. Neck muscles can become taut so working slowly on this area allows relaxation to take place, helping blood flow to other parts, including the head. Working from the shoulders to the head enables a sense of wellbeing for the client to be achieved. Personal presentation, hygiene, cheerfulness and a sense of calm is essential when performing this treatment. This will establish a good relationship with your client and yourself.

Attitude and state of mind

Posture

This is an important factor when performing massage. Your back must be relaxed but straight throughout the massage. When standing, bend your knees and tuck in your bottom, so the back works from the pelvis. Allow your thighs to do most of the work. It should be as relaxing and therapeutic to give a massage as it is to receive one. Bad posture can make you tired; so if you pay attention early to your posture it will become automatic later. Your state of mind should be calm. Tune into your client when performing massage. It may help to work with your eyes closed. Massage is an excellent tool for enabling us to become more aware of what is happening deep within us.

Initial consultation

The consultation is a very important part of the treatment. Sufficient time must be allowed, so that it is not rushed. The initial consultation will need detailed information, which must be accurately recorded on to a treatment card. The therapist must establish the outcomes and effects of previous treatments, if there is a need for changes to be made or further action to be taken.

- The client must be seated comfortably and the therapist seated alongside or opposite.
- The therapist must try to:
  - establish a rapport with the client
  - develop mutual trust and gain the client's confidence
  - identify contraindications
  - gain insight of particular needs and expectations of the treatment
  - explain the treatment fully to the client
  - agree a treatment plan
  - answer queries the client may have.
- Confidentiality is most important.
- Sometimes the therapist may have a client that has been referred by her GP. This would be classed as a referral. Medical record card and details must be strictly confidential.

Personal hygiene

Before carrying out this treatment, therapists must prepare themselves physically, taking into consideration high standards of professionalism and hygiene.

Points to consider:

- A daily bath or shower to remove stale sweat odours.
- Use of antiperspirant.
- Hair clean/tied back from the face.
- Nails must be kept short and well manicured; no nail enamel should be worn.
- Hands must be well cared for, smooth and warm.
- No jewellery worn on hands or arms.
- Underwear and tights should be changed daily.
- Uniform should be freshly laundered.
- Feet should be well cared for and comfortable shoes should be worn.
- Therapists suffering from colds and infections should not treat clients.
- Therapists must wash their hands before and after the treatment.

The benefits of Indian head massage

- Relieves eye strain.
- Relieves sinusitis.
- Increases the supply of oxygen and nutrients to skin, muscles and bones.
- Improves cellular activity.
- Relieves mental strain.
- Relieves tension and fatigue.
- Assists in relieving insomnia.
- Eases tinnitus.
- Soothes emotional imbalances.
- Balances energy levels.
- Improves concentration.
- Eases depression and anxiety.

to Indian head massage
- Neck injury.
- Head injury.
- Skin disorders/skin diseases.
- Cuts, bruises and abrasions.
- Recent surgery or fractures.
- Diabetes.
- Epilepsy.
- High/low blood pressure.
- Migraine.
- History of thrombosis or embolism.
- Spastic conditions.
- Dysfunction of nervous system.
- Pins and needles/numbness in fingers.

Indian head massage

Classification of massage movements

Effleurage
A light even stroking which prepares the tissues for deeper massage. Effleurage is used to link movements together during the massage sequence.

Petrissage
Compression movements using either the whole of the palm of the hand or the pads of the fingers and thumbs. Kneading, knuckling, rolling and pinching are all examples of petrissage.

Tapotement
Percussion movements which are performed lightly and briskly without compressing the skin. Stimulating movements, improving the blood flow and removal of waste from the skin.

Vibrations
These movements are used along a nerve path or through a nerve centre. The fingers or thumbs are used to perform a shaking or trembling which causes very little surface stimulation.

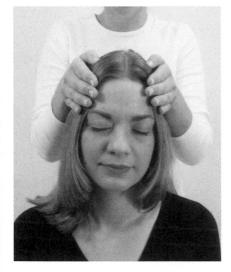

Effleurage

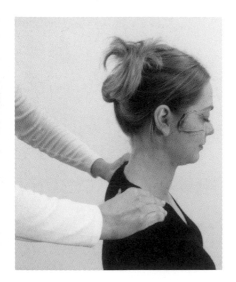

Petrissage

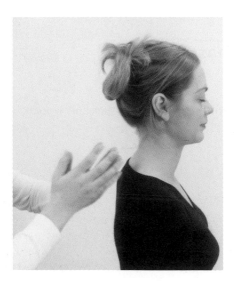

Tapotement

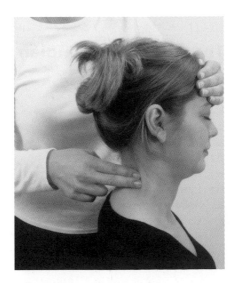

Vibrations

Frictions

These movements are used to relieve tension along the trapezius muscle of the back, to stimulate the lymphatic flow and to aid with desquamation. The thumb or fingers can be used to perform these small but firm rotary movements.

Pinches

Using the flat of the hands and lightly touching the skin squeeze a portion of flesh between index fingers pinch and release. If it is performed quickly it has an invigorating effect. Tones and stimulates muscles.

Pressures

Using either fingers or thumbs, use slight pressure over the nerve pathways or lymphatic pools. This can clear any blockage and increase circulation. Press and release action.

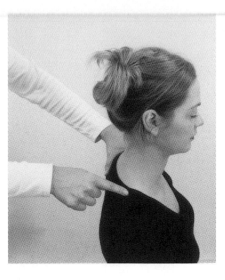

Frictions

Hair texture

Hair texture refers to the degree of thickness and feeling of the hair.

- Diameter of the hair: either coarse, medium or fine. Coarse hair has the greatest diameter. Fine or woolly hair the smallest diameter.
- Feel of the hair: either wiry, soft, silky or woolly.

The client's hair texture also depends on whether the hair is dry or oily, grey, dyed or bleached, and the amount of curliness it has. Careful observation and questioning of the client will help to detect these characteristics.

- Coarse hair texture: is the thickest or has the greatest diameter.
- Medium hair texture: found in hair of average diameter.
- Fine or very fine hair texture: requires special care when being treated. Usually only contains two layers, the cuticle and cortex.
- Wiry hair, whether coarse, medium or fine, has a hard glassy finish due to the imbrications which lay flat against the hair shaft. This type of hair is resistant to treatment and the penetration of chemicals.

Scalp flexibility

The condition of the client's scalp may be:

- Normal
- Flexible
- Tight.

A scientific analysis of the hair and scalp should cover the following:

- Form of the hair (curly, overcurly, straight).
- Length of the hair (long, medium, short).
- Texture of hair (coarse, medium, fine or woolly; feel – wiry, soft or silky).
- Elasticity of hair (normal or deficient).
- Shades of the hair (normal, faded or streaked or grey).
- Conditions of the hair (normal, brittle, dry or oily).
- Condition of the scalp (normal, flexible or tight).

Scalp treatments

The purpose of scalp treatments is to promote the health and beauty of hair and to stimulate the blood supply, which feeds the scalp and hair naturally. Scalp manipulation increases the blood circulation and soothes the nerves. It also increases the glands' activities, makes the scalp more flexible and promotes growth and health of the hair. Shampooing alone will clean the hair but will not prevent it from becoming dry and brittle. Scalp manipulations should be given with a continuous even motion. This will not only achieve a stimulating effect but also will have a soothing effect on the client.

Aromatherapy oils which can be used with Indian head massage

Mood enhancing oils

No matter who we are, sometimes we can be overwhelmed by uncomfortable feelings. Mood oils are a blend of various essences to give you on-the-spot relief from bad or sad moods, or to spice up good ones. Cooling sedating oils douse flaring tempers. Warm, calming oils ease panic attacks. Stimulating oils lift the spirits. These oils can be used to any Ayurvedic treatment that calls for essential oils.

Calming and warming (relieves anxiety):	3 drops Neroli and Lemon 2 drops Jasmine and Sandlewood 1 drop vanilla blend with 1 oz Jojoba oil base
Calming and cooling (relieves anger):	5 drops Sandlewood and Vetiver 1 drop Jasmine blend with 1 oz Jojoba oil base
Stimulating (relieves depression):	4 drops Bergamont and 3 drops Lavender and Basil Blend with 1 oz Jojoba oil base
Sedating (relieves insomnia):	6 drops Rose and 2 drops Jasmine and Chamomile Blend with 1 oz Jojoba oil base.
Grounding (strengthening, relieves fear):	4 drops Patchouli and 2 drops Sandalwood and Cardamon Blend with 1 oz Jojoba oil base

information point

Only qualified aromatherapists should attempt to blend their own oils for Indian head treatment.

Preparation of work and treatment area – a clean and tidy working station

- When greeting the client it is important to put her at ease immediately.
- Clients may be nervous or apprehensive; you may have to spend time calming and reassuring the client.
- Make sure the client is seated comfortably.
- Consultation with client – Name, Address, Medical History, Contraindications, etc.
- Ask the client to remove jewellery. Put them where the client can see them.
- Make sure the working environment is relaxing with no interruptions.
- Soft relaxation music may be played while performing treatment.
- Make sure the area is warm and comfortable and quiet. Lighting should be muted.
- If massage is performed with Indian oils clients must remove upper clothing. Bras for ladies may be left on.
- Make sure oil is removed before clients redress.
- Ensure adequate ventilation.
- Colour scheme should be tranquil.

Home after-care advice for your client

- Clients should avoid tea, coffee, alcohol and chocolate for 24 hours. They should drink water and anti-diuretic herbal teas.
- Eat a light meal.
- Try to relax and rest.

After-treatment care

- After the treatment ensure the client rests for a few minutes.
- Offer your client a glass of water.
- The client may want to talk and unburden their problems.
- Listen and smile.
- Do not give advice in a field you are not qualified in.
- Advise client about the healing crisis.

Healing crisis

This is also known as a contra-action to Indian head massage which can happen either during or after the treatment. Put simply, it means that a person may feel worse before they feel better due to the release of toxins and the rebalancing of the chakras from the effects of the treatment. Symptoms can include:

- Aching or sore muscles.
- Slight headache.
- Tiredness.
- Heightened emotional state – tearful.

Routine

- Prepare client.
- Wash hands.
- Grounding – breathing exercises with client to begin.

Shoulder massage

1 Hold hands on either side of the head, relax and wait for client to become acclimatised to your touch.

2 Slide hands down to your client's shoulders and effleurage from both sides of the neck over the shoulders and back six times.

3 Stand to the side of client. Place one hand on forehead and one under the occipital bone, gently move head back and fourth (rocking). If client cannot relax ask her to take three deep breaths.

4 Standing slightly away from the client, bend knees. Place hands on shoulders; using your thumbs and starting either side of spine in line with scapula draw thumbs up in a fan share to centre of shoulder working up the spine to the neck; repeat three times.

5 Place your thumbs on the middle of the trapezius muscle and your small, middle and index fingers on the clavicle, slide thumbs up to fingers six times, increasing pressure from light to medium to deep.

6 Reverse from 5. Slide fingers to meet thumb lifting the trapezius muscle. Repeat six times.

7 Using the thenar eminence muscle in the thumb (see p. 369) and closing the fingers together, use a hand friction either side of spine and top of shoulders.

8 Stand behind the client. Place one foot in front of the other. Place one hand on client's left shoulder. Using first and second knuckles of right hand, press either side of the spinal column at 2.5 cm (1 inch) intervals down the spine to the middle back. Repeat twice.

9 Place hands on shoulders; commence with sweeping effleurage and progress to deep kneading on the biceps, triceps and deltoids including the trapezius muscles; repeat three times.

10 Using the thenar eminence muscle of each hand, one hand after the other, use a hacking (tapotement) movement over the shoulder; repeat twice.

11 Using your arms, roll across the shoulders and down your client's arms to the deltoids; repeat three times (ironing).

12 Take your finger and thumb of each hand; starting from outer shoulders, working to the middle, lift trapezius muscle and squeeze outer inner/inner outer. Repeat twice.

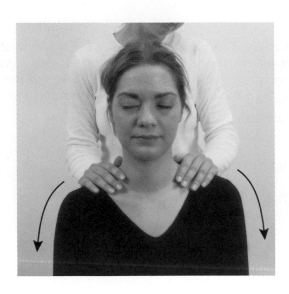

Iron down

13 Iron down. Finish shoulder movements with effleurage. Slide hands down the client's shoulders and effleurage from sides of neck over shoulders. Repeat six times.

Upper arm massage

14 Using your thenar eminence muscle on both hands, slide down biceps/triceps in rows of three. Repeat twice.

15 Bend the client's arms and rest them on her lap and work with friction movements around the elbow joints six times.

16 Squeeze and pluck with finger and thumbs of each hand starting from the top of the arm to the elbow. Repeat this routine down the arm, reverse back twice.

17 Stand behind the client, bend the client's arms, support the arm by holding the elbows, raise the arms and drop. Ask your client to relax. Repeat three times.

18 Standing in front of the client lift the client's right arm, support the client's right shoulder, then slowly rotate shoulder socket clockwise then anticlockwise with your left hand. Repeat on other arm using opposite arms.

19 Standing in front of your client, take client's right arm and effleurage from the wrist to the shoulder six times. Repeat on client's left arm.

Neck massage

20 Support the client's head with your left hand on the forehead. Grasp the back of the neck between your fingers and thumb drawing your fingers up the neck using small circular petrissage to the base of the occipital bone. Repeat three times.

21 Standing behind your client, place your elbow on the client's shoulders and slowly roll your client's head into the cupped palm of your hand. With your hand flat and using your thumb, glide from the base of the ear to the trapezius muscle working across the back of neck. Repeat on other side changing position.

22 Support your client's head with one hand on forehead. Place the other hand grasping the back of the neck slide up, grasp and pull back three times. Repeat procedure three times.

23 Place hands on either side of the client's neck. From the base of the neck apply pressure points up the thoracic vertebrae to the occipital bone; work along the occipital to the base of the ear; slide down neck and repeat three times.

24 Support the client's head and using the palm of your other hand perform large circular movements (heel rub) to the occipital bone, lift fingers and glide into the hair with a slight pull on the hair; repeat twice.

25 With the shoulder supported, use your forearm and slightly push the shoulders down. This stretches the neck muscles. Repeat on other side of the neck.

26 Stand at the side of the client. Support client's head with your left hand and using your fingers and thumb slowly massage in deep effleurage movements with your right hand working up the back of the neck. Repeat three times.

Scalp massage

27 Standing behind your client, using both hands start rotating small movements with your fingertips covering the entire scalp (petrissage).

28 Cupping the client's chin in your left hand, place the right hand at base of skull and rotate gently. Reverse positions of the hands and repeat three times.

29 Place fingertips on each side of the head, slide firmly upward spreading the fingertips until they meet at the top of the head. Repeat four times.

30 Same as 29, except that after sliding the fingertips, rotate 2.5 cm (1 inch) and move the scalp. Repeat four times.

31 Place fingers of both hands on the client's hairline, massage around hairline by lifting and rotating for 1 minute.

32 Place your left hand on forehand. Massage from right ear to the left ear along the occipital bone with heel of your hand using rotary movements.

33 Support and hold back of your client's head with left hand. Place stretched thumb and fingers of right hand on the forehead. Move hand slowly and firmly upward to top of the scalp. Repeat four times.

34 Place the palms of your hands firmly against the client's scalp. Lift scalp in rotary movements. First with your hand above the ears, second with hands placed at front of head, and third with hands at the back of the head moving the scalp (lifting petrissage).

35 Using the sides of your hands, one after the other use a gentle hacking movement, or with fingertips tapping over the entire scalp for 20 seconds.

36 Place left hand on forehead and stand at left of client. Rotate with right hand from base of neck along the client's shoulder and back across the shoulder blade to spine. Slide up spine to base of neck. Repeat on opposite side.

Facial massage

37 Support the client's head, standing from behind gently stroke the hair away from the face behind the ears. With the flats of your fingers start stroking the forehead until the client feels relaxed.

38 Place both thumbs in the centre of your client's forehead just above the eyebrows with your fingers around the sides of the head. Slowly but firmly draw your thumbs up to the top of the forehead; circle the eyes and repeat four times.

39 Using both thumbs stroke down the sides of the nose, unblocking the nasal passages. Repeat four times.

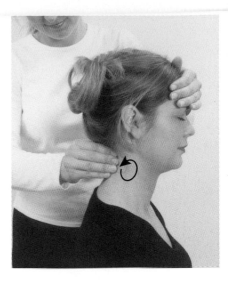

Finger and thumb circles to either side of neck

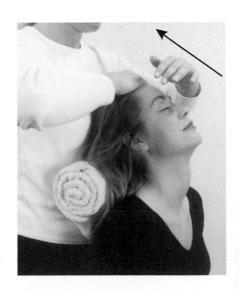

Effleurage to forehead

40 Place the thumbs of both hands either side of the bridge of the nose, glide outwards under the eyes working downwards; cover the whole cheek area. When you reach the ears massage them using your thumbs and first two fingers. Stretch and release ears gently. This will decongest the cheek bones.

41 Place your fingers under the chin and use pressure points along the mandible bone until you reach the ears. Repeat four times.

42 Place your fingers under the chin. Work outwards along the mandible applying pressure points. Work around the contour of the face, until you reach the temple. Work from the corner of the eyes up the bridge of the nose onto the forehead and up into the first inch of the scalp. Repeat this four times.

43 Using your fingertips massage the hairline from the top of the forehead around the base of the skull with deep circular friction movements firmly but slowly.

44 Completion of Indian head massage – stand behind your client, rest her head on your chest and gently stroke the hair from the roots to the tips to release the last remaining tension. Gradually allow your hands to rest on your client's temples and finish with a light pressure.

ACTIVITY

Perform four Indian head massage routines on a selection of clients (male and female), who display different conditions and age ranges. Keep a record of their condition both physically and mentally before and after the treatment as well as the choice of lubricant and the massage routine devised.

KEY TERMS

You will need to know what these words and phrases mean. Go back through the chapter to find out.

Aura

Ayurveda

Chakras

Contraindications

Grounding

Healing crisis

Holistic approach

SELF-CHECKS

1 Describe briefly the history of India head massage treatment.
2 Name and describe the three Ayurvedic principles.
3 Name and describe the seven main chakras and their colours.
4 List the three higher chakras.
5 Give three reasons why the massage treatment may be adapted.

Chapter 3 Aromatherapy

After working through this chapter you will be able to:

- define an essential oil
- outline the factors governing the quality of essential oils
- describe the effects of the main chemical categories of essential oils
- describe the main qualities of a selected number of essential oils
- describe the qualities of a number of carrier oils
- select the amounts of carrier and essential oil for massage
- carry out a consultation for an aromatherapy massage
- prepare a plan for an aromatherapy massage
- select oils which blend together well for aromatherapy massage
- prepare a client for aromatherapy massage
- adapt the principles of body massage to aromatherapy massage
- outline the basic principles of shiatsu pressures
- apply these principles to body massage
- apply these principles to face and scalp massage
- apply these principles to massage of selected parts of the body
- give home advice to clients following aromatherapy massage
- describe other therapeutic ways of using essential oils
- recognise how aromatherapy is being used in medical settings.

Aromatherapy is the name given to treatments that use essential oils – the pure, volatile portions of aromatic plant products. There has been a huge surge of interest in such treatments as part of the growing regard for holistic therapies and complementary medicine. There are many books and courses now for anyone interested in becoming an aromatherapist; beauty therapists, massage therapists and medical personnel such as nurses, occupational therapists and chartered physiotherapists are all becoming involved. It is a subject which can be studied to many levels, so that some people will call themselves aromatherapists who have only a limited knowledge of oils and others will have studied and practised for many years. As more people become aware of the benefits of aromatherapy, training standards will be raised and the levels standardised with a full qualification necessary to practise.

This chapter is meant to provide a starting point for the beginner and a basis for future development. As with other therapies, learning must start somewhere but should never stop. Aromatherapy becomes more fascinating the more you learn.

Skin absorption

There are many factors which determine how much of a chemical penetrates the skin. Some of these factors are:

- the amount and concentration of the chemical applied
- the length of time the chemical is in contact with the skin
- the skin's temperature and moisture content
- the concentration of hair follicles and sweat ducts in the skin in the area where the chemical is applied
- whether the skin is damaged in any way

All of these are likely to affect the absorption of substances such as aromatherapy oils.

Although there is little information on the absorption of essential oils as such, there has been research on the skin penetration of fragrance chemicals. This research shows that absorption is greater over areas of thinner, more delicate skin, such as that on the face and eyelids, and less on the thicker skin on the palms of the hands and soles of the feet. Children's skin is more permeable than adults' skin.

The two major factors governing the level of absorption of such chemicals by the skin appear to be the strength of the dose applied and the size of the area to which it is applied. Massage and heat may also encourage absorption as will covering the area with clothes or towels.

Allergy

Substances applied to the skin may cause the skin to react allergically against the substance. The reaction of some of the cells of the dermis is to release histamine, causing the tissue to become red, warm and swollen. The first contact with the substance may leave the tissue sensitised so that later contact can cause a more severe and generalised reaction. Once a person has become sensitised to a substance it must be completely avoided.

GOOD PRACTICE

- Clients should always be asked if they are allergic to any substances used in products being applied to the skin. If there is any doubt, perform a patch test. Apply some of the substance to a small patch of skin and check for any reaction after 24 hours.
- Aromatherapy products which contain the essential oils of plants are often considered safe because they are pure and natural. However, they are potent, concentrated, natural chemicals and some can be toxic. For example, the oil from the pennyroyal plant contains a liver toxin and cinnamon bark oil can cause allergic skin reactions. The contraindications of individual oils must be checked before use on the skin.
- The commonest way of applying these essential oils is by massage, which increases the flow of blood to the area and this may enhance absorption of the substances into the body.

Photosensitivity

Certain chemicals cause the skin to react more strongly than usual when exposed to sunlight. The best known of these used in perfumery and aromatherapy is oil of bergamot. The result can be 'sunburn' or a rash after a very short exposure to ultraviolet light. It follows that any product containing a photosensitiser should not be applied to the skin before exposure to natural or artificial sunlight (e.g. a sun-bed).

Because essential oils are said to be good for physical and mental conditions there is a temptation for the practitioner to regard aromatherapy as a form of medicine. If that were so, then beauty therapists and those without some medical training would not be using it. Aromatherapy is the use of essential oils to help maintain people in good health and to improve their wellbeing. Clients with medical conditions should always be referred to their doctor.

Essential oils

Essential oils are aromatic substances present at very low concentrations in different parts of plants: in leaves, flower petals, berries and even twigs. When they are extracted from plants and bottled as pure essential oils, their concentration is 100%. They are available for purchase in this form by the general public as well as aromatherapists and should always be adequately diluted for safe use.

Extraction

Oils are extracted from plants by several different methods.

Expression

A few essential oils, such as the citrus oils where the oil is contained in the outer part of the skin, can be obtained by simple pressure. (Examples: lemon, orange, bergamot.)

Distillation

Some essential oils are obtained by distillation. The plant parts are heated in water or steam and the vapour given off is cooled to produce a liquid which is a mixture of essential oil and water. The essential oil can then be easily separated and drawn off to leave perfumed water behind as a by-product.

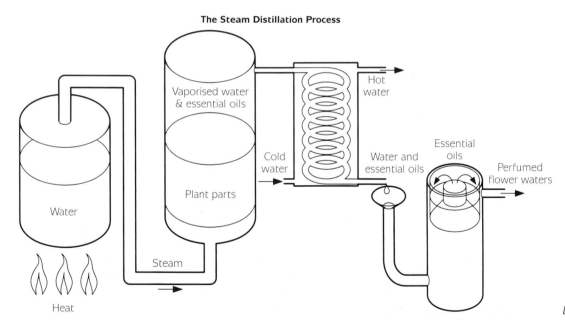

The Steam Distillation Process

Vaporised water & essential oils

Hot water

Cold water

Water and essential oils

Essential oils

Perfumed flower waters

Plant parts

Water

Steam

Heat

Distillation of essential oils

Solvent extraction

Solvent extraction is a method used to obtain some floral oils. The plants are immersed in hydrocarbon solvents to dissolve the essential oils. The solution is then distilled to leave behind a mixture of wax and oil known as a 'concrete'. The wax can then be dissolved in alcohol, which in turn can be evaporated off leaving an 'absolute'. Absolutes differ from true essential oils in that they are generally thicker and more viscous. They are more often used in perfumery than in aromatherapy.

More recently carbon dioxide has been used as a solvent to extract essential oils successfully. By using carbon dioxide in a state known as 'hypercritical' at high pressure, it becomes a very effective solvent that does not contaminate the oils. This method requires bulky and expensive equipment but the number of essential oils extracted by this method that are commercially available is increasing.

Enfleurage

Enfleurage is a traditional method of extraction that is only used today for some very expensive oils such as rose and jasmine. It involves spreading the petals of the plant on fat or oil which absorbs the essence and then extracting it from the fat by using solvents to separate them. However, even rose and jasmine these days are mostly extracted by the more commercial solvent or distillation methods.

Quality

The quality of essential oils is most important and care must be taken to use only oils which are pure and unadulterated. The best advice when starting is to deal only with a reputable supplier who is known to stock oils of the highest quality. Good suppliers are also the best source of advice on which oils to order; for example there are a number of different oils called lavender each with its own qualities and a good supplier will be able to advise you of the differences.

All plants have a common English name and a recognised scientific Latin name which identifies it more accurately and it is wise to become familiar with the Latin name to avoid mistakes when ordering and using the oils.

Factors which can affect the quality of oils include:

- choice of the best possible member of the plant species
- where the plant was grown
- whether it was grown organically
- how it was harvested and at what time of day
- what method of extraction was used
- how the oils have been stored.

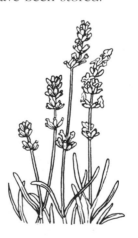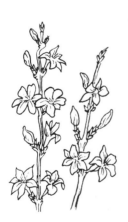

Lavender and jasmine

Categories of oils

There are a number of ways of classifying oils:

- By their volatility rate – that is, how quickly they evaporate into the air.
  Top notes evaporate the fastest, act quickly and tend to be stimulating. Examples: lemon and other citrus oils.
  Middle notes evaporate more slowly and are most often used to help the general metabolism. Examples: geranium and other floral and fruity oils.
  Base notes evaporate slowly and are relaxing and sedating. Example: sandalwood.

Some therapists will take this into account when mixing a blend of oils, using a base note oil to hold and 'fix' a top note oil. If you smell a mixture of oils containing different 'notes', you will smell the top notes first followed by the middle and base notes.

- By the eastern yin and yang philosophy. The terms yin and yang are descriptions of opposite 'energies' or qualities. Yin describes cool, moist, calming, feminine qualities (e.g. rose, geranium), whereas yang describes hot, dry, stimulating, masculine qualities (e.g. juniper). Many oils fall between these extremes and the nearer they are to the middle the more 'balancing' they will be (e.g. sandalwood). Some therapists take this into account when selecting oils for a particular client and when deciding what effects they need to produce – calming, balancing or stimulating.
- By the chemical constituents of the oils. This is a much more complex matter as each essential oil will consist of many chemical components which may even vary in oils of the same name depending on where the plant was grown and under what conditions.

Oils contain chemicals in varying proportions and tend to be classified according to which of the chemicals is predominant. These chemicals can be put in place on a chart according to their general yin or yang qualities. The chemicals also have general effects which can be described. The table below summarises the effects of certain chemicals and shows their relation to the yin and yang qualities.

YIN (calming)

Aldehydes – anti-inflammatory, antiseptic, anti-rheumatic, very calming and soothing.

Esters – the most widespread group of chemicals found in essential oils; anti-spasmodic, anti-inflammatory, anti-parasitic, cooling and soothing.

Ketones – healing, good for skin and scars, sedative, loosens mucous and softens fat, so often used for people with bronchitis and cellulite. **(Ketones should not be used for too long or in high concentrations when they may be toxic.)**

Ethers – anti-inflammatory, anti-spasmodic and anti-stress.

Sesquiterpenes – anti-inflammatory, anti-allergic, anti-parasitic; good for people with heart conditions and asthma.

—— Balancing line ——

Sesquialcohols – act as a general tonic.

Terpenes – antiseptic and anti-inflammatory; they can help to improve the blood and lymphatic circulation.

Alcohols – germicidal; some are very stimulating, but others are much less so.

Oxides – expectorant and decongestant, helping people to cough. Some are anti-parasitic, anti-viral and antiseptic.

Phenols – anti-bacterial, anti-viral, anti-fungal and anti-parasitic. **(Oils in the phenol category are very stimulating and are never used in aromatherapy massage.)**

YANG (stimulating)

The properties of essential oils

Selection of oils for use

Selection of oils for use with a particular client is the most important part of aromatherapy and can be very daunting for the beginner.

When starting, select from the limited list – between eight and ten oils should be enough, growing to 15–20 as experience increases. In the selection you choose include more calming and balancing oils than stimulating oils, select the more commonly used oils and be guided by a good supplier. Make sure you know if any of the oils have any contraindications or can have harmful effects.

A possible list might include the following oils. The oils are listed alphabetically along with their Latin names, predominant chemical category, their best known effects and some of the oils that can be used with them to make a good blend.

Yin oils

Basil (*Ocimum basilicum*) – top note, ether.

- Steadying, good for nervous clients, good for muscle aches and pains and for coughs and colds.
- Blends well with bergamot, geranium.

Bergamot (*Citrus aurantium borgamia*) – top note, ester.

- Uplifting; good for people who are anxious or depressed and having difficulty sleeping.
- Blends well with lavender, neroli, basil.

GOOD PRACTICE

- Bergamot has been shown to sensitise skin to ultraviolet so do not use within three hours of going out into the sun or using a sun-bed.
- Bergamot should not be used on children.

Clary sage (*Salvia sclarea*) – middle to base note, ester.

- Good for exhaustion and overwork, a good muscle relaxant, anti-depressant.
- Blends well with citrus oils, frankincense, geranium, juniper.

Chamomile (*Matricaria chamomilla*) – middle note, sesquiterpene.

- Soothing; a very gentle oil, good on the skin, very calming and good for people suffering from tension, anxiety and related conditions.
- Blends well with lavender, patchouli, geranium, benzoin.

Lavender (*Lavandula angustifolia*) – middle note, ester.

- Boosts the immune system, calming, balancing, healing (especially burns), muscular pain, problem skins. The most versatile and useful oil.
- Blends well with other oils especially floral and citrus oils.

Lemon grass (*Cymbopogon citratus*) – top note, aldehyde.

- Strengthening; good for muscle aches and pains, stomach upsets.
- Blends well with geranium, lavender.

Peppermint (*Mentha piperita*) – top to middle note, ketone.

- Cooling; traditionally used for stomach upsets, also for clearing the head and for coughs and colds. Very good for tired feet.
- Blends well with benzoin, rosemary.

Petitgrain (*Citrus aurantium*) – top note, ester

- Anti-stress, good for oily skins and stomach upsets.
- Blends well with rosemary, lavender, geranium, bergamot, clary sage.

Rose geranium (*Pelargonium graveolens*) – middle note, alcohol/ester.

- Balancing; good for dry and red skins, it stimulates the lymphatic system and can be used for cellulite.
- Blends well with most oils, especially citrus oils, lavender, bergamot and basil.

GOOD PRACTICE

Basil should not be used during pregnancy.

GOOD PRACTICE

Clary sage should not be used during pregnancy or the menopause.

GOOD PRACTICE

Lemon grass should not be used on children.

GOOD PRACTICE

- Peppermint can irritate sensitive skins.
- Avoid using peppermint during the first four months of pregnancy.

Rosemary (*Rosemarinus officianalis*) – middle note, ketone.

- Uplifting – after lavender, the most commonly used oil. It is useful for people with colds or other respiratory problems. Good for stiffness and discomfort in the muscles.
- Blends well with basil, citrus oils, frankincense, peppermint.

Yang oils

Black pepper (*Piper nigrum*) – middle note, terpene.

- Stimulating, good for the circulation and conditions related to poor circulation. Can stimulate the appetite.
- Blends well with frankincense, sandalwood.

Eucalyptus (*Eucalyptus globulus* or *radiata*) – top note, oxide.

- Decongestant, helping people with colds or bronchitis to cough. Also relieves muscular or rheumatic pain.
- Blends well with benzoin, lavender, pine.

Frankincense (*Boswellia carteri*) – basc note, terpene.

- Rejuvenating, very good on older skins, good for chest conditions – especially stress-related ones.
- Blends well with basil, black pepper, citrus oils, lavender, sandalwood.

Juniper (*Juniperus communis*) – middle note, terpene

- Diuretic, good for people with fluid retention or cellulite and can be helpful in cases of cystitis. Good on some problem skins, e.g. acne. Can be used as a disinfectant.
- Blends well with benzoin, lavender, sandalwood.

Lemon (*Citrus limon*) – top note, terpene

- Useful for clients recovering from viral-type illnesses. Also stimulates the circulation, so useful over areas of fat and cellulite and in rheumatic conditions. Refreshing.
- Blends well with lavender, neroli, ylang ylang.

Rosewood (*Aniba roseadora*) – middle note, alcohol.

- Gentle, very good for skin and stress-related conditions.
- Blends well with most oils, especially citrus and floral oils.

Sandalwood (*Santalum album*) – base note, sesquialcohol.

- Balancing; good on the skin and for stress-related conditions and nervous tension.
- Blends well with lavender, black pepper, bergamot, geranium.

Tea tree (*Melaleuca alternifolia*) – top note, alcohol.

- One of the best known of the essential oils and now being incorporated into creams and soaps for its anti-fungal, anti-bacterial and anti-viral qualities. Particularly useful in helping fungal conditions such as thrush and athlete's foot. It seems to stimulate the immune system and is particularly valuable if a cold or flu might be developing.
- Blends well with lavender, rosemary, clary sage.

Ylang ylang (*Cananga odorata*) – base note, sesquialcohol.

- Warming; soothes and boosts confidence, traditionally known as an aphrodisiac.
- Blends well with rosewood, bergamot.

Oils such as rose, melissa and jasmine are much too expensive to include in a starting list.

GOOD PRACTICE

- Rosemary is contraindicated in pregnant or epileptic clients and in those with high blood pressure.
- Rosemary should not be used for too long a period as it can be stimulating.

GOOD PRACTICE

- Lemon can cause skin irritation, so needs to be used in very low dosage.
- Do not use lemon during pregnancy.

GOOD PRACTICE

Note that some of these oils are contraindicated during pregnancy. Until fully qualified, it is wise to avoid using essential oils to treat children and women who are pregnant or breast-feeding.

SELF-CHECKS

Check that you remember the main effects of each of the chemical categories:

- Aldehydes
- Sesquialcohols
- Alcohols
- Ketones
- Sesquiterpenes
- Terpenes
- Esters
- Oxides
- Phenols
- Ethers.

Carrier oils

Essential oils are very concentrated and should never be used undiluted on the skin. For an aromatherapy massage they must be mixed with a carrier oil which will provide lubrication for the massage as well as carrying the therapeutic essential oils being used.

Although mineral oils such as baby oil are sometimes used for massage they are not suitable as carrier oils as they are not easily absorbed by the skin. You can use any vegetable oil so long as it is fairly light and does not have a strong smell which would overpower the essential oils. Just as a good cook will insist that the olive oil they use should be of the finest quality, so an aromatherapist will use only carrier oils that are organically grown, unrefined and cold pressed. Again, the advice of a reputable supplier is invaluable.

The carrier oil chosen can be used on its own with the essential oils or can have small amounts of other oils mixed with them. When beginning to mix oils, grapeseed oil is probably best used as a carrier oil as it is easily available and not expensive. Sweet almond oil is also an excellent choice. Other oils may be mixed with the carrier oils in small amounts before blending in the essential oils.

Examples are:

- Apricot/peach kernel oil contains vitamins A and minerals. It is beneficial to mature, dry skins but can be used on all skin types.
- Calendula oil has anti-inflammatory properties and is beneficial for cracked dry skin and as a base for treating dry eczema.
- Grapeseed oil contains a high percentage of linoleic acid and a small amount of vitamin E. It is light in texture and non-greasy, making it a very popular carrier oil.
- Jojoba oil contains vitamin E and has anti-inflammatory properties. It is beneficial for psoriasis, eczema, arthritis, rheumatism and dry skins. It is also an anti-oxidant useful for clients with wheat allergy.
- Sunflower oil contains vitamins A, B, D and E and is high in fatty acids. It is a light, non-greasy texture and is suitable for all skin types.
- Sweet almond oil is rich in protein, containing vitamins A, B1, B2 and B6 and a small amount of vitamin E. It nourishes and protects all skin types and has a calming effect on skin irritations.

information point

All of these carrier oils can be used on their own to make up 100% of the carrier oil mix or with other oils.

- Avocado oil contains vitamins A, B and D and is also rich in lecithin. It is rich and nourishing and is especially good for dry, dehydrated or ageing skins.
- Carrot oil contains vitamins A, B, C, D and E and fatty acids. It is beneficial for dry skins, psoriasis and eczema.
- Evening primrose oil is a rich source of gamma linoleic acid and vitamins. It is beneficial for dry scaly skins, psoriasis and eczema and mature skins.
- Wheatgerm oil contains vitamins, minerals and proteins and, in particular, it has a very high content of vitamin E and is beneficial for scarred or dry and mature skin. It is an anti-oxidant and so acts to prevent other oils going rancid.

Mixing the oils for aromatherapy massage

To prepare a blend for massage you will need:

- A glass measuring bottle that is marked in millilitres.
- A glass rod for stirring.

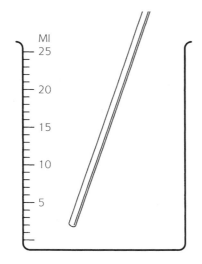

Mixing equipment

The amount of carrier oil needed for the massage is measured into the bottle and the drops of essential oils added. It is then stirred with the glass rod or shaken if there is a stopper, and then it is ready for use.

Amounts of oil needed for massage will vary but a useful 'rule of thumb' is: for a full body massage allow 10 ml for a small person, 14 ml for a medium size and up to 20 ml for a large person. In women, the dress size is a good indicator. Try not to mix too much oil as it will be wasted.

For body massage the essential oils should form 2% of the blend. It is not practical to measure the essential oils in millilitres as 2% of essential oil in 10 ml of carrier oil would be 0.2 ml. The essential oils are therefore measured in drops. 1% of essential oils in 10 ml of carrier is 2.5 drops and 2% in 10 ml of carrier is 5 drops. So if you divide the millilitres of carrier oil by two, the answer gives you the same number of drops of essential oils to give a 2% solution, i.e. up to 5 drops of essential oils can be added to 10 ml of carrier, up to 7 drops in 14 ml and up to 10 drops in 20 ml.

For facial massage the essential oils should form 1% of the blend, half the strength of that used for the body.

The scalp can be treated with a 2% blend and will need at least 5 ml of carrier oil as the hair tends to absorb some. Or, if face and scalp are being treated at the same time, a 1% blend can be used for both.

The oils selected for use are always the result of a careful consultation process which will take into account client preference. One, two or three essential oils may be used to make up a blend.

Factors to be considered in making up a blend

- Appropriate choice of essential and carrier oils for condition of client.
- Fragrance of individual oils acceptable to client.
- Fragrance of mix of oils acceptable to client.
- Oils with very strong fragrance used in small amounts so that they do not dominate, e.g. eucalyptus.
- Oils that complement each other.

The selection and blending of oils for use with a particular client is the most important part of the aromatherapy treatment. Some oils blend together well and are said to be acting synergistically as they seem to help each other's effects. Other oils may inhibit each other's effects and do not blend so well together. If a start is made by using the oils that the client is attracted to and which fit into the category that will help the main problems the client presents, then that is an excellent start.

Examples of oils that work well together are given in the lists of essential oils.

An example of selecting a blend may be for a client who has worries at work and gets constant cold-like symptoms:

- Select the general categories that suit the problems, i.e. an ester for the cooling, soothing qualities, an oxide to help the cold symptoms and maybe a ketone to loosen mucus if the cold is a chesty one.
- From the available oils, choose the ones that the client likes and that you think will go well together, e.g. lavender, eucalyptus and rosemary.

Experience will lead you to an instinctive blend of oils.

Consultation

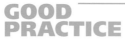

Read Chapter 9 on consultation procedures.

The consultation process is especially important in clients attending for aromatherapy massage. This is because the effects of massage and the effects of the essential oils have to be considered.

The purpose of the consultation is to find out, first, that it is safe to treat the client and secondly, how best to help the client.

Consultation should take into account:

- The medical background: contraindications, problem areas.
- Lifestyle.
- Personality: temperament, emotional state.

The consultation procedure to establish the medical background is fully covered in Chapter 9.

Lifestyle and personality

Information about lifestyle and personality helps to give an overall picture of the person and indicates how you may best help them. Questions should not be too

GOOD
PRACTICE

Check for contraindications to specific oils as well as to the massage itself.

direct or probing but should be open questions allowing the client to express themselves fully.

Examples of open questions are:

- What do you feel the problem is?
- How do you think aromatherapy can help you?
- What makes you feel good/bad?

Most questions beginning with 'how', 'why', 'where', 'what', 'when' will be open questions that will give the client the opportunity to talk. Any question that can elicit the answer yes or no is a closed question. Listen to what the client wants and how they perceive their problem.

One useful way of asking how a client feels emotionally is to ask them to consider how they feel on a scale of 1–10 on a bad day, a good day and at the present time.

GOOD PRACTICE

Consultation is an ongoing process which should continue throughout treatment.

Any counselling skills that you can acquire will be of real use here in dealing with clients who have problems.

CONTRAINDICATIONS

to treatment with essential oils
- Any condition requiring medical attention.
- Broken skin.
- Skin infections/diseases.
- Swellings.
- Severe bruising.
- Recent scar tissue.
- Fractured bones.
- Varicose veins.
- Alcohol in bloodstream.
- Fever/unwell.
- Thrombosis.
- Diabetes.
- Severe circulatory disease.
- Recent inoculations.
- Hepatitis/liver problems.
- Pregnancy (treatment should not be given in the early stages of pregnancy and care in latter stages should be taken on selection of oils as some are contraindicated during pregnancy).
- Young children (treatment of babies and young children is a very specialised area and should be given only by those qualified in advanced aromatherapy).
- Clients with nut or wheat allergies.
- Sunburn.

ACTIVITY

With a colleague acting as a client, carry out a consultation with the aim of selecting suitable oils for the client. Ask the colleague to explain how effective the questions were in eliciting relevant information.

AROMATHERAPY
CLIENT RECORD CARD I

Name of client: First .... Last .... Name of therapist ....

Address of client ....

Telephone .... Date .... Date of birth: Month .... Day ....

☐ Under 21
☐ 21–30
☐ 31–40
☐ 41–50
☐ Over 50

The following profile should be completed for all clients. This is to correctly evaluate the client's special needs in both salon treatment and home maintenance. This is completely confidential and to be used only for this analysis.

1.	MEDICATION: Are you taking any tablets or pills prescribed by a doctor? If YES, please give details. If NO, please indicate if you have had a need to visit a doctor in the last 6 months, or visit a dentist in the last 3 weeks.
2.	FEMALE: When is your period due? If your periods have stopped, please indicate whether naturally or surgically.
3.	CHILDREN: Please give ages.
4.	ALLERGIES: Any known allergies in your family (asthma, hayfever, etc.)? Do you smoke – or have you smoked in the past?
5.	OCCUPATION: Please give details/type of occupation (sitting, standing, driving).
6.	SLEEP: Please give details of your sleep pattern.
7.	EATING: Please give details of your eating pattern, times, etc., also amount of fluid intake daily.
8.	HEADACHES: Do you get headaches? Do you experience motion sickness or fear of falling? Do you wear contact lenses or glasses?
9.	EXERCISE: Do you take regular exercise?
10.	HABITS: Are there any habits you might be aware of (biting nails, biting lip, etc.)?

The above information will help us to recommend the correct essential oil blend and treatment for your personal needs

PLEASE INDICATE THAT THE ABOVE INFORMATION IS CORRECT BY SIGNING HERE

Signature .... Date ....

Aromatherapy client record card (1)

AROMATHERAPY
CLIENT RECORD CARD II

Client: ....

TREATMENT OBSERVATIONS

Therapist: ....

POSTURE   Standing   Hands/Arms
                      Sitting   Legs
                      Walking   Feet
                      Lying on couch   Back
                                                        Face
                                                      Neck

BLEND/FORMULATION RECOMMENDED

COMPARATIVE ANALYSIS

Foot chart

Right foot   Left foot

Aromatherapy client record card (2)

AROMATHERAPY CLIENT RECORD CARD III	Client:		
Date:			
Treatment given:			
Advice given to client after treatment:			
Essential oils recommended for use at home:			
Directions given on their use at home:			
Bathtime blends recommended:			
Complementary treatments recommended:			
Products purchased:			
Return treatment recommended:			
Therapist:			

Aromatherapy client record card (3)

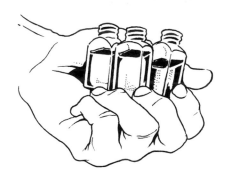

Let the client smell the selection

Treatment plan following full consultation

- Decide on the aims of treatment, focusing on the client's main and secondary problems.
- List the essential oils suitable for use with these problems.
- Select two or three compatible oils from this list.
- Ask the client to smell and approve each individual oil.
- Ask the client to smell and approve the oils together.
- Decide treatment method:
  Full body massage.
  Full body massage with facial massage.
  Part body massage.
- Agree time scale and charges with client. Many clients may feel uncomfortable if the therapist assumes that there will be a series of treatments. Always ask if a client wants to book a series or individual treatments.

Once the treatment method and time scale have been decided the treatment plan is carried out.

Complementary home-care advice should be given with the opportunity to purchase aromatherapy products. Advice might include the use of a bath oil that will complement the treatment or the use of an aromatic burner with appropriate oils.

Example

Following full consultation with a middle-aged, female client you decide the aims of treatment are:

- General relaxation (very busy, tense lifestyle).
- Improve sluggish circulation (cold hands and feet).

Time scale/financial constraints:

- Ideally over a period of six weeks.
- Full body aromatherapy massage every other week alternating with an aromatherapy facial treatment.
- Costs will be as per clinic price list.

Suitable oils to use for relaxation are:

- Lavender.
- Rose geranium.
- Bergamot.

Suitable oils to use to stimulate the circulation are:

- Rosemary.
- Juniper.
- Black pepper.

Ask the client to smell each oil briefly and reject any not liked.

Select two oils the client has approved, one from each group, say lavender and rosemary, and let client smell them together. If the combination is approved by the client the oils can be mixed.

- For the full body massage, in 15 ml carrier oil mix 5 drops of lavender and 2 of rosemary.
- For the facial massage, in 6 ml of carrier oil mix 2 drops of lavender and 1 of rosemary.

More than two essential oils can be used but not more than four. If three oils are preferred for the body massage the blend may be: 4 drops lavender, 2 drops rosemary, 1 drop bergamot.

Offer to mix oils or products for home use or take the opportunity to sell aromatherapy products. When the client returns for the next treatment always discuss the effects of the previous treatment and be ready to adjust the oils and method of application to suit the client's needs.

REMEMBER

Bergamot must not be used on skin to be exposed to natural or artificial sunlight.

GOOD PRACTICE

Keep a record of the blends you use, the clients they were used on and the results of the treatment.

Other useful essential oils

Less common essential oils are listed here in alphabetical order along with their Latin names, predominant chemical category and the effects they are best known for.

Aniseed (*Pimpinella anisum*) – middle note, ester.
- Warming, antiseptic, expectorant.

Benzoin (*Styrax bensoin*) – base note, ester.
- Anti-inflammatory, warming, good for joint conditions, colds and the skin.
- Blends well with sandalwood.

Cedarwood (*Cedrus atlantica*) – base note, terpene.
- Antiseptic, astringent, expectorant, bronchial and urinary infections, catarrh.
- Blends well with rosewood, bergamot, ylang ylang.

Cinnamon (*Cinamomum zeylanicum*) – middle note, aldehyde.
- Astringent, stimulant (circulatory, cardiac and respiratory), poor circulation, rheumatism.
- Blends well with ylang ylang, mandarin, benzoin.

Clove (*Syzygium aromaticum*) – middle note, ketone.
- Anti-histamine, anti-oxidant, antiseptic, nausea, rheumatism.
- Blends well with rose, clary sage, bergamot.

Cypress (*Cupressus sempervirens*) – middle to base note, terpene.
- Anti-rheumatic, vasoconstrictor, diuretic.
- Blends well with juniper, lavender, pine.

GOOD PRACTICE

Avoid using aniseed on sensitive skin, especially allergic or inflamed skin.

Fennel (*Feniculum vulgare*) – middle note, ether.

- Eases wind and stomach upsets, traditionally used for obesity.
- Blends well with geranium, lavender, sandalwood.

Fennel, sweet (*Foeniculum vulgare*) – top note, terpene

- Diuretic, detoxifying, cellulite, nausea, odema, amenorrhoea.
- Blends well with geranium, rose, lavender.

Geranium (*Pelargonium graveolens*) – middle note, ester.

- Anti-depressant, antiseptic, acne and oily skin, premenstrual tension, eczema.
- Blends well with lavender, patchouli, neroli.

Immortelle (*Helichrysum angustifolium*) – middle note, ketone.

- Expectorant, good for aches and pains, skin conditions and breaks in the skin.
- Blends well with chamomile, clary sage, geranium and lavender.

Jasmine (*Jasminium grandiflorum*) – middle note, ester.

- Relaxant, anti-depressant, sedative, coughs, muscular spasm.
- Blends well with rose, sandalwood, citrus.

Mandarin (*Citrus reticulata*) – top note, ether.

- Antiseptic, sedative.
- Blends well with other citrus oils such as neroli.

Marjoram (*Origanum majorana*) – middle note, alcohol.

- Warming, sedative, soothing, good for joint conditions.
- Blends well with lavender, rosemary, cypress and eucalyptus.

Melissa (*Melissa officinalis*) – middle note, terpene.

- Asthma, coughs, menstrual problems, eczema and skin problems.
- Blends well with lavender, geranium, citrus.

Myrrh (*Commiphora myrrha*) – base note, sesquiterpene.

- Healing, good for the chest, sedative.
- Blends well with frankincense, sandalwood, benzoin, juniper.

Myrtle (*Myrtis communis*) – middle note, oxide.

- Good for catarrh, slightly sedative, soothing.
- Blends well with begamot, lavender, rosemary and clary sage.

Neroli or orange blossom (*Citrus aurantium*) – base note, alcohol.

- Calming, anti-stress, good for shock and depression.
- Blends well with most oils.

Niaouli (*Melaleuca viridiflora*) – top note, terpene.

- Antiseptic, acne, respiratory problems, poor circulation.
- Blends well with lavender, rosemary, clove.

Orange, sweet (*Citrus sinensis*) – top note, terpene.

- Anti-depressant, digestive problems, oily skins, cold, flu.
- Blends well with lavender, geranium.

Patchouli (*Pogostemon cablin*) – base note, sesquialcohol.

- Good for depression, anxiety, healing skin.
- Blends well with vetiver, sandalwood, geranium, neroli.

Pine (*Pinus sylvestris*) – middle note, terpene.

- Good for colds and chest infections, stimulating.
- Blends well with tea tree, rosemary, lavender, juniper.

Rose otto (*Rosa damascena*) – middle note, ester.

- Astringent, thrush, labour pains, period pains, menopause, anxiety, insomnia.
- Blends well with jasmine, bergamot, lavender, clary sage.

Sandalwood (*Santalum album*) – base note, terpene.

- Astringent, expectorant, catarrah, coughs.
- Blends well with black pepper, clove, jasmine.

Thyme (*Thymus vulgaris*) top note, terpene.

- Coughs, sinusitis, poor circulation, bruise, cellulite.
- Blends well with lemon, rosemary, melissa.

Valerian (*Valeriana fauriei*) – top note, ester.

- Anti-spasmodic, bactericidal, sedative, insomnia, nervous indigestion.
- Blends well with pine, lavender, rosemary.

Vetiver (*Vetiveria zizanoides*) – middle note, sesquialcohol.

- Calming, stimulates the circulatory system.
- Blends well with sandalwood, patchouili, lavender and clary sage.

SELF-CHECKS

1 What is an essential oil?

2 Give five factors governing the quality of an essential oil.

3 Select pairs of oils that would be suitable for use with clients who:

   a have a very stressed lifestyle

   b have problems sleeping

   c have weight and cellulite problems

   d tend to get stiff and sore after an activity such as gardening.

Aromatherapy massage

Although essential oils can be used in many ways, massage is the most important and commonly used method of applying them in aromatherapy. This is because massage combines the therapeutic power of touch with the properties of the oils. Massage provides a very effective way of introducing the oils into the body. As the skin absorbs the oils, a useful amount will be taken into the bloodstream in the relatively short time that a body massage takes.

In general the conditions and legislation that cover the practice of aromatherapy will be the same as those covering the practice of massage.

The effects of aromatherapy massage will consist of:

- the effects of the massage
- the effects of the oils used.

Aromatherapy oils can be administered to the body using a typical body massage routine and different aromatherapists will have quite different techniques depending on their training and experience. However, in general the massage used in aromatherapy treatments is a relaxing massage using mainly effleurage and stroking movements and omitting the percussion and more vigorous petrissage movements. Instead of these more vigorous movements many therapists integrate finger pressures into their massage which may be called acupressure, shiatsu pressures or neuro-muscular techniques.

to aromatherapy massage will consist of:
- contraindications to massage
- contraindications to the oils to be used
- contraindications to acupressure.

Acupressure

Acupressure refers to many treatment systems that manipulate the acupuncture points on the body by pressure rather than by needles, as is the case with acupuncture. The acu points are found along twelve pairs of meridians, or channels, which pass down the body. It is said that energies flow along these meridians which govern the body's systems.

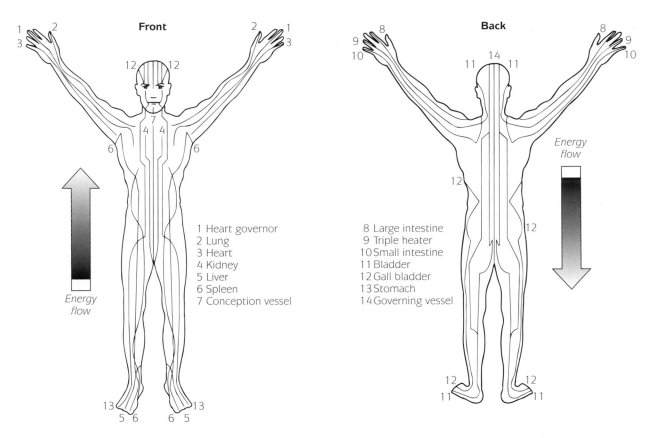

Front

Back

1 Heart governor
2 Lung
3 Heart
4 Kidney
5 Liver
6 Spleen
7 Conception vessel

8 Large intestine
9 Triple heater
10 Small intestine
11 Bladder
12 Gall bladder
13 Stomach
14 Governing vessel

Energy flow

The meridian system

When pressure is applied to a point on a meridian, it stimulates local nerves and tissues and also influences the flow of energy through that and other meridians. The basic philosophy of acu points comes from traditional Chinese systems of healing, however most Eastern societies will have pressures in their massage therapies.

Shiatsu

The Japanese word shiatsu (*shi* – finger, *atsu* – pressure) describes pressures on the acu points which may be applied with the fingers, other parts of the hand and even the elbows or feet. The massage itself is just one part of a whole philosophy of treatment attempting to return the energy, or chi, of the body to a state where yin (negative) and yang (positive) qualities are in balance.

A shiatsu treatment is very different from the usual Swedish-style massage. No oil is used and there are no smooth, flowing strokes; just pressure and stretching are used. However, some shiatsu-type pressures applied with the fingers or the thumb can be integrated into a Western-style massage very successfully and more can be used as a knowledge of the meridian lines is gained. Sliding pressures applied with the thumb or the hand along meridians are particularly useful as oil is being used.

Pressures

The thumbs are the usual tools used for applying pressures as the acu points are mostly placed in thumb-sized hollows. In some areas a finger may be used, often supported by the adjacent finger. The heel of the hand may be used over larger areas such as the side of the buttocks.

Pressure should be applied in a firm, controlled manner with body weight controlling the amount of pressure. No poking or roughness should be used and pressure should be moderate to light. When sliding pressure is applied it should be even and the sliding movement steady with care being taken not to cause discomfort by pulling on hair or skin.

The client should breath out when pressure is applied to the back or chest and breath in between pressures.

Pressures are usually performed only once over the area whereas the traditional massage movements will be repeated a number of times depending on the time available and the speed of the strokes.

GOOD PRACTICE

- Contraindications to pressures are the same as those for massage; don't press over any tender or fragile areas and if pain occurs, use very light pressure. Take care that nails do not dig in.
- Use your eyes to check the client's responses to the pressure applied.

Routine for an aromatherapy treatment

- Consultation – which should take at least half an hour in the first instance.
- Complete consultation card.
- Obtain the client's signature.
- Check for contraindications to massage and oils.
- Select appropriate oils and check acceptability with the client.
- Mix oils and check acceptability with the client – mix enough 5% mixture for the body and 1% mixture for the face.
- Check that all necessary oils, creams, towels, cotton wool and tissues are close to hand.
- Suggest the client empties the bladder.
- An infrared treatment may be given to warm the client, but saunas and steam baths are not suitable.
- The client should be lying supine, warm and well covered by towels.
- Cover the hair with a light, loose cloth or towel unless the scalp is to be included.
- If the scalp is to be included ask the client if oil may be used on the hair.
- Deep cleanse the face if facial massage is to be included.
- Place a little of the 1% oil mixture on the client's hands and ask them to inhale and lightly stroke the cheeks with the oil mixture. If there is only 2% mixture available apply a little to the client's upper lip.

GOOD PRACTICE

Always take care to avoid getting oils in the eyes or on the eyelids.

The following aromatherapy routine is reproduced courtesy of the Eve Taylor Institute of Clinical Aromatherapy. Note the diagrams are for guidance only.

Back of legs movements

1   Start with the left leg. Using the base of your hands and commencing with your left hand, stroke up the back of the whole leg and follow through with your right hand to the popliteal area only. Repeat 3–6 times.

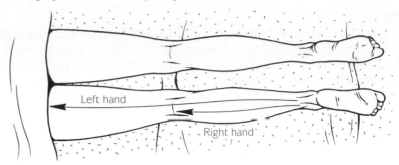

Movement 1

2   Lift (about 15 cm/6 in) and support the client's ankle and using the palma pad of your hand, slide up the centre of the calf to the popliteal area. Repeat 3–6 times.

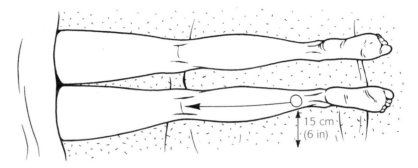

Movement 2

3   Tilt your thumbs upwards and thumb slide from the ankle to the knee. Repeat 3–6 times.

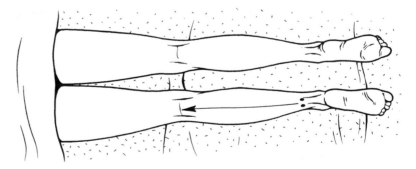

Movement 3

4   Slide your fingers up and finger slide over the calf to the popliteal area.

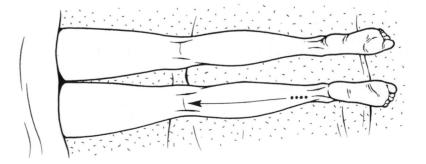

Movement 4

5   Repeat movement 2.

6   Repeat movement 1.

Repeat movements 1–6 on the client's right leg.

Back movements

Group one: searching and finding

1   Using cushioned fingers, perform a figure-of-eight movement up and out over the client's back using both hands. Repeat 3–6 times.

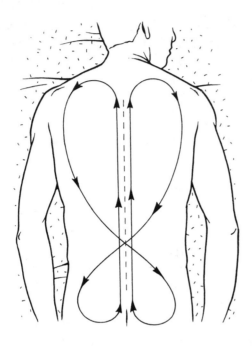

1 Figure-of-eight

2   Using your thumbs, work down each side of the spine separately using a press and release movement. Repeat 3–4 times.

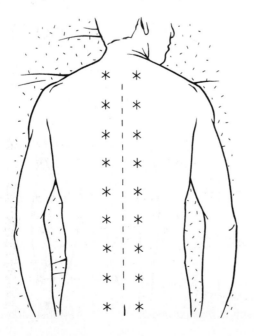

2 Thumb press, release and move

3   Using your thumbs, work down each side of the spine separately using a press and slide movement. Repeat 3–4 times.

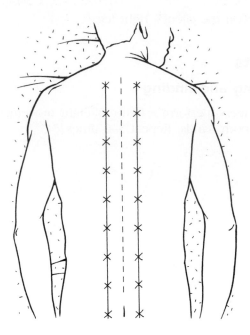

3 Thumb press and move

Group two: heat movements

1   Using cushioned fingers and working both hands simultaneously on either side of the back, work up the upper back area. Repeat 3–4 times.

2   Using cushioned fingers, work one hand followed by the other up over one side of the upper back then repeat on the other side. Repeat 3–4 times.

3   Place one hand cupped like a pyramid over the base of the elimination area of the back whilst the other hand operates like a corkscrew twisting up and out over the upper back and shoulder area. Repeat on the other side. Repeat 3–4 times.

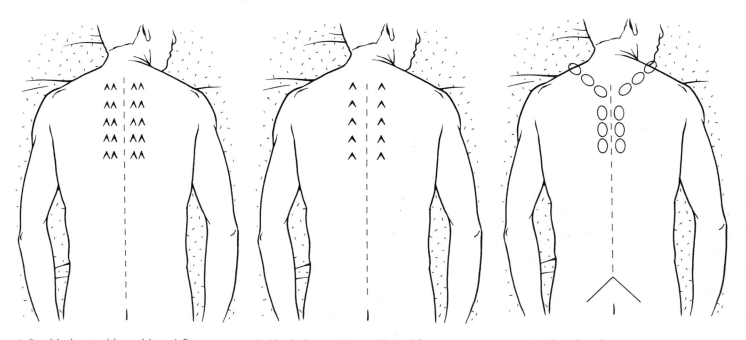

1 Double heat with cushioned fingers   *2 Single heat with cushioned fingers*   *3 Pyramid and corkscrew movements*

Group three: erase, loosen and drain

1   Using the sides and base of your hands, loosen the connective tissue working by pumping from the spine out to the side of the body then repeat on the other side. Repeat 3–4 times.

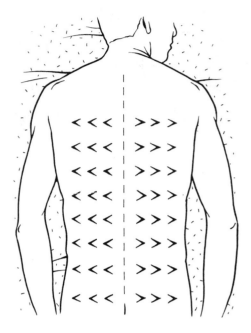

1 Loosen connective tissue

2   Using cushioned fingers, drain from the spine out to the outside of the body, then repeat on the other side. Repeat 3–4 times.

3   Spread your hand to make a fan shape and use your fingers to stroke up and out over one side of the lower back, quickly followed with alternate hands. Repeat this over the other side of the lower back. Repeat 3–4 times.

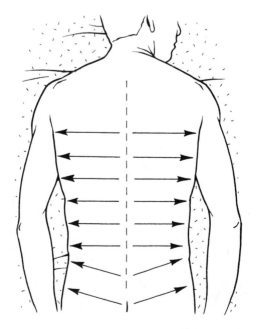

2 Slide out with cushioned fingers

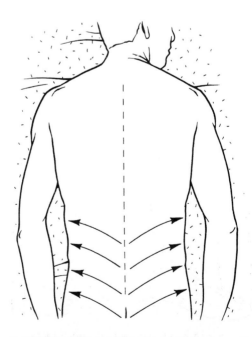

3 Repeated fan movements

Movements on the neck

Support the client's head and check the five points on the base of the skull for sensitivity using the fingertips in a gentle pumping action. If there is any sensitivity, work the area gently.

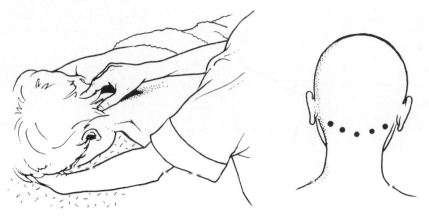

Movements on the neck

Foot movements

Part one: wake up routine

1 Using your knuckle on the solar plexus point, press in and up on both feet simultaneously. Then start work on the client's right foot.

2 Work the pituitary area using your thumb and a pumping technique.

3 Work the neck area using your thumb and a pumping technique.

4 Work the reproductive area using your thumb and a pumping technique.

5 Massage the spinal reflex area from the inner foot to the reflex area followed by massaging the heel to the kidney area using your thumb and a pumping technique.

6 Using the thumb pumping technique, massage from the kidney reflex to the bladder reflex.

Repeat movements 2–6 on the left foot.

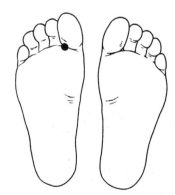

Movement 1

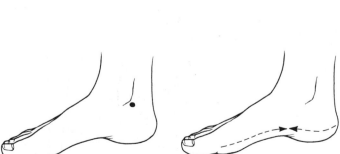

Movement 3

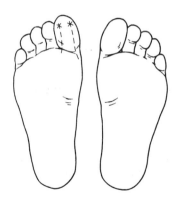

Movement 2

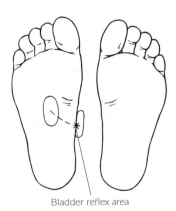

Bladder reflex area

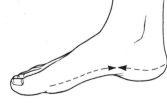

Movement 4   *Movement 5*   *Movement 6*

Part two: wake up technique

1   Using your left hand to hold the sole of the right foot, your right thumb massages the solar plexus area whilst your fingers rotate the toes three times. Repeat on the left foot.

2   Placing your thumbs on the solar plexus points and your fingertips on top of the feet, push up on the plexus and drain out with your fingers. Repeat by moving your fingertips out slightly.

3   Rotate the client's foot outwards with your left hand gently gripping the foot, then grind out over the sole of the foot with the thumb of your right hand. Repeat on the other foot.

4   Using your thumbs, apply pressure to both solar plexus points. Close your eyes and as your client breathes in push up gently. Release as the client breathes out.

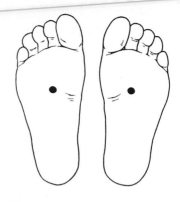

Movement 1

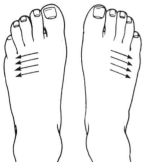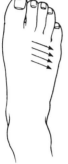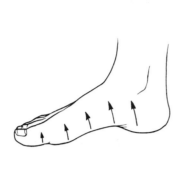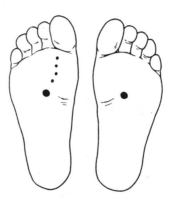

Movement 2　　　　　　*Movement 3*　　　　　　*Movement 4*

Face and décolleté movements

Wash your hands and apply appropriate oil for this area.

NB All the following movements are repeated 3–4 times.

1   Place your fingers just above the client's ears and your thumbs between the eyebrows. Using your thumbs press, release and repeat gliding back to the hairline.

2   Keeping your fingertips in the same position, use your thumbs to press and slide using a gentle pumping action until you reach the hairline.

3   With your fingers still resting over the ears use your thumbs to press and slide out from eyebrows to temples.

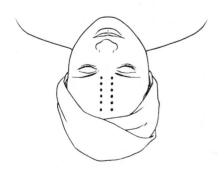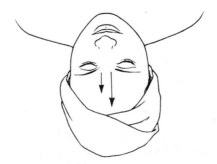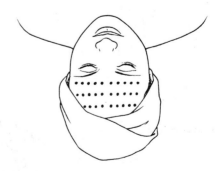

Movement 1　　　　　　　　　*Movement 2*　　　　　　　　　*Movement 3*

4   Using the palma pad of your hands slide out over the forehead and drain down towards the ears.

5   Place your thumbs between the eyebrows and use cushioned fingers to drain out from the nose towards the ear, first above the bone, then below the bone.

6   Using two fingers, drain with both hands simultaneously from the centre of the jawline out towards the ear.

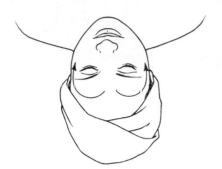

Movement 4

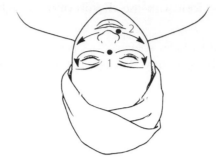

Movement 5

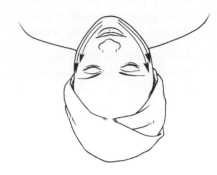

Movement 6

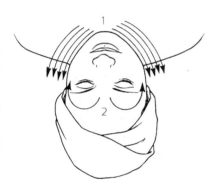

Movement 7

7   Drain with your fingertips with both hands simultaneously up the jawline to the face and use the palma pad of your hands to drain out over the forehead back down the face.

8   Using your fingers of both hands simultaneously drain down to the clavicle, release the pressure in your fingers, press down and back on the shoulders three times, and push down on the shoulders towards the client's feet three times.

9   Slide your fingers from the shoulders to the neck along the trapezius until they meet at the spine and flow up into the neck, and release.

10 Place one hand under the client's neck on the occipital area, the other gently cupping the jaw (mandible) area on the front of the face. Very gently, move the head from side to side. This slightly stretches the spine. Bend your knees to gain the correct posture and support the client's head and neck by resting their neck on your hands and head on your wrist and arms. Tell the client which way you are going to move and slowly move your leg rather than your body from side to side.

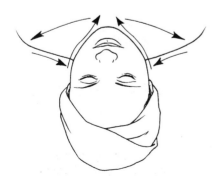

Movement 8

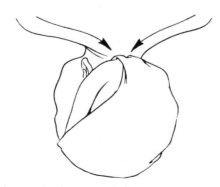

Movement 9

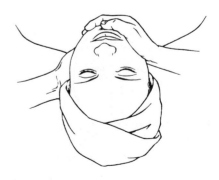

Movement 10

HEALTH AND BEAUTY THERAPY: A PRACTICAL APPROACH

Arm movements

1 Support the client's arm by gently resting their fingers on your wrist and your fingers on their wrist. Using the side of your hand slide and glide using a pumping action working up the arm. Repeat 3–4 times.

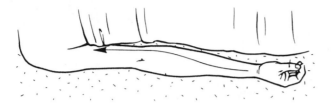

Movement 1

2 Using the same supportive technique and action, work up the inner forearm, then the outer upper arm, then the inner arm. Repeat 3–4 times.

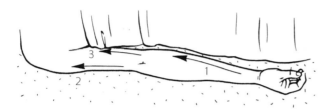

Movement 2

Repeat movements 1–2 on the client's left arm.

Clavicle and abdominal movements

1 Using three fingers above the bone, drain out over the clavicle and slide your thumbs down into the axillary groove. Repeat 3–4 times.

2 Using the fingers of your left hand, make a large circle moving up the ascending colon, across the transverse and down the descending colon, immediately following through using your right hand to make a small circular movement over the intestines. Repeat 3–4 times.

3 If the client's abdomen is distended with air, place your hands over the abdomen and ask the client to breathe in and push their stomach up, hold for 7 seconds and then breathe out. As the client breathes out, gently press down. Repeat 3–4 times.

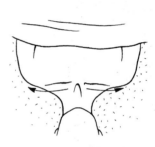

Movement 1

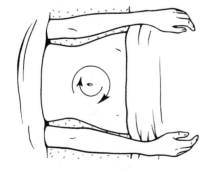

Movement 2   *Movement 3*

4 Resting your fingers gently on either side of the rib cage, use your thumbs at the base of the sternum to drain lightly down over the transversus to the umbilicus. Then repeat using finger and thumb sliding. Repeat 3–4 times.

5 With overlapping hands, drain out around the diaphragm in light pumping movements then repeat on the other side. Repeat 3–4 times.

information point

Eve Taylor's routine is available on video through Eve Taylor Institute of Clinical Aromatherapy, 9 Papyrus Road, Werrington Business Park, Werrington, Peterborough, Cambridgeshire PE4 5BH.

6 From the waistline, use strong draining movements over to the pubic zone using alternate hands. Repeat on the other side.

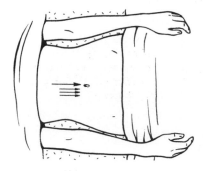

Movement 4

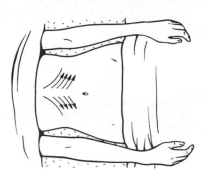

Movement 5

Middle finger of left hand

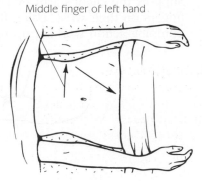

Movement 6

ACTIVITY

Practise the back routine until you are able to perform it fluently.

A whole body massage may not be required or appropriate. Individual parts of the body may be treated by aromatherapy massage taking less time and costing a proportional amount, for example:

- back massage – 30 minutes
- feet and lower legs – 15 minutes each leg
- face and scalp – 30 minutes
- face, chest and shoulders – 30 minutes.

If only a small part of the body is to be treated the essential oils may be used in slightly stronger concentrations. 3% to 5% mixes may be used on the body, but not the face, and only if the safety of the oil has been checked.

ACTIVITY

Consider what types of client would benefit most from an aromatherapy massage consisting of:
a full body
b feet and lower legs
c face and scalp
d face, chest and shoulders.

After-care and home-care advice

Following a body massage a client should be advised to leave the oils on the body for a few hours in order to maximise the effects. It is also wise to tell the client whether the oils used could have a sedative or stimulating effect, especially if the client is driving.

The following advice should be given to the client.

1 Drink 6–8 glasses of water.

2 Do not sunbathe or use sun-beds for 24 hours.

3 Avoid heat treatments such as sauna or steam.

4 Where possible avoid using machinery or driving for 12–24 hours.

Further uses for essential oils

Essential oils can be used effectively in ways other than massage. They can be used in skin care by mixing them with a bland cream or adding them to a basic facial mask, in compresses, baths and diffused into the atmosphere.

Compresses

Compresses can be hot or cold. For a hot compress, a few drops of oil can be added to a bowl of hot water and a cloth or flannel dipped in and wrung out. This can then be placed on the affected area. They are useful to place on the back, for instance, while the rest of the body is being massaged.

A cold compress is prepared in the same way using ice cold water and is suitable for the forehead if the client has a headache.

Baths

Essential oils can be added directly to bath water just before getting in or can be mixed with a little carrier oil first. If added directly to the water, mix the oil well in to the water before sitting in the bath to avoid them coming into direct contact with the skin. If used with a carrier oil, be careful not to slip.

Suggested oil for the bath:

- Relaxing – 6 drops lavender with 4 drops of geranium or 7 drops chamomile with 3 of basil.
- Colds – 6 drops of pine with 6 of eucalyptus.
- Aches and pains – 4 drops of rosemary with 3 of chamomile.

Diffusion

Oils can be diffused into the atmosphere in a number of ways. The commonest way is to use a pottery burner which contains a tea light candle. A few drops of oil are placed in warm water in a saucer shaped bowl above the candle. The heat from the tea light speeds the evaporation of the oil into the atmosphere.

Specific oils can be chosen for their effects, e.g. frankincense and lavender for a relaxed atmosphere and eucalyptus or sweet myrtle when people have colds.

A more effective way of spreading oils into the atmosphere is to use an electrically operated nebuliser which propels the oil into the air in a very fine mist.

All these methods can be used to enhance and complement aromatherapy massage.

Massage and aromatherapy in a medical setting

The recent growth in popularity of complementary therapies is reflected in the number of healthcare professionals who are showing an interest in training and in using these therapies in the treatment of patients. There is a real desire among nurses, physiotherapists and occupational therapists to return to their caring role rather than the medical model that has been the trend for many years. The term 'holistic approach' is being used more and more where all aspects of the individual being treated are considered rather than just the physical. Some recent examples of massage and aromatherapy being used in such a way follow.

Labour ward

Midwives at the John Radcliffe Maternity Hospital in Oxford wanting to find a way of relieving pain and calming women in labour set out to evaluate the use of essential oils for the purpose. The project lasted six months and the oils used were lavender,

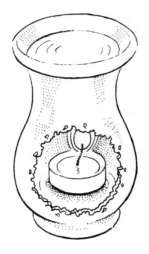

Pottery oil burner

clary sage, peppermint, eucalyptus, chamomile, frankincense, jasmine, rose, lemon and mandarin.

The oils were used in baths, footbaths, inhaled or massaged. The most effective oil used was lavender. Peppermint and clary sage also showed good results. There was a high degree of satisfaction from the women and the midwives and the use of essential oils has been retained in the labour ward.

Intensive care

Research in the intensive and coronary care unit of the Royal Sussex County Hospital showed that massage and the use of essential oils reduced the heart rate and breathing rate in most of the patients tested and seemed to be more effective than massage alone.

The feet were massaged with lavender in a carrier oil and comparison was made with patients who were massaged with carrier oil alone. The drop in the heart rate was significantly greater in the lavender group.

Occupational therapy

Aromatherapy and massage are currently being used by many occupational therapists in a variety of settings to develop relationships, relieve anxiety and to help physical function. One example is where the occupational therapist massages the hands of children using lavender oil to relax and mobilise the hands before exercise. Other uses may be to diffuse into the atmosphere to promote concentration or relaxation.

Sleep patterns

A trial to evaluate the effects of lavender diffusion on the sleep patterns of patients with dementia was carried out in 1993 at Newholme Hospital, Bakewell. The trial ran over a seven-week period using an electric diffuser. The results showed a significant improvement in the sleep patterns of the patients.

KEY TERMS

You need to know what these words mean. Go back through the chapter to find out.

Acupressure

Anti-inflammatory

Anti-oxidant

Antiseptic

Base note

Compress

Diffusion

Distillation

Expression

Middle note

Sedative

Shiatsu

Solvent

Synergistically

Therapeutic

Top note

Volatile

ACTIVITY

Try to carry out a literature search in professional journals and collect references to the use of massage and aromatherapy in a variety of medical settings.

Chapter 4 Electro-epilation

After working through this chapter you will be able to:

- list what electro-epilation is and why it is used
- understand why clients might need electro-epilation
- identify the procedures to follow in an electro-epilation treatment
- state the hygiene procedures to follow
- perform safe working practices for electrical equipment
- prepare the working area
- greet clients
- conduct consultations
- identify contraindications for each of the treatments
- prepare the client
- understand the procedures for diathermy treatments
- understand the procedure for galvanic treatments
- perform blend treatments
- identify the after-care procedure and instructions
- name the different methods of electro-epilation
- understand the alternative methods of hair removal
- describe the structure of the hair and follicle
- name and describe the hair growth cycle
- briefly describe the endocrine system.

Introduction

Electro-epilation is a permanent method of removing excess or unwanted hair by a variety of different techniques.

The different methods of electro-epilation are:

- **Short-wave diathermy** (high frequency alternating current). Also known as high frequency or thermolysis, it causes destruction of the dermal papilla by the production of heat within the tissues of the follicle.
- **Galvanic** (direct current). This method brings about the permanent destruction of the dermal papilla by a chemical action that occurs within the follicle.

- **The blend technique** (combined galvanic and diathermy currents). This method combines the effects of both short-wave diathermy and galvanic giving thorough and more effective treatment than either can do alone.

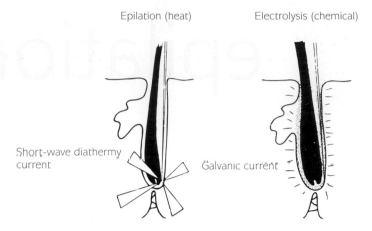

Epilation (heat)   Electrolysis (chemical)

Short-wave diathermy current   Galvanic current

Comparison of the areas of tissue destruction when using diathermy and galvanic currents

information point

Normally clients use electro-epilation for the following reasons:
- To remove excess or superfluous hair.
- For a permanent professional treatment.
- For a long lasting effect.

Electro-epilation is the only way hair can be permanently removed. People with hyper-trichosis, women with hirsuitism and sex change clients tend to benefit more from electro-epilation.

It is important to understand the following terms:

- Superfluous hair – this is unwanted hair that grows in addition to hair that is considered normal. Superfluous hair can grow anywhere on the body.
- Hyper-trichosis – this is excess hair growth.
- Hirsuitism – this is the growth of excess hair in the male hair pattern, i.e. on the face, neck, chest and abdomen.

The main causes of superfluous hair

- Hormones – some females have low levels of oestrogen and progesterone (the female hormones) and high levels of androgens (the male hormones).
- Hereditary and racial background – all ethnic groups are different; for example, northern European people from Britain and Scandinavia have less hair than Mediterranean or Semitic types. Negros have relatively little hair, Mongolian and Oriental races have least body hair.
- Stress – this makes hair grow heavier due to the adrenal glands being very active in times of crisis and produce androgens, the male hormones.
- Puberty – the androgens can briefly become dominant.
- Pregnancy – the androgens can briefly become dominant.
- Menopause – the female hormones can be reduced due to the degeneration of the ovaries.
- Drugs – steroids can affect the adrenal cortex; cortisone and the Pill can lead to excess hair.
- Illness and disease – for example, Cushing's Syndrome and Stein Leventhal Syndrome.
- Increased blood supply to the area.
- Disease.
- Injury.

The causes of superfluous hair

- Congenital or hereditary
- Topical
- Systemic.

Congenital causes

This hair growth has been with the person since birth and, although the client may consider it 'abnormal' or excessive, it is in fact considered normal for the race of the individual.

FUNCTION OF THE HAIR		
Hair	Region of body	Function
Cilia	Eyelashes	To shade, prevent dust, dirt, etc. entering the eyes.
Supercilia	Eyebrows	To shade, prevent dust, dirt, etc. entering the eyes.
Vibrissae	Nostrils	To screen incoming hair and prevent a build up of particles in the lungs.
Capilli	Scalp	For protection against ultra violet and to maintain body temperature.
Hirci	Body hair	To retain body heat and protect against friction.

Abnormal congenital hair patterns

Congenital hyper-trichosis may appear at birth or emerge later in life. The hair growth may be very excessive and is only due to the unusual genetic structure. This is a very rare condition but requires many years of treatment.

Topical causes

This is hair growth in response to any potential threat to the epidermis by rubbing or some other cause of irritation. Hair grows deeper and coarser to protect the skin in the immediate area, as the blood supply has been stimulated. Moles and birthmarks are frequently a cause of excessive hair growth due to the unusual development of capillaries near the surface of the skin.

Systemic causes

This is hair growth as a result of a change in the chemical structure of the endocrine system. There can be normal systemic causes and abnormal systemic causes.

Normal systemic causes of hair growth

Androgens are the only hormones capable of stimulating target follicles to produce hair; a woman's system usually produces smaller quantities than a man's. Certain times of a woman's life can disturb the normal hair growth pattern; these include puberty, pregnancy and menopause, where hormone levels are apt to increase. There is no set pattern of how the hair grows during a hormone imbalance, it will vary according to the individual.

- Puberty: the gonads and adrenal cortex excrete large amounts of steroid hormones causing the production of hair patterns in the male and female.
- Pregnancy: the possibility of the production of excess androgens can cause hairs to appear on the upper lip, chin and sides of the face. After the birth, when the endocrine balance is restored the hairs usually return to normal.
- Menopause: This marks the end of a woman's reproductive life, a gradual process occurring over a number of years after about the age of 40.

Abnormal systemic causes of hair growth

This is an endocrine imbalance caused by unnatural circumstances as a result of hereditary or glandular defects, acquired disease or infection, a tumour or diet deficiency. The conditions known to disturb the normal hair growth patterns are:

- Cushing's Syndrome
- Adrenogenital Syndrome
- Archard Thiers Syndrome
- Stein Leventhal Syndrome (Polycystic Ovary Syndrome)
- Acromegaly
- Dietary deficiency
- Anorexia nervosa.

Procedure to follow in an electro-epilation treatment

1 Prepare the work area for treatment.

2 Greet the client.

3 Escort the client to the treatment area.

4 Carry out the consultation.

5 Prepare the client for the treatment.

6 Position the lamp.

7 Wash your hands and wear disposable gloves.

8 Load the needle and begin the treatment.

9 Carry out the treatment.

10 Carry out and explain the aftercare.

11 Explain to the client when they should have the next appointment.

Deciding on the needle size to use

The needle diameter should equal the hair diameter. The treatment is affected by the diameter of the needle, a smaller needle has a larger surface area making a diathermy current more localised and intense, but with a galvanic current the needle with the greatest area transmits the largest amount of current.

Scale = 100 : 1

Needle diameters

002 003 004 005 006 010

Deciding on the type of needle to use

This is a matter of personal opinion for the electrologist, unless the client has an allergy to a specific type of needle.

Needle types

- **A one piece needle**. This needle is constructed from a solid piece of stainless steel wire in varying diameters. The tapered shape concentrates the current at

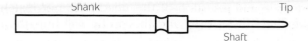
the base of the needle, preventing over-treatment of the surface area thus making it good for the blend and diathermy. This type of needle is particularly good for deep strong hairs.

- **A two piece non-tapered needle**. This needle bends easily, as the point of attachment at the shank is weak. The tip of this needle is rough with scratches from grinding, and is unpolished.
- **Two piece tapered needles**. The shank of this needle is made of brass, providing good conductivity. The well-tapered rounded end allows easy insertion.
- **Insulated needles**. Approximately three-quarters of the needle is insulated, leaving the last quarter free, therefore the current is only spread around the tip of the needle. It has been found that the insulation may break off from around the needle, but many clients find less pain with insulated needles.

Deciding on the current strength

The correct current is the lowest current needed to successfully remove the hair, without causing any skin damage or unnecessary discomfort to the client.

The treatment must be started with a low current, which is increased gradually until the hairs can be removed from the follicle without any force.

An accurate treatment

The definition of an accurate and correct treatment is defined by the following criteria:

- The amount of current discharged.
- The position of the needle.
- The length of time that the needle is inserted for.

Insertion of the needle into the follicle

Looking through the magnifier it is possible to see exactly where the hair enters the skin, the needle should be lined up parallel with the hair and slid into the follicle just under the hair itself. The insertion must be slow and precise so it is possible to see and feel the base of the follicle and so know when to stop the insertion.

The angle of insertion of the needle

Hairs grow at different angles all over the body. On the legs the insertion is much flatter than on the chin for example. Short hairs which have regrown after shaving give much less indication of their true angle under the skin. The section of the shaft closest to the skin gives guidance as to the likely angle of the root under the surface.

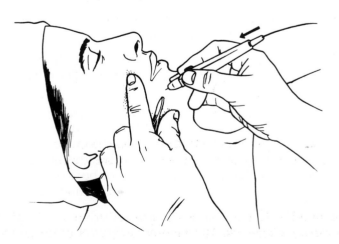

Correct elbow and wrist position

If the angle of the follicle and insertion of the needle do not match exactly the needle will not enter the follicle easily and the probe will hurt the client.

Inserting the needle

Stretching the skin slightly will allow the needle to enter the follicle easier. The skin must not be over-stretched as this will be uncomfortable for the client and make insertion less accurate. When the needle is in the follicle either press the finger button or foot pedal to discharge the current into the follicle. The needle must be kept perfectly still while this is being done. The length of time that the needle is left in the follicle will depend on how high the current is; the lower the level of current the longer you will need to keep the current on for. When enough current has been given, release it before removing the needle gently from the follicle.

The electrologist

The electrologist should work in a comfortable position, with the back straight and not bent. The height of the stool should be adjusted until the operator is able to reach the treatment area easily and without strain. Then the trolley and equipment should be positioned on the electrologist's working side, so that the flex does not trail across the client. Fidgeting and repositioning during application must be avoided. Uncomfortable positioning often results in inaccurate probing, damage to needle holders and needles, physical and mental fatigue, eyestrain and a slow rate of work.

The client

The client should be made as comfortable as possible without prohibiting the operator. The client should be asked to move into the best position for the work to be carried out. Pillows can be used for extra client support.

Care when probing the needle

If the electrologist's hand is not kept steady the current will not reach the dermal papilla or matrix of the hair and the desired destructive effect will not be achieved.

Movement of the needle may cause too much current to seep through to surrounding skin tissue leaving too little to treat the dermal papilla. This can result in a burn or even scarring and ineffective treatment.

If too fine a needle is used it may pass through the follicle wall or base of the follicle, thus making the probe inaccurate. The operator's sense of touch and the client's reaction give the guidance as to whether the insertion is accurate.

If the hair does not come out after the treatment

The follicle should be treated again, checking that:

- probing is accurate
- level of current is suitable
- length of current application is suitable
- the needle did not move while in the follicle.

On the second insertion the current should not be turned up, but should be applied for a longer period of time. If this does not remove the hair a third treatment can be applied.

The third treatment should be the last one. If the hair does not come out properly after this treatment then it should be removed because you cannot just leave it in the follicle as it will cause infection and it will cause too much trauma to the skin to probe the follicle again. The therapist should realise this is a definite indication that the current is too low. (This procedure must not be a common occurrence, it is something that is only likely to occur when initially finding the correct level of current.)

The current should now be increased to successfully remove the remaining hairs.

Types of scars that can be caused by electro-epilation

- Keloid scarring.
- Pitting.
- Hyper- or hypopigmentation.

Keloid scarring

This is an unusual thickening of the skin due to over-multiplication of its constituent cells. It is a skin reaction due to damage or injury, and the keloid is a permanent lesion which will occur only on certain individuals who have congenital predisposition to keloid. The operator should take care to notice if these scars are already present, as the over-treatment of the follicle may result in keloids in some instances. If none of these are present there is no danger that the client will keloid from your treatment. Negroid skin is especially prone to keloid scars. If some are already present before the treatment the client should be advised that the same might happen either from treatment or if any infection develops.

Pitting

This is a form of scarring that causes the skin to drop below the surface level of the rest of the skin.

Hyperpigmentation/hypopigmentation

Hyperpigmentation is when extra pigmentation develops in the area that has been worked on. Asian skins are particularly prone to this type of reaction with diathermy but less so with the blend or galvanism. Hypopigmentation is when the area of skin being treated loses its colour.

Hygiene

It is necessary to keep all working surfaces disinfected, any working implements sterilised and any areas of the body that you will be working on sanitised.

Sterilisation

This is the absolute destruction of all forms of microbial life, including spores. A sterile object or environment is free of all living organisms.

Disinfection

Usually a chemical destroys the growing forms of infection and infectious microbes, but not the spores. To disinfect is to destroy the growing forms but only inhibit the growth of non-pathogens. When the effect wears off the organism regrows (disinfectants should not be used on the skin).

Antiseptic

This is a chemical which is the same as a disinfectant but safe to use on living tissues. It kills bacteria and fungi completely, but not the spores.

Sanitiser

This is a substance which reduces microbes to a level considered safe by the Public Health Authority. Disinfectants and/or antiseptics act as effective sanitisers.

Bacteriostatic

This is an environment in which growing forms of bacteria are temporarily inhibited.

Bacteriocidal

This is a condition in which growing forms of bacteria are killed.

Methods of sterilisation/sanitisation

- Alcohol.
- Autoclaves.
- Boilers/Steamers.
- UVC Sterilisers.
- Chemicals (Cidex, Formaldehyde).

Alcohol

Alcohol, or a suitable alcohol-based disinfectant (e.g. chlorahexidine/alcohol), can be used in certain circumstances, to sanitise or disinfect not sterilise. 70% alcohol is the recommended concentration. When used for instruments care should be taken that:

- Only one or two instruments at a time are disinfected.
- The alcohol should cover the instruments completely.
- Period of immersion is timed for 30 minutes (recommended), 15 minutes at the minimum.
- That the alcohol should be discarded after one use.
- Containers used for disinfecting with alcohol should be washed regularly with hot water and detergent, rinsed thoroughly and left to dry. Alcohol impregnated wipes, available commercially are recommended.
- Discard used alcohol down the sink in running water.

Autoclaves

An autoclave is a steriliser that puts instruments and other articles under steam pressure: if the correct temperature (higher than boiling) and pressure (higher than atmosphere) are used for the correct length of time (varying from 15 minutes at 121 °C to 3 minutes at 134 °C) then the instruments will be sterilised (which boiling cannot do). For medium to large salons especially, an autoclave is highly recommended. It is still the most efficient method of sterilising objects. All metal objects as well as some plastics can be sterilised in this way. Autoclaves are easy to use and cheap to run.

Boilers and steamers

Boiling water or steam does not sterilise, it only disinfects. However, they are useful for cutting down the risk of spreading infection, and they are good as a temporary method. The unit should be heated by electricity, with a lid, a perforated removable shelf for raising and lowering instruments, and an automatic timer. Instruments should be boiled or steamed for 10 minutes and then removed with clean forceps; for boilers timing should commence from the point at which the water begins to boil after the instruments have been immersed in it. Clean distilled or deionised water should be used and replaced completely once a day.

UVC sterilisers

Ultraviolet light has disinfectant properties only. This would not be recommended to replace any of the previous methods.

Chemicals

The utensil must be immersed in the chemical for at least 20 minutes. The container holding the chemical and implements should be covered to prevent further particles infecting it, and the chemical must be changed at regular intervals according to the manufacturer's instructions. Bear in mind that the more implements put into the chemical the sooner it will require changing.

Complete sterilisation can only be achieved in the salon using an autoclave.

Keeping surfaces, furniture and floors clean

Basins can be cleaned using any proprietary cleanser. Other surfaces may be wiped with 70% surgical spirit or similar alcohol-based disinfectant wipe three or four times a day. These surfaces should also be washed at the end of each day with a solution of household detergent in hot water. Floors and chairs should be kept clean with a regular wash down.

Preparing the work area

- Always ensure that the working area has been prepared before the client arrives.
- Cover the bed with bed roll.
- A new bed roll should be used for every client.
- Put a pillow under the bed roll for the client's comfort if it is not going to get in the way.
- Place two stools under the bed.
- Cover both shelves of the trolley with tissue.
- Place the following items on your trolley:

Epilation machine	Cotton wool
Needle holder	Tissues
Selection of needles	Disposable gloves
Tweezers in a pot of hibitane	Mirror
Sharps box	Bowl for jewellery
Antiseptic skin cleanser	Consultation card and pen
Cosmetic skin cleanser	Hand towel.
After-care lotion	

- Place a waste bin protected by a bin liner underneath the trolley, ready for any waste. The bin should have a lid on it so the waste is covered up.

Greeting the client

When a client enters the salon the therapist should greet her politely and with a smile. The manner should be cheerful but not overpowering as this can put the client off.

The therapist should:

- Introduce herself to the client.
- Escort the client to the treatment area.

Consultation

This is a set of questions and a possible examination carried out at the beginning of a treatment to check it is safe to do the treatment.

A consultation is used for the following reasons:
- To find essential information from the client:
  - Name
  - address
  - telephone number
  - Age
  - Doctor's name
  - Doctor's address
  - Doctor's telephone number.
- To find out if the client has any contraindications.
- To find out information on medical history:
  - The date of the last pregnancy
  - If everything ran smoothly in the pregnancy
  - If everything is normal with periods
  - Any operations and details
  - How long has the hair been present?
  - Did anything start the hair growth off?
- To find out about any previous methods of hair removal, e.g.
  - Has epilation been carried out in the past?
  - What method of epilation was used?
  - How long ago and for how long?

- How did the area react to the treatment?
- Are any temporary methods being used?
- How often is the hair being removed?
- How long has the method been used for?
- To gain information on the area to be treated, e.g.
  - What area needs working on?
  - What is the hair growth like?
  - What is the skin condition like?
  - What is the healing like?

Although these are the main questions to ask clients, as the consultation progresses there may be other areas that become evident that you need to know more about, so ask the client about them and note them on the card.

The consultation should always be carried out:

- At the beginning of a treatment.
- In a private place
- With both therapist and client comfortably seated:
  - Near enough so that questions and answers do not have to be shouted or repeated
  - Arranged facing each other but not across a table or desk
  - At the same height.

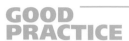

Introduction
The client may be tense and nervous, so the therapist's manner and appearance are vital.

The environment should be welcoming to put the client at ease.

Effective communication
This depends on using all the senses, and adapting interview techniques depending on the motivation, attitude, age, sex, etc. of the client.

Case history
Essential information is asked in a logical sequence, with the aid of a pre-planned record/consultation card. It checks that the treatment is not contraindicated, and the information should also be helpful if another therapist needs to take over.

Motivation
The therapist must be enthusiastic to the client and give her confidence where necessary.

The purpose of keeping records and information
- Record specific particulars about clients.
- Contact clients if you need to.
- Record how often the client has treatments.

Explanation of treatment
Explain how the treatment is carried out, the benefits and the after-care. Do not use too much jargon.

Throughout the consultation the therapist should give the client the chance to ask any questions that they may have as well as covering in detail the treatment procedure being carried out, as follows.

How the treatment will be carried out
- The skin is cleansed with an antiseptic such as hibitane.
- A new sterile disposable needle is used each time so there is no risk of cross-infection.
- The needle size is chosen to match the size of the hair or follicle.

- The needle is inserted into the hair follicle alongside the hair. This is the pore the hair sits in the skin. This involves no piercing of the skin.
- When the needle is in the skin a slight heat sensation is felt when the machine is brought into action. The hair is then removed from the follicle without being plucked with a pair of tweezers.
- The reaction in the follicle gradually cauterises the blood supply that the hair receives nourishment from, until the hair has no supply to grow from, and destroys the hair germ cells that produce the hair.
- This process causes a gradual reduction in the strength and colour of the hairs until they are totally reduced.

The number of hairs that can be removed per treatment
- There is no set speed an electrologist should work at, accuracy is far more important than speed.
- Some areas are more difficult to work on, which will slow down the pace of the treatment, while others are easily treated.
- The skin reaction will also dictate how much work can be carried out in one area, as the skin will react badly if there is over-treatment.
- All the answers to these points will only be found out when the electrologist works.

How often will the client need to have appointments?
- Again this will depend on how large the treatment area is and how well the skin heals between treatments.
- The client must understand that it is much better to have regular appointments initially to make any progress, maybe weekly, fortnightly or monthly.
- The frequency of the appointments will reduce as the client responds to the treatment.

Length of time for the treatment
It is difficult to determine the length of time required for the treatment as everyone responds differently to the treatment, so all the therapist can give the client is an estimate based on the following points:

- How much hair is present.
- How thick and dark the hair is.
- The condition of the skin.
- The healing of the skin.
- How frequently the client can attend the clinic/salon.
- How long the treatment sessions are.
- The method of electro-epilation chosen.

It is vital the client understands that you are only estimating and that neither you nor anyone else can guarantee accurately a date.

Skin appearance after the treatment
- Immediately after the treatment the skin usually looks pink/red. If the after-care instructions are followed this will disappear quite soon, within an hour.
- Occasionally clients with poor skin healing may notice slight scabs appearing, in which case they should let them heal without picking and no long-term problems will be encountered. Scabs usually occur on the body where healing is slower than on the face.
- When the treatment is carried out properly the skin looks normal after completion of the treatment.

The cost of the treatment
- The client pays for the length of time she is worked on, and this price will vary from clinic to clinic and area to area.
- Some clinics sell courses where it works out cheaper for the client to prepay in bulk, and this is recorded on the consultation card.
- Other clinics simply charge separately for each appointment.

Contraindications

This is anything which indicates to you that you should not do the treatment or you should proceed with extreme caution. Depending on what you find, you will need to decide whether to proceed with caution or ask the client to visit his/her doctor for their opinion on the matter. It is very important that you do not try and diagnose any condition you feel the client may be suffering from no matter how sure you are of what it is.

CONTRAINDICATIONS

to electro-epilation treatment
- Areas of inflammation, cuts, sores or open wounds.
- Any abnormal skin condition.
- Signs of infectious and contagious diseases.
- Hairy moles (unless a doctor's written consent is supplied).
- Women in final months of pregnancy should not have treatment on the abdomen or breasts, but areas such as the face can be treated. Superfluous hair during pregnancy often disappears after the birth of the child.
- Clients who are emotionally disturbed. Their pain threshold is usually too low to tolerate any discomfort.
- Young people under 16 years of age. They should not be treated except in conditions agreed with the client's doctor, since any hormonal imbalances may correct themselves as the youngster matures.
- Clients with:
  - Diabetes. There is very poor skin healing and a doctor's note is required.
  - Epilepsy. Epileptic attacks might be triggered by the sensation of the treatment. A doctor's note is required.
  - Heart conditions. These seldom offer problems but pace-makers are a contraindication because the high frequency current can speed up the pace-maker.
  - Asthmatic clients. If they have a nervous disposition they should be treated with care.
  - Clients receiving medical treatment of systemic disorders.
  - Hepatitis or AIDS. The electrologist will have to decide if she/he wishes to work on this client. If so, gloves must be worn.
  - Negroid skin. There is a risk of keloid scarring, hyperpigmentation and problems with curved follicles so extreme care should be taken.
- Clients displaying abnormal fear of the treatment. All the aspects of the treatment should be explained to the client as their cooperation is essential.
- Work around bruises, bites, stings, varicose veins, and care should be taken in areas of dilated capillaries.
- No treatment inside ears, nose, very close proximity to the pubic region, directly in the nipples.
- Warts, moles, unless doctor's permission and written consent is supplied. Blood spots, skin tags, must not be attempted unless training has been received, and then a doctor's consent is still required in most cases.

Checklist for client to read through of possible contraindications
- Heart condition
- Pacemaker
- High or low blood pressure
- Epilepsy
- Diabetes
- Haemophilia
- Thyroid problems
- Thrombosis
- Phlebitis
- Hepatitis B
- HIV Positive
- Asthma
- Acne vulgaris

Preparing the client

1 Ask the client to remove any necessary clothing and hang it up.
2 Help the client onto the couch.
3 When the client is in position protect any clothing with towels or tissue, then assess the hair and decide the needle size.
4 Wash your hands.
5 Wipe over the area to be treated with a square of cotton wool with skin cleanser/hibitane on it, then blot the area dry with a tissue. Use a fresh piece of cotton wool for each area.
6 Using neat hibitane/alcohol wipe over the probe.
7 Position the lamp in a suitable position.

Loading the needles

1 Select a suitable needle.
2 Loosen the chuck on the probe.
3 Unwrap the needle without touching it.
4 Using the wrapping or tweezers, place the needle in the probe.
5 Use the tweezers to move the needle to the correct height in the probe.
6 Tighten the chuck until it is gripping the needle tightly.
7 Remove the plastic covering over the needle with the tweezers.

The therapist should have two pairs of tweezers – one for loading the needle, the other for working with.

Disposing of the needles at the end of the treatment

- Loosen the chuck.
- Tip the probe into the sharps box allowing the needle to fall into the box.
- The needle should never be touched or used on anyone else.

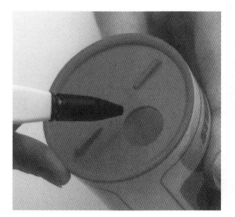

Sharps box

The procedure for diathermy treatment

1 Prepare the work area as described above.
2 Carry out the consultation as described above.
3 Prepare the client as described above.
4 Load the needle as described above.
5 Turn the machine on to a low current.
6 Probe the follicle and apply the current for a couple of seconds according to how strong the hair growth seems and what the condition of the skin is.
7 Stop applying the current and remove the probe from the follicle.
8 Try removing the hair from the follicle with the tweezers.
9 If the hair will not be removed easily, probe the same follicle but apply the current for a longer period of time.
10 Try the hair again with the tweezers, if it comes out after the second probe then you will know that you only need to increase the current a little, to be at the right working level.
11 If the hair will not come out after the second probe then a third should be applied again applying the current for a longer period of time. This should allow the hair to be removed with the tweezers, and the current increased accordingly.
12 If at this stage the hair still will not come out, it should be removed with the tweezers and the current increased enough for the next hair treated.
13 The current should now be suitable to work on the area, although there will be times when strong hairs require further treatment or increased current.

The length of current time and the effect on the heating pattern

The longer the current is left on, the larger the heating pattern becomes, so destroying more of the follicle, to the point of destroying parts that should not be touched. The stronger the hair the longer the current will have to applied for.

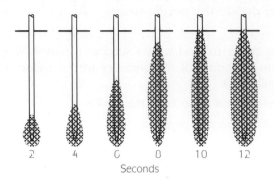

Effect of time on heating pattern

2   4   6   8   10   12
Seconds

The strength of current and the effect on the heating pattern

Lower currents will take longer to spread out over the necessary parts of the follicle, while higher currents will treat more quickly. It is not advantageous to work with the current too high however as it will over-treat the follicle and disfigure the skin. The strength of the current and the length of time it is applied for must be considered together.

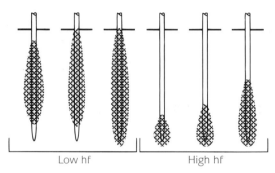

Effect of intensity on heating pattern

Low hf   High hf

The needle diameter and the effect on the heating pattern

Larger needles cause a stronger and more concentrated heating pattern that will have greater destruction in a smaller area, making them suited to very strong hair growth. The thinner the needle the less dense the heating pattern is and the more spread out it is, which is more suited to finer hairs. Needles that are either too large or smaller than the hair diameter will not give the correct amount of current and it will not be applied in the correct places of the follicle. For the most successful treatment the needle diameter must equal the hair diameter.

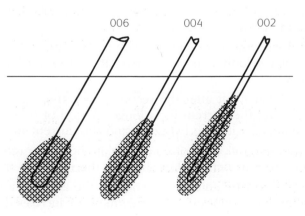

006   004   002

Effect of needle diameter on heating pattern

The depth of insertion and the effect on the heating pattern

If the insertion is shallow, the current distribution is affected, often resulting in the current being spread out over the surface of the skin. If the insertion is too deep, again the heating pattern misses the necessary part of the follicle. Unless the insertion is completely accurate the current will not be able to treat the necessary part of the follicle and so treatment will not be totally successful.

The procedure for a galvanic current

1   Prepare the work area.

2   Carry out the consultation.

3   Prepare the client.

4   Load the needle.

5   Turn the machine onto a low current.

6   Probe the follicle and apply the current for a number of seconds according to how strong the hair growth seems and what the condition of the skin is. A galvanic current needs applying for far longer than a diathermy current to have any effect, as this is a much slower process.

7   Stop applying the current and remove the probe from the follicle.

8   Try removing the hair from the follicle with the tweezers.

9   If the hair will not be removed easily turn up the level of the current and probe the follicle again.
   A balance must be achieved between the level of the current and the length of time each probe is taking, for example:
   –   the current must not be so high that the skin is being unnecessarily affected
   –   the current must be high enough to have an effect within a reasonable period of time
   –   the level of current and period of time required will be different for different clients.

The procedure for a blend treatment

1   Prepare the work area.

2   Carry out the consultation.

3   Prepare the client.

4   Load the needle.

5   Turn the diathermy current so it is just on, then turn on the galvanic current to a low level.

6   Probe a follicle and apply the two currents for a suitable period of time according to the hair strength and skin type. While this treatment will not take as long to react as the galvanic treatment, it does usually take longer than diathermy.
   The galvanic current can be increased as necessary and the length of time the currents are applied for can be increased but the diathermy current does not need to be increased.
   It is possible to treat a follicle with the blend current and the hair not slide out of the follicle immediately but be easily removed a couple of seconds or minutes later. This method is suitable as long as you know which hairs you have treated.

After-care instructions for the client

●   Do not have any hot baths or showers for the next 24 hours.
●   Do not use any perfumed products for the next 24 hours.
●   Do not sunbathe or use sun-beds for the next 24 hours
●   Avoid wearing tight clothes that might rub or chaff.
●   Do not use deodorant or antiperspirant for the next 24 hours.
●   Try to avoid touching the area.
●   No saunas or any form of heat treatment for the next 24 hours.

Normal skin reaction

The therapist should advise the client that if red colouration/blotches are evident, these should fade within a few hours.

Abnormal skin reactions

- Swelling. The most common cause for swelling is over-insertion, too much work in one area or an allergy to the treatment. Antiseptic soothing creams and an ice pack will soothe and cool the area, which will reduce the swelling.
- Bleeding. A bad insertion or bent or blunt needle pierces the follicle causing bleeding.
- Crusts/scabs. Either blood or lymph can accumulate in the area and when it dries out it forms a crust or scab. These should be left to fall off in their own time.
- Scarring. This may be caused by one of the following:
    operating too quickly and not taking enough care
    - using a faulty machine and not being able to control the exact level of current
    - using a bent or blunt needle as the current gathers and builds up at this point
    - using a current which is too strong so over-treating the skin and tissue
    - concentrating the treatment too much in one area, over-treating the skin
    - probing at the wrong angle so piercing the follicle wall
    - probing and removing the needle from the follicle with the current. This burns the surface of the skin
    - not giving the skin long enough to heal between treatments, over-treating the skin
    - the client not following the after-care instructions and causing infections
- Bruising. This can be caused by using a needle which is too big for the follicle, or a bad insertion that pierces the follicle wall or base. Too much pressure in an area or over-working can also cause bruising.

Regrowth hairs

These are hairs which grow after epilation has taken place and partial destruction of the follicle has occurred. These hairs are finer than the original hairs, also paler in colour and shallowly placed in the skin.

Regrowth of superfluous hair

Regrowth, if at all, is modified on areas of superfluous hair, and these hairs usually react quickly to treatment. If the hairs are growing from abnormally active follicles and are resistant to treatment, this should be kept in mind when the treatment is applied.

The effect of hormone imbalance on regrowth

Hormone imbalance or steroid therapy may make regrowth more persistent, sometimes making further medical advice necessary. The client and the therapist need to know what other factors are affecting the hair growth besides the treatment so that they have a good idea of what to expect.

Previous treatments and the effect on regrowth

Any previous treatment will affect the rate of regrowth. Any distortion of the follicle affects the accuracy of probing and hence the success of the treatment. Where previous methods have involved a certain amount of topical stimulation the results will also be far slower. As plucking is regarded as a form of topical stimulation, the client must not pluck out hairs during her course of treatment as it will reduce the effectiveness and speed of success.

Condition	Symptoms	Cause	Outcome
Honey-coloured scab/crust	Lymph or plasma seeps through capillary walls and accumulates in the follicle.	Mild over-use of current or over-treatment in area.	Fluid eventually hardens and soon drops off leaving perfect skin.
Reddish scab/crust	Slow seepage of blood into follicle, causing disintegration of large sections of skin.	Over-use of current Over-treatment Inaccurate insertions.	Scab should not be picked off or a pit may result taking a number of months to heal. If the scab is left to fall off the skin, the skin will appear pink, but will revert to normal in time.
Pustule	Inflammation. Heat swelling and pain.	Bacteria invading the follicle after treatment.	If the body does not destroy the bacteria pus will develop forming a pustule, this disappears after 1–2 days, leaving a honey-coloured crust. If the crust falls off naturally, the skin will be normal, if the crust is picked off, a pit will be left behind and take longer to heal.
Folliculitis	Large pockets of pus in the skin. Superficial folliculitis is found under the stratum corneum. Deep folliculitis affects the entire follicle.	Secondary infection of the follicle.	Heals without any mark. Often leaves a pit upon healing.
Gas/vapour blister	Hydrogen-filled gas blister, which develops quickly: usually at one side of the needle. Hydrogen and water-filled blister, develops as above.	Possible result of galvanic treatment. Possible result of blend treatment.	On removal of the needle the blister is pressed with a sterile tissue so it will go down and not cause any problems. Care must be taken to prevent bacteria entering and causing a pustule.
Vapour blast	Extreme heat quickly converts moisture in the tissue to vapour, sometimes the tissue can be seen to move.	High intensity diathermy current.	If the epidermis does not turn white due to over treatment, there will be no harm to the tissue, if it does the condition is called blanching and it will take much longer to heal and may result in a pitted scar.
Bruising	A blue/black discolouration that may swell. Usually appears upon insertion.	Incorrect insertion. Over-sized needle.	Tissue will heal perfectly.
Pitting	Formation of crust. Region of damaged tissue that sits below the level of the surrounding skin.	Over-treatment of follicle. Picking crusts.	Pitted scar which will improve with time depending on the degree of damage.
Keloid scarring	Raised scar with a shiny stretched appearance.	Some people, particularly negroids, have a predisposition to keloid scars. In epilation the damaged tissue would result from inaccurate probing or over-treatment.	Fibroblasts proliferate in the dermis resulting in over-healing of the tissue and formation of a raised scar.
Hyper- and hypo-pigmentation	Changes in the pigmentation of the skin. Black skins show the colour change more with either very dark or very light areas.	Inaccurate probing. Excessive diathermy current.	Excess skin colour. Loss of skin colour in the area just around the follicle which will not fade.

Diathermy	Blend	Galvanic
Alternating current short-wave high frequency current.	Alternating current and direct current.	Direct current.
Produces heat in skin.	Produces heat and chemicals in the skin.	Produces chemicals in the skin.
Allows quick removal of each hair, but this is thought to be the least thorough of the methods per treatment.	Allows hair to be removed in a medium length of time with thorough results.	Hair removal is very slow but this is a very thorough process.
The sensation felt is a sharp quick sting.	The sensation is a quite mild sting for a medium amount of time.	The sensation is mild for a relatively long period of time.
The skin reaction varies with each individual, but can cause a lot of redness.	The skin reaction varies with each individual, but is milder than just diathermy.	The skin reaction varies with each individual but is usually the least of all the three.
Treatments can be as regular as the skin will allow to ensure full healing has occurred.	Treatments can be as regular as the skin will allow, but as they are more thorough you do not usually require as many as with diathermy.	Treatments can be as regular as the skin will allow, usually quite a lot of treatment sessions are needed as only a few hairs can be worked on each time.

Alternative methods of hair removal

Bleaching
Bleaching can be an effective way of disguising unwanted hairs, by removing the colour in the hair.

The chemical ingredients
3% Hydrogen peroxide

Possible reactions to bleaching
Nausea, hives, burned skin, severe life-threatening allergies and swelling of the face.

Chemical depilation
Creams or pastes applied to the skin to dissolve the hair above the level of the skin.

The chemical ingredients
Hydrogen sulphide was the most effective chemical, but this has an unpleasant odour which is hard to mask. Most sulphides have been replaced with salts of thioglycolic acid, which take more time to act but smell better and are not as irritating.

Ingredients of a typical depilatory cream
Calcium thioglycolate, calcium carbonate, calcium hydroxide, cetly alcohol, sodium lauryl sulphate, water and a strong perfume.

Possible reactions to depilatory creams
Irritating to the skin and any ingestion may cause gastrointestinal irritation.

Shaving
Removal of hair at skin level by cutting it off with a blade.

Equipment required
A razor and shaving cream for a wet shave, or a lady shave for a dry shave.

Possible reactions to shaving

The skin can appear grazed and therefore red or may develop a shaving rash.

Cutting

Removal of hair at skin level using scissors.

Equipment required

Scissors.

Possible reactions to cutting

Nothing unless the skin is cut by accident.

Plucking

Removal of hair from root level by pulling out with tweezers.

Equipment required

Tweezers.

Possible reactions to plucking

Small spots can occur in the follicle (folliculitis), if any dirt enters the follicle.

Waxing and sugaring

Removal of hair from root level with the use of either hot or cool wax.

Equipment required

Wax pot, hot or cool wax, spatulas, strips for removing cool wax and the relevant before and after products.

Possible reactions to waxing

The skin will turn pink or red immediately after the treatment, but this will fade quickly. Some clients can be prone to in-growing hairs as a result of waxing, then they should use a loofah and moisturiser or body exfoliant.

A COMPARISON OF DIFFERENT METHODS OF DEPILATION

Method	Duration	Process	Pain intensity	Treatment area	Effect
Waxing	Lasts about 6 weeks	Hair removed from root	Semi painful	Used on large or small areas	Causes skin to go red and after-care must be followed
Shaving	Lasts a few days	Hair removed at skin level	Only painful if skin is cut	Used on large or small areas	The skin is easily cut or grazed
Cutting	Lasts a few days	Hair removed at skin level	No pain	Small areas	A slow process that needs repeating regularly
Plucking	Lasts about 6 weeks	Hair removed from root level	Semi painful	Small areas	A slow process not suitable for large areas
Chemicals	Lasts a few days	Hair removed at skin level	No pain unless allergy occurs	Used on large or small areas	Smelly and messy to use
Electro-epilation	Permanent	Hair removed from root	Semi painful	Used on large or small areas	Takes a long time and can be expensive, skin goes red and after-care must be followed
Bleaching	Lasts a few days	Hair not removed	No pain unless allergy occurs	Used on large or small areas	Can be messy to use. Satisfactory results depend on colour of hair
Sugaring	Lasts about 6 weeks	Hair removed from root level	Semi painful	Used on large or small areas	Time consuming process but the hairs can be removed when they are very short

Hair

- Hairs are dead structures made up of the protein *keratin* found situated in tube-like indentations called hair follicles.
- Hairs are found on nearly every part of the body, except the palms of hands and soles of the feet. Hairs vary in length, thickness and colour in different parts of the body and in different races.
- The hair follicle grows out of the epidermal cells, but it extends into the dermis.
- Over most parts of the body the hairs are fine and downy, giving the appearance of hairlessness.
- In furry mammals the function of the hair was for temperature control and the sensation of touch, and they still have these functions in man.
- Arrector pilli muscles are attached to each hair follicle and when they contract they make the hair stand up on end, giving a goose pimple effect, i.e. in temperature control
- The duration of the life of a single hair varies from about four months on the eyelashes and axillary to about four years on the scalp, after which it is shed and replaced by new cells from the matrix of the hair.

The different types of hair

Almost the entire skin of the human during foetal life is covered with a fine hair called *lanugo*. These hairs, which are classed as primary hairs, are mostly shed by birth and are replaced by fine hairs called *vellus* hairs in the early months of postnatal life. These are retained in most regions, but are replaced by *terminal* hairs of the eyebrows, axillary and those on the face and chest of the male which appear at puberty, their development and growth being under hormonal control.

Lanugo hair

These hairs are only found on the unborn child. They are shed soon after or before birth.

Lanugo hairs are very soft and lack pigmentation. They grow from the sebaceous gland and do not become terminal hairs unless stimulated by topical or systemic conditions. If the hair is stimulated, it may grow down, first becoming an accelerated lanugo hair, i.e. longer than its neighbours but with no bulb, then a shallow terminal hair. This change may take from a few months to a few years.

Lanugo hairs shed and replace slower than terminal hairs.

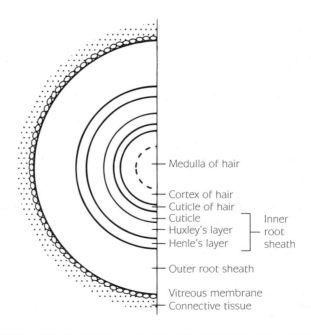

The layers of the hair and follicle

Vellus hair

- Soft fine hairs covering most areas of the body except:
  - palms of hands
  - soles of feet
  - lips
  - genital areas.
- Replaces lanugo hair.

Terminal hair

- Replaces lanugo or vellus hair.
- Deep root, well-developed coarse hairs found
  - on scalp
  - underarms
  - pubic region
  - some other parts of body.
- Terminal hair has three layers.

The structure of the hair

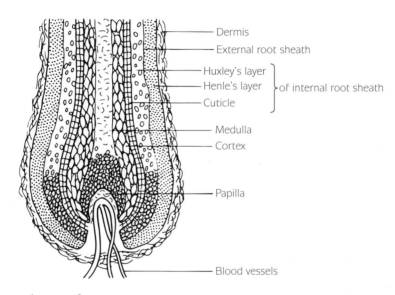

Dermis
External root sheath
Huxley's layer
Henle's layer } of internal root sheath
Cuticle
Medulla
Cortex
Papilla
Blood vessels

The hair structure

The hair is made up of:

- The inner medulla – the centre part of the hair. It is made up of large loosely connected cells containing keratin. The medulla is sometimes not continuous within the same hair. This creates air spaces which determine the sheen and colour tones of the hair.
- The outer cortex – this is the layer of the hair outside the medulla. The cortex is composed of elongated cells containing keratin that are cemented together. Melanin, the colour pigment, is found in this layer; if the melanin is absent then the hair appears white or grey.
- The cuticle – this is a single layer of overlapping cells with the free margins directed towards the tip of the hair. These cells interlock with the cells of the cuticle of the inner root sheath. The function of the cuticle is to anchor the hair in the follicle, and provide elasticity to the hair. The outside of the cuticle is surrounded by an insoluble lipid and carbohydrate layer which is thought to protect the hair from chemical and physical agents.

The growth cycle of hair

Anagen

- This is the first stage of the hair growing cycle.
- Normally 90% of scalp hairs are in anagen stage.

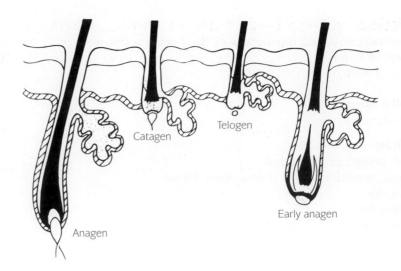

Telogen

Catagen

Early anagen

Anagen

Stages of hair growth

- During anagen the hair is firmly attached within its follicle, to dislodge it a force must be applied which is usually sufficient to fracture the hair in its non-keratinised zone, leaving a portion of the root behind in the follicle. Such a hair will have a ragged end where the fracture occurred.
- Anagen hairs if pulled intact will be encapsulated by a sheath around the end of the hair.

Catagen

- This is the second stage of the growth cycle, when the hair is already fully grown and the mitotic activity in the matrix stops.
- The hair moves up the follicle so moving away from the papilla. At this stage the hair has to receive its nourishment from the surrounding follicle.
- As the hair moves up the follicle, the part of the follicle that is left behind degenerates and disappears. As this part of the follicle is capable of disappearing and being reformed, it is called transient or temporary.
- The transient part of the follicle never disappears totally, instead it forms the dermal cord, which is a chain-like structure that maintains some contact with the dermal papilla.

Telogen

- This is the third and final stage of the cycle, known as the rest phase.
- The length of time the hair spends in this stage varies according to the type of hair and the nature of the individual.
- The hair is not receiving nourishment from anywhere during this stage and the inner root sheath dries out and shrivels up.
- The hair continues to move up the follicle until it falls out.
- Sometimes before one hair has fallen out another starts to form at the base of the follicle, and grows and pushes out the old hair.

Endocrine system

A wide variety of physiological processes are carried out unconsciously by the endocrine system through chemical messengers called 'hormones'. The endocrine system is a collection of glands that produce these hormones, which are necessary for normal bodily functions. The hormones regulate metabolism, growth and sexual development. These glands release the hormones directly into the bloodstream, where they are transported to organs and tissues throughout the entire body.

The function of the endocrine system

The endocrine system controls the slower processes and reactions in the body, such as growth and development, digestion, excretion and sexual activity. (The quicker reactions are controlled by the nervous system.)

Endocrine glands

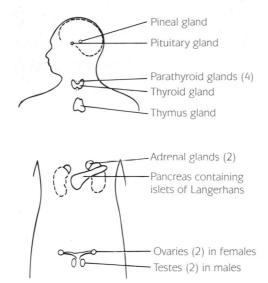

- Pineal gland
- Pituitary gland
- Parathyroid glands (4)
- Thyroid gland
- Thymus gland
- Adrenal glands (2)
- Pancreas containing islets of Langerhans
- Ovaries (2) in females
- Testes (2) in males

Location of the endocrine glands

An endocrine gland has no duct leading from it linking it to another part of the body, so it is often called a ductless gland. These glands produce hormones and release these hormones directly into the blood stream to be carried round the body.

Main endocrine glands of the body

These are:
- Pituitary gland – found in the middle of the brain and also referred to as the master gland because this gland controls the secretions of all the other endocrine glands.
- Thyroid gland – made up two lobes found in front of the throat and above the voice box.
- Parathyroid glands – four small glands found on the posterior of the thyroid gland.
- Thymus gland – situated in the central chest region behind the sternum.
- Adrenal glands – two glands found on top of each kidney.
- Islets of Langerhans – small endocrine cells found within the pancreas.
- Testes/Ovaries – the male and female reproductive endocrine organs.

Hormones

A hormone is a chemical messenger made by an endocrine gland from protein, which is put into the blood and carried in the blood to the target organ that it will affect. Hormones help regulate internal growth and development, and contribute to the reproductive processes.

The production of hormones

The hypothalamus in the brain can detect if the body needs a particular hormone, it then stimulates the pituitary gland of the endocrine system to cause the production of the necessary hormone. When the hormone level in the body reaches the required amount, the hypothalamus is stimulated by a process called negative feedback. It then stimulates the pituitary to inhibit the further production of the hormone. Hormones are specific, which means they will only carry out one type of reaction, therefore there is only one place for them to go.

Perform a course of four short-wave diathermy treatments and then four blend treatments on the same client and chosen area. Note the effectiveness and responses to treatment.

KEY TERMS

You will need to know what these words and phrases mean. Go back through the chapter to find out.

Abnormal skin reactions

Anagen

Blend technique

Catagen

Congenital

Galvanic

Heating pattern

Hirsuitism

Hyper-trichosis

Lanugo hair

Short wave diathermy

Superfluous hair

Systemic

Telogen

Terminal hair

Topical

Vellus hair

SELF-CHECKS

1 Describe what electro-epilation is and why it is used.
2 List the main reasons why clients might need electro-epilation.
3 Identify the procedures to follow in an electro-epilation treatment.
4 State the hygiene procedures.
5 State the safe working practices for electrical equipment.
6 How would you prepare the working area and greet clients?
7 Explain the importance of conducting a consultation.
8 Identify contraindications for the treatment.
9 State the procedure for diathermy treatments.
10 State the procedure for galvanic treatments.
11 Describe blend treatments.
12 Identify the after-care procedure and instructions.
13 Name the different methods of electro-epilation.
14 Compare and contrast the alternative methods of hair removal.
15 Describe the structure of the hair and follicle.
16 Name and describe the hair growth cycle.
17 Briefly describe the endocrine system.

Chapter 5 Facial and body electrotherapy treatments

After working through this chapter you will be able to:

- identify the different types of electrical treatment for the face and body
- list the contraindications to electrical treatments
- describe the effects of electrical treatments
- understand the preparation required for a variety of electrical treatments
- competently carry out a variety of electrical treatments for the face and body on clients.

Electrical equipment

A variety of equipment is manufactured internationally to meet the demands of the fast expanding beauty industry. The majority of companies produce a full range of electrical equipment, though some specialise in one area. Each company offers equipment at differing prices according to the development and design on offer and the back-up services available.

When selecting equipment, the therapist should carefully consider the treatments that can best be offered by the salon within their available budget. Once these have been decided on it is wise to attend exhibitions, read trade journals and liaise through professional associations with other therapists before deciding which manufacturer's items to purchase. If possible it is advisable to visit and view equipment showrooms to compare choice, range and availability of equipment.

There are a number of key questions that should be considered before any decisions are made:

- Is the therapist to offer salon-based or home visiting services?
- Where is the equipment to be used and stored?
- How much space is available for equipment presentation and storage?
- Would a multi-purpose unit be more beneficial if there is a shortage of storage space? (A multi-purpose unit could also be used as a point of sale for other treatments. However, if it is the only piece of equipment, what happens when it breaks down or has to be serviced?)

- If the equipment has to be carried in and out of cupboards, is it light-weight?
- How are the electrodes stored – with the machine in a purpose-designed area or separately? How will this suit the salon environment?
- What is the durability of the equipment? How often will the equipment need servicing? Where will this occur – on- or off-site? How long will it take? What will it cost?
- What training is offered by the company? Is this included in the price? Where will it take place?
- What back-up services are offered by the company? Do they provide training manuals, telephone support? Do they charge for these services?
- What is the reputation of the company? Are they long standing? Do they attend the major international exhibitions? Are they active in more than one country?
- If purchasing from overseas, always check that equipment is compatible for use in the UK, e.g. check the wiring and voltage, repair and replacement of accessories, etc.
- Ensure items of equipment have been manufactured in accordance with current European directives (EU countries only) and are CE labelled.

Two of the major points that therapists do tend to consider when choosing electrotherapy equipment are the aesthetic appearance and the overall cost, but these should not be the only points that are considered!

Having purchased equipment, the therapist will want to use it to its maximum potential for the benefit of their clients. The services should be marketed well and full use of existing and passing clientele should be made, including displaying information on the new services in the reception area, perhaps offering a discount for a course of treatments and an open evening to demonstrate the treatment and explain its effects.

Electrical treatments are generally given as a course. When used on the body, face, neck and décolleté, a number of treatments are often combined together to gain the maximum benefit for the client. If the aim is for figure improvement, home-care advice on diet and exercise should be given, and if it is to improve the skin condition, home-care advice on the use of professional skin care products should also be given.

Care of electrical equipment

- Hygiene is of the utmost importance so the machine and accessory items must be kept clean. (Check cleaning instructions before using solvents. Alcohol-based products are not recommended for cleaning plastic surfaces/cases, but sun-bed cleanser for acrylic Perspex is often suitable.)
- Leads and plugs should be regularly checked to ensure there are no loose wires.
- The equipment should be serviced regularly (portable appliance tested – PAT).
- The therapist should ensure that all machines are maintained in good working order and kept in a safe place and that they are familiar with its operation.

Safety precautions to be observed when using electrical equipment

- Ensure the correct care and maintenance has been given to the equipment. (Look for any signs of wear and tear, etc.)
- Check the machine is placed on a sturdy trolley or where the equipment has its own built-in trolley, ensure the castors are firmly in place and that it is easily accessible for use. Never push trolleys or items on wheels, always pull.
- Do not place water near or on top of the unit. Do not attempt to operate the machine with damp hands.

If the equipment is not under a guaranteed service warranty, take out a service contract with a local electrician who is familiar with beauty equipment. Ask the manufacturer or the local wholesaler if they can recommend one.

- Make sure that there are no trailing leads that the client or other therapists (including yourself) could trip over.
- Ensure that the machine is working correctly before applying to the client. Carry out simple self-tests.
- Ensure all accessory items, including products, are at hand before greeting the client.
- Do not allow the client to touch any machine unless you specifically direct them to do so.
- Test the equipment on yourself, explaining the procedure, its effects and sensation the client will experience.
- Check for contraindications and where necessary test the client for skin sensitivity.
- Before commencing the treatment, ensure all dials are at zero and that the machine is switched off.

Skin sensitivity test

When using electrical currents that pass through the body, it is paramount that a skin sensitivity test is carried out to check the accuracy of the client's sensation in the area to be treated. It is usually performed by first testing the client's interpretation of different temperature extremes, by placing hot and cold water in glass containers, such as test tubes, and touching the area to be treated intermittently; then the client's sensation of touch is tested using a harsh and smooth surface, such as the pointed tip of an orange wood stick and the other end wrapped in cotton wool. Both these tests should be carried out with the client's view obstructed.

ACTIVITY

Research the number of equipment manufacturers available through your local wholesalers or main centres of electrotherapy supply. Compare their ranges, prices and back-up services on offer.

information point

Electrotherapy treatments
Therapists use the term 'electrotherapy' to refer to electrical treatments where low currents are passed through the client's body for their therapeutic effects.
   The four main electrotherapy treatments used by therapists are:
- High frequency.
- Neuro-muscular electrical stimulation (NMES), sometimes referred to as electrical muscular stimulation (EMS).
- Galvanic.
- Micro-current.

Micro-electrotherapy

Micro-current electrotherapy is a staple part of beauty therapy these days, but what is it and how exactly does it work?

Micro-current machines use a modified direct current usually with a low frequency range and relatively long pulse width 'on' time (compared to neuro-muscular electrical stimulation [NMES] devices) which is measured in micro-amps (a micro-amp being a millionth of an amp). A micro-amp (mA) is a thousand times smaller than a milliamp (which is a thousandth of an amp). In beauty therapy the milliamp is the scale of amplitude usually used for measuring the output ranges of traditional galvanic devices.

As micro-current is so small, the client should feel little, if any, sensation – it is virtually subsensory and it does not stimulate motor points or nerve pathways as does NMES. It bypasses the surrounding structures and enters the belly of the muscle to stimulate the muscle. Micro-current works in harmony with the body's own bio-electrical field.

More than 20 years ago, in the USA, Dr Thomas Wing carried out pioneer work using micro-current to treat sports injuries and Bell's palsy and stroke victims. During his work he discovered that by using micro-current he could realign the damaged muscle tissue to the healthy side of the face. He noted that during these treatments the damaged muscle tissues were actually lifting higher than the healthy side and he realised the beneficial effects this current would have on the cosmetic industry.

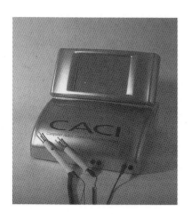

Micro-current machine

From Wing's research, the CACI™ machine (computer-aided cosmetology instrument) evolved and was introduced into the UK for cosmetic work. Once CACI™ was launched around 1993, most other electrotherapy manufacturers added micro-current into their range of equipment.

By using micro-current via cotton-tipped probes or roller bars – which work along the origin and insertion to grab the belly of the muscle – on a healthy muscle where there is no nerve damage, the nerve pathway is clear and the effects obtained are quite significant. It has other healthy effects since it not only works on muscles but also on skin.

The main effects are that:

- Fine lines and wrinkles are softened and reduced.
- It helps to normalise sebaceous secretions so it is good for dull, sallow skin tones, oily skins and sluggish complexions.
- It is extremely beneficial for photo-damaged skin, acne pitting, stretch marks, keloid scarring and cellulite.
- It refines, remoisturises, rejuvenates and retexturises skin.

As micro-current uses a modified direct current, it will basically have the same physical and physiological effects of the direct current used in galvanic treatments, but because of the relatively short pulse width 'on' times (compared to galvanic continuous direct current) and usually much lower levels of amplitude these effects are significantly reduced.

- Where the current passes through tissues, stimulation of the metabolism encourages lymphatic and venous drainage.
- Where the electrodes are in contact with the skin there will be the effects of both poles. The negative pole causes deep cleansing; dilation of blood and lymph; exfoliation of the stratum corneum; stimulation of nervous response. The positive pole creates tightening of the pores; firming of the tissues; soothing of the nervous response; and constriction of blood and lymph flow.

Micro-current is generally considered safe, with some top athletes using it to treat muscle and soft tissue injuries. The muscles cannot be harmed, and if a client does not keep up the maintenance, the muscles will never be worse than when the client started their course, they will merely return to the original condition. As the basic principle of treatment is to re-educate muscles, lifting and toning the facial or body contours, a course of treatments is necessary, followed by a monthly maintenance programme. A course of treatment will vary slightly depending on the condition of the client's muscles, but an average course is between ten and 14 treatments that are carried out preferably two to three times a week for the first few weeks, decreasing to once a week as the lift on the muscle lasts.

There are some conditions that are contraindicated to treatment including epilepsy, skin disorders, pregnancy, recent scar tissue, pacemakers, heat conditions, metal pins and plates in the immediate area, and silicone implants and collagen ridges. It is always wise to ask clients with high blood pressure and spastic conditions for a letter of approval from their GP before considering treatment.

As with all therapy treatments, it is essential to carry out a thorough consultation and prepare a treatment plan for the individual client.

This should include personal dietary and medical details and should be reviewed by the therapist. Keeping photographic evidence at varying stages throughout the course is useful since many clients tend to forget the original condition of their muscles as they become more used to their new look. Like all records these must be kept confidential.

Micro-current treatments for the face are very popular but they can also be used on the muscle of the body or for cellulite. An average facial treatment lasts between 60 and 75 minutes.

Waveforms

information point

- A micro-current machine has a waveform (whereas traditional galvanic machines do not). The waveform is the 'shape' of the current (as can be seen on an oscilliscope – a special device to visualise and measure electrical current). Most machines produce a selection of waveforms. These are often selected for use according to the client's needs, for example a sharp waveform may be recommended for a client with a severe ageing condition, and a gentle waveform for a younger client with good muscle tone. The waveform is created by interrupting the direct current and controlling the actual build-up, duration and decline of the pulses.
- The selection of frequency indicates the number of pulses per second emitted from the machine (the number of waves that pass any fixed point in a second) and are measured in hertz (Hz). The higher the frequency, the shorter the wavelength (the intensity shows the strength of the current and is shown in micro-amps).
- Some manufacturers generate the pulses as direct current, then reverse each alternate pulse electronically. Some enable the operator to select the options of pulse, frequency, intensity and waveforms, while others pre-set them.

Example of a micro-lifting treatment for the face

1 A very detailed consultation is carried out with the client, checking for any contraindications and discussing appropriate products to be used.

2 The skin is thoroughly cleansed ensuring that all traces of the medium are removed.

3 A specialised gel/solution is normally applied. This often contains essential oils and prepares the area for lifting by increasing the circulation and stimulating the lymphatic system. The probes are gently worked over the area.

4 A lymphatic programme is normally applied with the probes being used to follow the direction of lymphatic drainage.

5 A lifting programme is used with the machine being set on a low frequency to work the muscles, stretching and shortening as appropriate.

6 Further programmes may now be used depending on the individual manufacturer's machine. These may include more lifting, working on the lymphatic system or working on softening fine lines and wrinkles.

Facial toning treatment

7 The treatment is normally concluded by wiping over the area to remove any residue and applying a moisturising product.

8 Relevant home-care and future treatment advice should be given.

Treatment time per session for micro-electrotherapy is approximately 45 minutes to 1 hour.

Note: As with any toning programme, it is essential that a course of treatment is given and regular maintenance is given thereafter.

SELF-CHECKS

1 State the main effects of micro-electrotherapy treatments.

2 List the contraindications to micro-current treatments.

3 What safety precautions should be carried out when performing micro-current treatments?

information point

- As the skin ages it becomes less able to regenerate itself. On average old skin needs twice as long – as much as eight weeks – before it has renewed itself. This is because the sebaceous and sweat glands no longer exercise their function efficiently, the natural acidic protective coating changes. The skin becomes drier and thinner and as a consequence cannot retain enough moisture and grease.
- One of the main causes of skin ageing is the reduction of the body's hormone production. Hormones like testosterone or melatonin are only produced in great quantity until a person reaches 20 years of age. These hormones encourage physical fitness, an efficient immune system and the regeneration of cells. Due to the decline in the hormone level, the functions of the body's tissues, cells and organs start to break down.
- *Free radicals* are a contributing factor of skin ageing. These are parts of molecules, e.g oxygen molecules, that are found in the body. As a result of external factors like ultraviolet radiation, nicotine or unhealthy food, the free radicals become prone to react. This means that they are constantly looking for other chemical substances to bond with. Hence they attack the collagen fibres, cellular membranes and lipid layer of the skin. Free radicals change the inherited properties stored in the cell nucleus, so that the quality of newly formed skin cells deteriorates. The body protects itself against these aggressors through anti-oxidant enzyme systems (anti-oxidants), but from the age of 20 onwards, these natural defence mechanisms gradually decline, so that the skin can no longer defend itself.

Ultrasound

Ultrasonic sound waves have been used for cosmetic purpose since the early 1980s. Wide therapeutic use, easy control, and great results has made ultrasonic instruments for aesthetic use a natural. Ultrasonic sound waves are at a frequency of more than 20,000 Hz and are not heard by the human ear.

For skin care, most machines are created at 1 MHz with continuous and pulsed frequencies.

Mechanical function

Ultrasonic sound waves act on the body in the following way – they stimulate body cells, the tiny massage it produces expands the space in which the cells exist, causing movement of the cytoplasm, the rotation of mitochondria, and the vibration of the cell nucleus; it stimulates and expands the cell membrane. It improves local blood and lymph circulation, and increases the penetration of skin tone enhancing products.

Ultrasound helps to improve the metabolism and regeneration of body cells.

Warming and heating action

Warming and heating action is one of the most important therapeutic factors of ultrasound. It is a kind of internal heat, of an increase of about 79–80% – this heat is carried away by the blood circulation and is not perceived by the client. This warming action can change the blood circulation and helps reduce inflammation.

It is of great benefit prior to plastic surgery to reduce swelling and after the healing process is well on its way to reduce puffiness. It produces a relaxing and comforting feeling for the client.

Chemical function

The biochemical function of ultrasound comes from the reaction to anabolism and catabolism.

- Anabolism – the process that converts substances into other components of the organism's chemical architecture.
- Catabolism   the metabolic process by which cells convert substances into excreted compounds. In other words, the process of cell metabolism.

Small doses of ultrasound treatments can promote the synthesis of protein inside the cells, help to regenerate the wounded tissues and promote the synthesis of fibre cells in the body. In the process of anabolism and catabolism, the induced product is being absorbed and utilised by the cells. The accelerated metabolism of the cells changes the pH level of the skin to a more alkaline state and facilitates the absorption of the induced product. The skin lightens and smoothes visibly.

Ultrasonic exfoliation

A new way to clean the skin is by ultrasound. The skin is wetted with a de-ionised solution and the spatula is glided over the skin to 'split off' dead cells. The result is remarkable; an instant clearing and smoothing effect can be observed. This process is totally non-invasive and can be used on most skin types. You can also spot induce (deep lines and wrinkles are treated) product into the skin by either a pulsed method – to increase the fibroblast within the skin – or the continuous cycle.

Therapeutic and cosmetic benefits of ultrasound treatment

- Increases anabolic and catabolic process.
- Reduces puffiness.
- Helps to smooth lines and wrinkles.
- Exfoliates the top layer of the skin.
- Improves blood circulation.
- Increases cell regeneration.
- Soothes inflammation and speeds wound healing.
- Increases moisture retention of the skin.
- Softens the thrombus (a blood clot within a vessel that partially or totally obstructs circulation).
- Improves acneic skin and reduces pore size.

CONTRAINDICATIONS

to ultrasound treatment
- Never use on dry skin.
- Do not use on stomach of pregnant women.
- Do not use on people with pacemakers or electrical implants.
- Avoid using on people with heart conditions.
- Always use ultrasonic electrodes with sufficient media (herbal spray or serum on the skin).
- Ultrasonic treatment can be received by *all* skin types. The massage time and machine setting is varied for different skin types: most sensitive – least amount of time (3–5 min) and the setting is at its lowest.

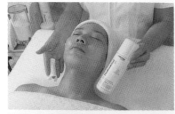
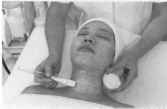
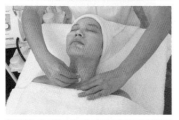
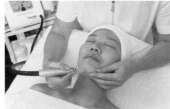
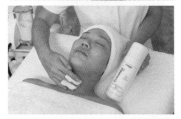
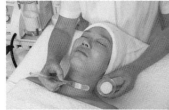
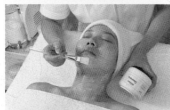
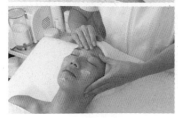

Combining the use of ultrasound treatment with other treatments

Ultrasonic exfoliation lends itself perfectly as an after-treatment for micro-dermabrasion, glycolic and other peels. It removes dead cells and any left-over crystals better than most cleansing techniques. If you want to speed up the healing and rejuvenation process of your client's skin, induce a water-soluble product into the client's skin with ultrasound after you complete the cleansing process.

Micro-dermabrasion

Micro-dermabrasion is becoming increasingly popular in the beauty therapy industry. It is a skin resurfacing treatment designed to correct or improve a range of skin abnormalities that originate in the epidermis or superficial layers of the dermis.

The treatment evolved from dermabrasion, which has been used by dermatologists in the medical profession for a very long time. This form of treatment is correctly known as open dermabrasion and uses wire brushes and diamond fraises to deeply remove the epidermis down to the lowest levels; it is very invasive but effective.

Micro-dermabrasion, or closed dermabrasion, on the other hand, is less invasive but will work much more deeply than any exfoliating product or treatment currently offered in the beauty therapy clinic. It can be used to treat stretch marks, post-acne scars, post-surgical scars, wrinkles, hyperpigmentation and inactive keloids.

Micro-dermabrasion equipment consists of a vacuum pump, compressor, crystal canisters and a delivery hand-held unit with pipework. Most systems operate in a similar fashion using a device which allows the projection of a flow of inert corundum crystals onto the skin via a controlled vacuum unit. This is achieved by placing the hand unit onto the skin, which normally has a 3–6 mm diameter hole, so the vacuum automatically generates a flow of crystals towards the skin. When the micro-crystals hit the skin's surface they cause billions of micro-traumas which in turn remove small fragments of skin cells. The micro-crystals and removed skin particles are then simultaneously sucked up towards a disposable flask. It is important to look for a machine that is totally hygienic, that is, one which has a disposable container for the contaminated crystals and where the hand-held unit can be sterilised. Machines can be set at different levels to allow for the required depth of abrasion needed. Most machines have about three levels of peeling.

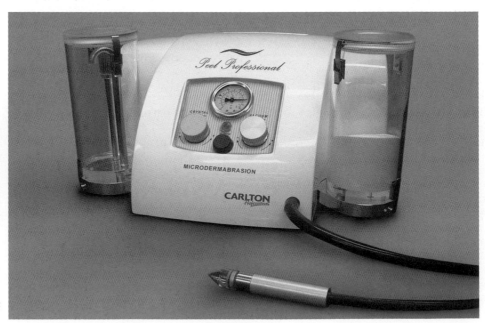

Micro-dermabrasion machine and an example of a routine

The treatment programme

- Level 1 involves the peeling of the stratum corneum of the epidermis which is suitable for fine lines and wrinkles and as a hydration pre-treatment to improve the penetration of products.
- Level 2 involves peeling more of the epidermis for thicker skins, scar tissue, pigmentation and acne scarring.
- Level 3 involves deep peeling all of the epidermis until blood appears. This is for medical application and only to be carried out by a physician.

The crystals that are used in the treatment are composed of aluminium oxide (corundum) and pointed like diamonds. They are completely non-toxic so totally safe when they come into contact with the skin. Micro-dermabrasion is suitable for most skin types from oily/acne to dehydrated and mature. It can also help with stretch marks. The treatment offers other benefits such as increased circulation, oxygenation of the skin, increased cell renewal, refining open pores and pigmentation and improving the skin's absorption of other products.

CONTRAINDICATIONS

to micro-dermabrasion
- Eczema.
- Psoriasis.
- Broken skin.
- Over moles.
- Diabetes.
- Retin A users.
- Keloid scarring.
- Scarring under six months.

After-care and home-care advice

- Following treatment, it will be necessary to advise the client to wear a sun block at all times and not to wear make-up for 24 hours afterwards. The client should also be advised that the skin may peel for a few days afterwards (this is because the treatment speeds up cell regeneration) and any flakes of skin can be gently removed with a warm face cloth.
- Home-care products should complement salon treatments.
- Some micro-dermabrasion equipment incorporates an infrared laser that emits monochromatic pulsating light. This is designed to speed up healing of the skin following treatment, regenerating the skin's surface through high stimulation of the fibroblast cells which increases the production speed of elastic fibres and collagen, whilst also creating faster absorption of liquids through the capillaries with reduction in swelling. The laser application reduces the number of micro-peeling treatments needed and accelerates the skin's repairing process.

information point

A number of ultrasound skin peeling systems have been successfully introduced for beauty therapy where frequencies of usually 28,000 Hz are transferred via a flexible actuator which passes over the skin with a fluid medium, to effect impressive low trauma peeling.

Mechanical massagers

There are three types of mechanical massager available to the therapist: audio sonic massagers, percussion massagers and gyrators. These can be chosen according to the desired effects of treatment and the space available for storage within the salon.

Audio sonic

An audio sonic massager is generally used to help relieve nodules of tension in the muscles. It is a small, hand-held vibrator that emits sound waves which produce a humming noise. These waves will penetrate 6 cm or more into the body's tissues

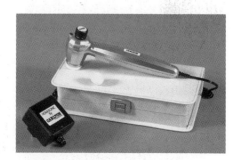

Audio sonic equipment

- The audio sonic unit has its own transformer to reduce the mains voltage to 12–14 volts.
- The audio sonic vibrator uses an electromagnet which causes the fixed magnet of its arm to vibrate when the alternating current from the mains supply is switched on.

Ball massage head

Plate massage head

and as the effects penetrate deep down it is ideal for sensitive skins. The action of the massager appears very gentle as it does not move up and down on the skin. It can only be used in small areas at a time due to its size.

The audio sonic unit is shaped like a small hammer. The external applicator head is directly attached to an internal electromagnetic coil or vibrator, whose action causes the applicator to move 'in and out' at frequencies in the audio spectrum, e.g. 30–20,000 Hz. The adjustable knob on the back or top of the unit is designed to restrict the distance that the applicator travels, thereby controlling the intensity of the massage application. A rocker on/off switch makes or breaks the electric circuit.

The are generally two massage head attachments sold with the unit:
- Ball massage head – used to intensify the actions of the vibrations in small areas.
- Plate massage head – used to evenly apply the vibrations over the largest possible area.

Percussion

The percussion type of mechanical massager is a small, hand-held unit which comes with a variety of massage heads, creating similar effects to manual percussion massage movements. A number of percussion vibrators have an intensity adjustment dial to enable the therapist to increase or decrease the vibration produced according to the depth or tissue being treated; they all have a main switch for turning the unit on or off. Percussion vibrators are generally used on the fine tissues of the face, neck and shoulders.

Different heads supplied are:
- Sponge head – used for gentle stimulation of the tissues.
- Spiky head – a rubber head used to create a more stimulating tapotement effect.

information point

- The intermittent alternating current causes the electromagnet of the vibrator to create an intermittent magnetic effect on the iron bar magnet within the unit which vibrates creating a tapping effect in the massage head attachments.
- The current alternates at 50 Hz releasing a tapping effect every half cycle (100 taps per second are emitted).
- If using audio sonic, a heat treatment such as sauna or steam bath may be given to relax the tissues prior to treatment.

CONTRAINDICATIONS

to audio sonic and percussion
- System conditions.
- Skin disorders/diseases.
- Bruised areas.
- Recent scar tissue.
- Highly vascular conditions.
- Varicose veins.
- Thrombosis or phlebitis.
- Over bony areas.
- Recent fractures.

Effects of audio sonic and percussion
- Increase blood circulation.
- Aid desquamation.
- Increase metabolism.
- Promote relaxation through warming the tissues.

Reasons for using audio sonic

- Where use of other massagers such as percussion is contraindicated due to skin sensitivity.
- To help break down nodules of tension and relieve tightness in muscle areas, e.g. the trapezius.
- For clients suffering with arthritis to create heat in the tissues which may help ease their aches and pains.

Reasons for using percussion

- To stimulate blood circulation and sebaceous flow in dehydrated or dry skins.
- To produce warmth in the tissues to promote relaxation.

Preparation for audio sonic and percussion treatment

1 Observe general safety precautions for using electrical equipment.

2 The machine is placed on a stable trolley.

3 The machine is checked and tested to ensure it is working correctly.

4 The products required for treatment are selected and placed on the trolley.

Audio sonic and percussion treatment

1 The client is greeted at reception and escorted to the treatment area.

2 A consultation is carried out to check for any contraindications and to explain the effects of the treatment.

3 The client removes their jewellery and is helped onto the couch.

4 The therapist ensures the client is warm and comfortable and prepared for treatment.

5 The appropriate massage head for the desired effects is selected and fitted firmly to the unit.

6 A suitable product medium is selected and applied to the area to be treated, e.g. talcum powder for oily skin and cream for dry.

Method

1 Check massage head is firmly attached.

2 Ensure that the unit is switched off and the mains lead is plugged into the mains.

3 The machine is tested on the therapist in front of the client.

4 The massage heads are cleaned with appropriate disinfecting fluid.

5 The unit is switched on by turning the main switch (on/off).

6 The adjustment dial is altered as necessary.

7 Apply the massage head to the treatment area working in a methodical manner throughout the treatment either using circular movements or working in straight lines. Treatment time will vary between 5–15 minutes according to the area being treated and the effect required.

8 The unit is removed from the client's skin, the machine is switched off and where needed the massage head changed and the treatment routine completed.

GOOD PRACTICE

- Avoid very bony areas.
- Ensure the tapping action is not too strong as this can lead to bruising.
- Do not use too close to the ears.

information point

- Remember to avoid applying directly to bony areas such as the zygomatic arch or frontal bone when working on the face or vertebral column on the back.
- The therapist may apply the vibrator indirectly over more sensitive bony areas by placing the massage head on to their hand and working across the area to reduce the stimulation achieved.

9 The medium used is removed and further treatment may be given if appropriate, e.g. massage.

10 The client is helped from the couch, the record card completed, appropriate home-care and further salon treatment advice is given, along with samples of the skin-care products used if applicable, and their next appointment is confirmed.

11 The therapist tidies the treatment area and cleans the massage heads used with hot water and wipes them with disinfectant.

ACTIVITY

With a colleague, perform on each other an audio sonic and percussion massage treatment. Discuss the physiological and psychological effects.

Gyrators

This is the most widely used mechanical massager and is commonly found in health spas and salons offering body treatments. It creates a much deeper massage effect within the tissues than the audio sonic and percussion vibrators. It is ideal for large muscular areas of the body and sometimes preferred by men with large muscle bulk to manual massage. There are a number of makes of electrical massage apparatus but the specific 'gyratory' action distinguishes this equipment.

The trademark G5™ is synonymous when describing gyratory massagers – the French manufacturer Monsieur Henri Cuiner created the very successful range of G5™ massagers over 30 years ago; the trademark derived from G for Gyratory and 5 from the number of accessory heads. Gyratory massagers are usually best used on a free-standing base with castors as this enables easier use and movement of the long flexible drive shaft, which runs from the body and motor of the unit, into which alternative massage heads can be attached.

A rotary electric motor inside the unit causes the crank and peg to fit into the massage head of the machine creating a gyratory (eccentric) movement.

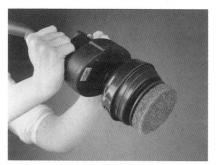

Guidance control handle

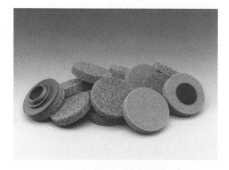

Disposable sponge heads

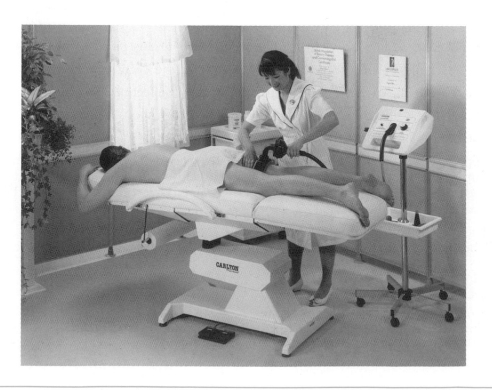

Gyratory massage

There are a variety of massage head applicators available, the traditional ones tend to be made from rubber or polyurethane. The most commonly used or 'standard' accessory heads are:

- Round and curved sponge heads – used to create an effleurage effect. The curved head is used on curved areas of the body, e.g. arms, shoulders and legs. Used at the beginning and end of treatment. Increases blood circulation and produces hyperaemia in the area being treated. It also promotes relaxation.

Round and curved sponge massage heads

- Single and double ball heads – used to create a deep petrissage effect on large muscle bulk, e.g. trapezius and gluteals.
- Egg box head (four half-domed heads) – used to create a deep petrissage effect on fatty tissues, e.g. quadriceps and gluteals.

Single and double ball massage heads

- Multi-pronged head – used to create a deep petrissage effect on fatty tissues.
- Spiky or brush heads – used to create stimulating tapotement effects.

GOOD PRACTICE

- Plastic covers for the massage heads can be purchased which will help improve their life span and are better for hygienic practices. They also enable the therapist to work with oil.
- Some therapists use disposable plastic bags to cover the massage heads, which detracts less from the aesthetic 'feel' of the massage head and is ideal for hygienic use. It is important that a new cover is used for every client.

'Egg box' massage head

Multi-pronged massage head

Additional accessories

- Water massage heads can also be purchased. Warm or cold water is placed inside the soft rubber head.
- There are a number of more specialist heads available for the traditional gyratory apparatus which are very useful to the experienced therapist.
- A Directional Stroking™ adapter allows the applicator head to move in a simultaneous stroking and patting movement.
- A variable speed controller on a gyratory massager alters the massage effect and offers the therapist greater choice of application.
- New gyratory massage heads have been designed for specific use with oil mediums (without deterioration) and can also be autoclave sterilised.

Brush massage head

A hand-held unit is ideal for the therapist who offers a home visiting service or in a salon that has little storage space. This can operate on the same principles as the larger, heavy-duty, free-standing gyrator (but an electrical motor is housed directly in the body of the unit and no drive shaft is attached). Traditionally small, less powerful hand-held massagers are usually two-handed and the massage heads are larger and often fit over the massage plate.

Water massage head

Effects of gyrators

- Increase blood circulation.
- Aid desquamation.
- Increase metabolism.
- Promote relaxation through warming the tissues.
- Repeated electrotherapy pressure massage may help the more efficient dispersal of fatty deposits, particularly when the client is on a weight-reducing diet and exercise programme.

CONTRAINDICATIONS

to gyratory massage

- Skin disorders/diseases.
- Infected acne conditions.
- Bruised areas.
- Cuts and abrasions.
- Recent scar tissue.
- Sunburn.
- Sensitive and fine skin.
- Loose crepey skin.
- Oedema.
- Glandular swelling.
- Highly vascular conditions.
- Varicose veins.
- Thrombosis or phlebitis.
- Over bony areas.
- Very hairy areas.
- Over the abdomen during menstruation and pregnancy.
- Epilepsy.*
- Diabetes.*

* Only to be carried out with medical consent.

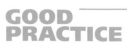

GOOD PRACTICE

A heat treatment such as sauna or steam may be given to relax the tissues prior to treatment. It is important that the area to be treated is sufficiently warmed before petrissage type massage is applied.

Reasons for using gyrators

- To help break down nodules of tension and relieve tightness in muscle areas, e.g. the trapezius.
- For general relaxation.
- For improvement of poor circulation.
- To assist as part of a weight reduction programme for spot areas, e.g. quadriceps and gluteals.
- To assist in the improvement of the texture of dehydrated and dry skins.

Preparation for gyratory treatment

1 Observe general safety precautions for using electrical equipment.

2 The machine is placed on a stable trolley where necessary.

3 The machine is checked and tested by the therapist to ensure it is working correctly.

4 The products required for treatment are selected and placed on the trolley.

Gyratory treatment

1 The client is greeted at reception and escorted to the treatment area.

2 A consultation is carried out to check for contraindications and to explain the effects of the treatment.

3 The client removes their jewellery and is helped onto the couch.

4 The therapist ensures the client is warm and comfortable.

5 The appropriate massage head to begin the treatment is selected and fitted correctly to the unit.

6 A suitable medium is selected and applied to the area to be treated if necessary, e.g. talcum powder.

Method

1 Check massage head is correctly attached and will not loosen during treatment.

2 Ensure unit is switched off and mains lead is plugged in.

GOOD PRACTICE

When using massage heads with screw threads, care should be taken not to cross thread.

3 The machine is tested on the therapist in front of the client.

4 Clean massage heads are selected.

5 The unit is switched on by turning the main switch (on/off).

6 If the unit has a variable speed control, this is adjusted accordingly.

7 Apply the massage head to the treatment area working in a methodical manner.

With the effleurage heads, follow the contours of the client's body and the direction of the venous return.

To create a kneading effect to the tissues the therapist selects a petrissage-type head. This is applied in a circular motion allowing the kneading of the tissues. It is important to lift and support the client's tissues towards the head.

For a desquamating, stimulating effect the therapist selects a tapotement-type head and works in circular movements supporting the client's tissues with their hand. The treatment is always completed with the effleurage head.

The treatment time will vary according to the area being treated and the effect required, e.g. spot reduction or full body massage treatment. In some cases only a few massage heads will be selected, particularly if performing a full massage routine.

8 The medium used is removed (if appropriate) and further treatment may be given if indicated, e.g. neuro-muscular electrical stimulation.

9 The client is helped from the couch, the record card completed, appropriate home-care advice given, e.g. diet and exercise, along with further salon treatment advice and the next appointment is confirmed.

10 The therapist tidies the treatment area and cleans the massage heads with hot water and detergent and then, according to the massage head used, wipes with a suitable disinfectant.

GOOD PRACTICE

- Ensure continuity is maintained whilst performing the treatment.
- Pressure should not be too heavy as bruising can occur.
- Support tissue areas as necessary during the treatment.
- Ensure the pressure from the head is kept flat and even to prevent damage.
- Massage heads must be stored only when thoroughly dry.
- As a safety precaution switch the unit on below the level of the couch in case the head is not firmly fitted and flies off.
- Care must be taken when selecting heads for the abdomen as there is no natural protection to the area from a bony superstructure, i.e. only the muscles and tissues of the abdomen itself.
- Mechanical massagers have been used by therapists for a long time. However in the past few years there has been a strong movement towards manual massage due to the psychological benefits gained from treatments that offer clients the warmth and understanding of the personal touch.

ACTIVITY

Describe suitable gyratory massage treatment programmes for the following clients and conditions:

a   30-year-old active male for relaxation

b   45-year-old female office worker with hard fat deposits on thigh areas.

1 Give six examples of questions that a therapist should consider before purchasing electrical equipment.

2 List the general safety precautions that should be observed when using electrical equipment.

3 Describe how a skin sensitivity test is carried out.

4 **a** What are the three types of mechanical massager available for salon use?

   b Give three reasons for using each type of massager.

   c List four common contraindications for the three types of mechanical massage.

5 Describe the preparation and treatment for one type of mechanical massage.

Vacuum suction massage

This treatment is used by therapists to assist in the movement of lymph fluid to the main lymph nodes, thus aiding the removal of waste products in the body. It also increases the efficiency of the circulatory system. It is generally given as part of a course of treatments and often combined with other treatments such as manual massage or dietary home-care advice, depending upon the area of the client being treated and the effect required. Treatment of the body using vacuum suction is often used for spot reduction in specific areas such as the thighs and buttocks rather than a full body treatment.

In order to perform this treatment effectively it is essential that the therapist has a knowledge and understanding of the lymphatic system (see Chapter 12).

Vacuum suction machines can be purchased for facial or body treatments. However, the majority of manufacturers produce mainly body or combined face and body units. These units generally consist of an electrically driven vacuum pump, a mains switch control, a gauge (which registers the amount of 'negative' or 'reduced' pressure produced) and a control dial for increasing or decreasing the amount of pressure required to treat the different tissues of the face and body. Accessory items to the unit are plastic tubing and an assortment of different sized ventouses or cups, which are generally made from Plexiglas or clear Perspex for the body and glass for the face. Some cups have a small hole in the side which the therapist places their finger over to maintain the pressure in the cup or to release the pressure when they want to. If there is no hole in the side of the cup the therapist has to release the pressure by gliding their finger under the cup. Some machines also have an outlet for blowing air out of the unit which can be attached via a nozzle to a bottle which will emit a fine spray. These can be used for a variety of preparations such as rose water for refreshing the client's skin.

Most vacuum suction machines available offer the therapist the single cup method of application. The multi-cup systems can be used for the body area enabling the therapist to work with a number of cups at the same time, thus reducing the treatment time. The method of application for this treatment is different but the effects achieved are the same. However, these systems are not widely used in the salon environment.

The most widely used method of vacuum suction is referred to as the gliding cup method whereby the therapist glides the chosen ventouse in a selected pattern and direction towards the nearest lymph nodes. Some units are designed to offer an additional pulsating action where intermittent pressure levels within the ventouse lift

information point

The gauge on a vacuum suction machine registers the height of mercury on a sphygmomanometer. This was incorporated into the unit by manufacturers to meet the tuition requirements of some examining bodies who state the approximate measure that should be registered during use. The majority of therapists judge the intensity required by the percentage of tissue in the ventouse and how it actually feels to the client.

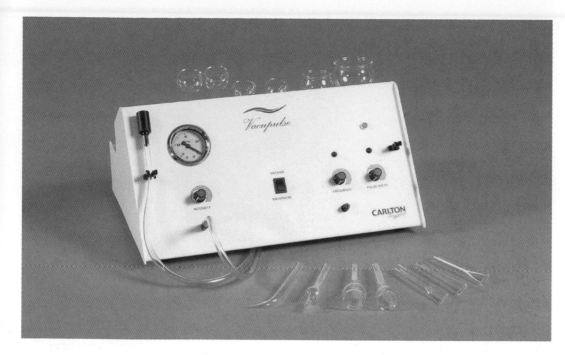

Vacuum suction machine

and drop the skin and body tissues as the therapist glides towards the lymph nodes. This method produces a gentle tapping effect on the skin producing stimulation in the area of treatment.

In body therapy treatments the therapist may select the gliding cup method for general lymph drainage, the pulsating gliding cup for further stimulation of the tissues along with lymph drainage or the static cup method for spot treatment in areas of fatty deposits, e.g. the thighs.

The static method can be used to lift the tissues in a specific area and generally involves the multi-cup method of application, but can be performed by the therapist with a single cup outlet. The therapist selects the appropriate size cups and applies to the treatment area ensuring the cups are moved around the area to prevent over-stimulation and possible bruising. After treatment the gliding cup method is used to drain the lymph to the nearest node.

Vacuum applicators

- Lymph drainage. This ventouse can be used for most vacuum treatments. It has a flat, thin head and is useful for working in the fine facial expression lines.
- Facial cups. These vary in size and are generally used for general cleansing or lymph drainage.
- Comedone applicator. These have a small, round opening which is used over the site of comedones, exerting even pressure on the surrounding issues.
- Body cups. These vary in size depending on the amount of adipose tissue in the area being treated.

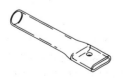

Lymph drainage applicator

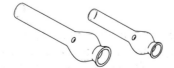

Facial cups

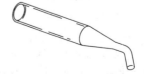

Comedone applicator

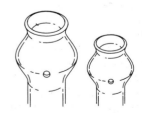

Glass body cups

to vacuum suction massage
- Skin diseases/disorders.
- Bruised areas.
- Cuts and abrasions.
- Varicose veins.
- Highly vascular conditions.
- Recent scar tissue.
- Sunburn.
- Sensitive or fine skin.
- Loose, crepey skin.
- Epilepsy.*
- Diabetes.*
- Any glandular swelling.
- Infected acne conditions.
- Bony areas.
- Very hairy areas.
- Thrombosis and phlebitis.
- Oedema.
- Heart conditions.*

* Only to be carried out with medical approval.

> **information point**
>
> The larger the diameter of the ventouse, the greater the reduced pressure will be at the same setting of depression.

> **information point**
>
> - The vacuum pump inside the unit is driven by an electric motor which produces suction in the ventouse by reducing the amount of air available, thus causing the client's skin to be drawn up into the cup.
> - The degree of reduced pressure produced by the vacuum pump can be increased or decreased according to the density of the client's body tissue by altering the intensity control allowing more or less air to leak, which affects the amount of vacuum produced.

> **information point**
>
> The amount of reduced pressure being exerted on to the body tissues is registered on the vacuum gauge.

Effects of a vacuum suction massage treatment
- Increases blood circulation.
- Increases lymph circulation thus aiding removal of toxins and waste products.
- Aids desquamation.
- Improves general skin texture.
- Stimulates metabolism.
- Promotes cellular regeneration.
- Scar tissue may be softened.
- May help in the utilisation and movement of fatty cells when combined with diet and exercise.

Reasons for using vacuum suction treatment
- To assist in reducing cellulite.
- To assist in reducing areas of oedema (non-systemic).
- For sluggish lymph circulation in specific areas, e.g. legs.
- To assist in a weight loss programme combined with diet, exercise and other salon treatments.
- To stimulate dry skin. The treatment time would be approximately 8–12 minutes.
- For deep cleansing very oily skins. The treatment time would be approximately 10–15 minutes.
- As a general skin cleanser on all but sensitive skin types. The treatment time for this would be approximately 5–8 minutes.

General preparation for vacuum suction treatments
1 Ensure the unit is switched off and connect the mains lead.
2 The therapist selects the size ventouse required for the treatment area and attaches it to the plastic tubing which connects onto the outside of the unit.

GOOD PRACTICE
- When working on the delicate tissues of the face, the amount of reduced pressure exerted on the tissue will be a lot less than when working on the more dense body tissues.
- The ventouse should be inspected for cracks as these will affect the pressure.
- The therapist should ensure that the working ventouse surfaces are smooth and even so as not to damage the client's skin.

Preparation for vacuum suction treatment

1 Observe general safety precautions for using electrical equipment.

2 The machine is placed on a stable trolley.

3 The machine is checked and tested by the therapist to ensure it is working correctly.

4 The products required for treatment are selected and placed on the trolley.

Facial vacuum suction treatment

1 The client is greeted at reception and escorted to the treatment area.

2 A consultation is carried out to check for contraindications and to explain the effects of the treatment.

3 The client removes their jewellery, which is kept safely by the therapist until the end of the treatment.

4 The client is helped onto the couch and their clothing and hair protected accordingly.

5 The therapist ensures the client is warm and comfortable.

6 The skin is cleansed with appropriate products.

7 A steam treatment may be given to soften the tissues.

8 A suitable product medium is selected and applied to the client's face and neck.

Method

1 Select a suitable ventouse to suit the treatment area and the desired effects.

2 Check the ventouse is correctly fitted.

3 Ensure the mains lead is plugged into the mains supply and that all switches are off and all dials are at zero.

4 The machine is tested on the therapist in front of the client.

5 Check the ventouse is recleaned with appropriate disinfecting fluid.

6 The unit is switched on by turning the main switch (on/off).

7 The intensity dial is adjusted to achieve the appropriate reduced pressure in the ventouse.

8 The cup is held in a perpendicular way to apply the ventouse to the skin. Remember not to draw more than 20% of the skin and tissues up into the cup.

9 Following the contours of the client's face and neck glide the cup slowly, to allow time for the effects of the treatment to be achieved, to the nearest lymph nodes.

10 The suction in the ventouse is released before the cup is removed from the skin by the therapist releasing their finger from the hole on the side of the cup or where there is no hole, by the therapist gliding their finger under the cup.

11 Following the pattern shown in the figure, repeat the sequence to each area 4–8 times depending on the skin reaction.

12 If the desired effect of the treatment is to loosen stubborn comedones the appropriate cup is used in small circular movements over the problem areas which tend to be the nose, upper lip and chin.

13 The product medium is removed and either further treatment such as massage and/or a face mask may be given or the skin is toned and moisturised with appropriate products.

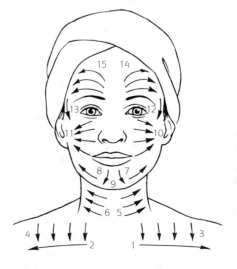

Direction of flow to the lymph nodes of the face, neck and décolleté

14 The client is helped from the couch, the record card completed, appropriate home-care and further salon treatment advice is given along with samples of the skin-care products used and the next appointment is confirmed.

15 The therapist tidies the treatment area and washes the cups and tubes used in hot water and detergent and then soaks them in an appropriate disinfectant.

GOOD PRACTICE

- The loosening of blockages can be combined with the general cleansing treatment.
- When using the comedone applicator, cotton wool may be placed in the top of the ventouse to prevent waste matter entering the plastic tubing.

ACTIVITY

Select two clients with differing skin conditions and carry out a minimum of six facial vacuum suction treatments. Describe the consultation, products selected, method of treatment and home care advice and evaluate the effectiveness of the programme.

Body vacuum suction treatment

1 The client is greeted at reception and escorted to the treatment area.

2 A consultation is carried out to check for contraindications, to explain the effects of the treatment and decide on the desired effects required from the treatment.

3 The client changes, showers and may have a heat treatment to soften and/or another salon treatment, e.g. a mechanical massage.

4 The client is helped on to the couch.

5 The therapist ensures the client is warm and comfortable.

6 A suitable product medium is selected and applied to the treatment area.

Method

1 Select a ventouse(s) to suit the treatment area and the desired effects.

2 Check the ventouse is correctly fitted.

3 Ensure the mains lead is plugged into the mains supply and that all switches are off and all dials are at zero.

4 The machine is tested on the therapist in front of the client.

5 Check the ventouse is recleaned with appropriate disinfecting fluid.

6 The unit is switched on by turning the main switch (on/off).

7 The mode of use is selected, e.g. pulsating method or static cup.

8 The intensity dial is adjusted to achieve the appropriate reduced pressure in the ventouse(s).

9 The cup is held in a perpendicular way to apply the ventouse to the skin. Remember not to draw more than 20% of the skin and tissues up into the cup.

10 **a** If using the gliding cup method the contours of the client's body are followed gliding the cup slowly (to allow time for the effects of the treatment to be achieved) to the nearest lymph nodes. The pattern shown in the figure indicates the movement sequence for working on the body with the gliding cup. The sequence is generally repeated to each area 4–8 times depending on the skin reaction.

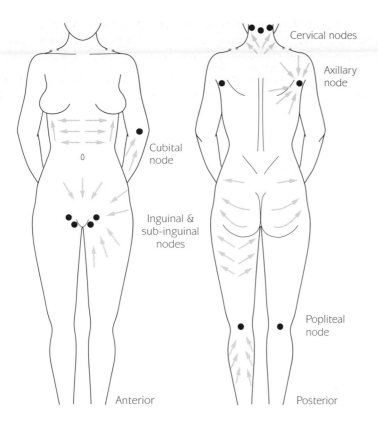

Direction of flow to the lymph nodes of the body

Labels on figure: Cervical nodes, Axillary node, Cubital node, Inguinal & sub-inguinal nodes, Popliteal node, Anterior, Posterior

b If using the spot treatment static or pulsating cup method, the appropriate size ventouse for the amount of adipose tissue is applied to the area. The suction in the ventouse is released before the cup is removed from the skin by the therapist releasing their finger from the hole on the side of the cup or, where there is no hole, by the therapist gliding their finger under the cup and placing it in another area.

Note: Trainee therapists sometimes combine the two methods of use, e.g. first using the gliding cup to loosen the tissues and stimulate the blood circulation prior to using the multi-cup spot treatment, which may help to loosen fatty deposits, before completing the treatment with the gliding cup to drain toxins and waste to the nearest lymph nodes.

11 The oil is removed and further treatment may be given, e.g. massage.

12 The client is helped from the couch, the record card completed, appropriate home-care and further salon treatment advice is given and the next appointment is arranged.

13 The therapist tidies the treatment area and washes the cups and tubes used in hot water and detergent and then soaks them in a disinfectant.

> ### information point
>
> Although traditional body vacuum suction is not the most common salon treatment, there is an increasing use of pressure massage equipment, which promotes lymph drainage, and new aspiration devices (such as Cellu M6 and Celluloss) incorporate the basic principles and direction of flow of body vacuum.

GOOD PRACTICE

- When applying the multi-cup static or pulsating method, a rocking action is used to roll the cups onto the skin at the same time to ensure the suction in the cups is equal.
- Care must be taken not to use too high a reduced pressure in the ventouse or to pull the cup off without releasing the pressure or to work in an area too long as all these can lead to dilated capillaries and bruising of the skin.
- Drain to the lymph node, not over it.

Plan a course of body vacuum suction treatments for a client with sluggish lymph circulation. Clearly outline the treatment objectives, describe the consultation, treatment methods and products to be used along with the client home care advice. Evaluate and justify your findings on the effectiveness of the programme.

High frequency

The term 'high frequency' traditionally applies to the high frequency apparatus used to stimulate blood flow and uses a rapidly alternating electrical current in the region of 100,000–250,000 hertz. It is a high voltage, but low current treatment. As the pulses of the current are short, they do not stimulate motor points to contract muscles – instead they pass directly into the skin via the electrode applicator at the point of contact, producing warmth in the tissues which creates a heating effect. The therapist can apply high frequency in two ways depending upon the client's skin condition. Each method creates different effects on the tissues:

- Direct method.
- Indirect method (often referred to as the Viennese massage).

High frequency equipment may vary in general appearance as manufacturers develop equipment to appeal to therapists from an aesthetic and economical view, but the basic operations of the equipment will be similar. There are generally two main control switches: the on/off switch and the intensity control. A mains lead connects the unit to the power supply. A flex leads from the unit to the handle, which is used to house the glass electrodes. There is a variety of electrodes that the therapist can select to use depending upon the method of application and the area to be treated and the desired effects.

Electrodes

The glass electrodes have metal conducting caps (ends) which connect with the metal plate found in the handle allowing the current to flow from the machine to the electrode. The electrodes fit firmly into the holder but not tightly, otherwise the therapist would be unable to change electrodes.

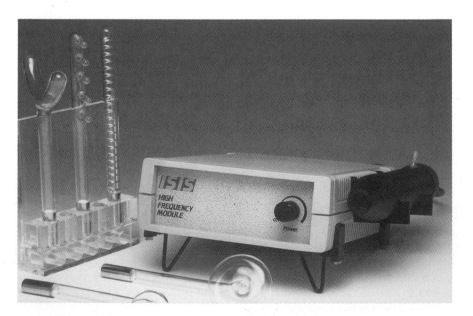

Isis modular high frequency unit

- **Large head surface electrode (large mushroom)**. This is used for facial and body work when using direct high frequency. It can also be used for 'sparking' treatments to intensify the current by using only on a side edge lifted on and off the skin with small movements.
- **Small head surface electrode (small mushroom)**. Used for direct high frequency. This electrode is useful for working on small, difficult areas such as the nose. It can also be used for sparking.
- **Roller electrode**. Used for face and body direct high frequency treatments. It rolls easily over the skin and can be used without gauze or a sliding medium.
- **Neck electrode**. Used for direct high frequency application to the neck area or other curved areas of the body, e.g. arms.
- **Sparking electrode**. Used for application of direct high frequency for sparking to specific areas and cauterising individual pores. Care should be taken to use a low current with this electrode.
- **Rake electrode**. Used for direct frequency to the scalp area.
- **Intensified saturator electrode**. This electrode is used for indirect high frequency and is known as a saturator. It usually contains a metal spiral running through the inside of the glass which intensifies the effect and ensures that only a low current is required to give maximum effect.

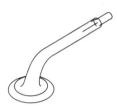

Large head surface electrode

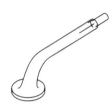

Small head surface electrode

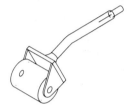

Roller electrode

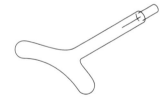

Neck electrode

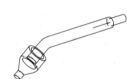

Sparking electrode

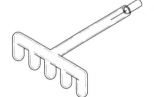

Rake electrode

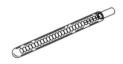

Intensified saturator electrode

CONTRAINDICATIONS

to high frequency
- Cuts or abrasions to the skin in the area to the treated.
- Skin diseases or disorders.
- Highly vascular conditions.
- Sensitive skin.
- Highly nervous clients.
- Excessive metal in the area of application, e.g. plates or fillings.
- Swellings in the area.
- Very hairy areas.
- Sinus blockages.
- Heart conditions.*
- Epilepsy and diabetes.*
- Circulatory conditions.*
- Pregnancy.*
- Asthmatics.*
* Only to be carried out with medical approval.

information point

Within each electrode is sealed a small quantity of inert gas, usually argon. As the current flows through the gases a coloured glow is produced. The electrodes glow either blue–violet if they contain argon or red–orange if they contain neon.

The indirect method

This method of applying the high frequency current involves creating a circuit of current that flows from the saturator to charge the client. The therapist massages the client, thus discharging the current from the client's face to the therapist's massaging finger or hand.

Effects of indirect high frequency

- Increases circulation.
- Increases metabolism.
- Warms and relaxes the tissues.
- Improves the skin texture.
- Improves the moisture balance of the skin.
- Calms the sensory nerve endings.

Reasons for using indirect high frequency

- To improve dry or dehydrated skins.
- To improve tired skin.
- To help improve fine lines.
- To help relax the tissues.
- To help improve poor circulation.

Preparation for indirect high frequency treatment

1   Observe general safety precautions for using electrical equipment.

2   The machine is placed on a stable trolley.

3   The machine is checked and tested by the therapist to ensure it is working correctly.

4   The products required for treatment are selected and placed on the trolley.

Indirect high frequency treatment

1   The client is greeted at reception and escorted to the treatment area.

2   A consultation is carried out to check for contraindications and to explain the effects of the treatment and a skin sensitivity test is carried out.

3   The client removes their jewellery, which is kept safely by the therapist until the end of the treatment.

4   The client is helped on to the couch and their clothing and hair protected accordingly.

5   The therapist ensures the client is warm and comfortable.

6   The skin is cleansed with the appropriate products.

7   A suitable product medium is selected and applied to the client's face and neck, e.g. massage or nourishing cream.

Method

1   Ensure the mains lead is plugged into the mains supply and that all switches are off and all dials are at zero.

2   The therapist tests the machine in front of the client and reassures them where necessary about the buzzing noise it makes.

3   Talcum powder is applied to the client's hands to absorb any perspiration.

4   The saturator is wiped with disinfectant and placed firmly in the holder.

5   Depending upon the apparatus used, the saturator is held firmly by the client at the free end, taking care not to hold over the point of electrode insertion into

the handle. The handle can also usually be held by the client with their second hand, but check the intended use with the manufacturer as in some cases this is not advised, and the handle is supported by a towel.

6 The therapist places one hand in contact with the client's skin and begins to massage using small circular effleurage movements whilst with the other hand turning the intensity dial slowly, to suit the client's tolerance.

7 Place the other hand on the opposite side of the client's face and without losing contact, massage using both hands. The therapist should feel warmth in their fingers.

8 The treatment time will vary between 8 and 20 minutes depending upon the client's skin condition.

9 At the end of the treatment the therapist keeps one hand in contact whilst using the other to turn the intensity dial to zero before switching off the machine.

10 The cream is removed and either further treatment such as a face mask may be given or the skin is toned and moisturised with appropriate products.

11 The client is helped from the couch, the record card completed, appropriate home-care and further salon treatment advice is given along with samples of the skin-care products used and the client's next appointment is confirmed.

12 The therapist tidies the treatment area and cleans the electrode used by carefully wiping with hot water and then disinfectant. Special care must be taken not to wet the metal and connector of the saturator. All electrodes should be dry before being stored for later use.

GOOD PRACTICE

- Care should be taken when working around the hairline as sensation will usually intensify because hair is a conductor of electricity.
- Contact must not be broken. If the circuit is completely broken and then remade without turning the intensity dial to zero, the client may feel a stronger tingling sensation, which may make them apprehensive of further treatment. However, if the therapist wishes to intentionally create a stimulating effect on the skin they can slowly lift the fingers slightly off the skin and return them.
- Rings must not be worn by the client on the hand that holds the saturator (and preferably not at all).
- Care must be taken to ensure any belts with metal buckles are kept away from the saturator or removed.
- The client or therapist must not touch any metal conducting material whilst the indirect high frequency treatment is in progress, e.g. couch, trolley, etc.

information point

- The intensity dial may need to be reduced when progressing to areas of finer skin, e.g. the forehead.
- The intensity of the current in the tissues will be increased when lifting one hand off the skin during the massage.
- Tapotement movements such as tapping will intensify the current in the area being treated.
- In the past, talcum powder was used as a medium to create a stimulating effect, but its drying effects are not beneficial for a dry or dehydrated skin.

ACTIVITY

Research the variety of portable high frequency units suitable for use by a home visiting therapist. List the company names, cost, features of the equipment and back-up service. State and justify which unit you would recommend for purchase.

Direct high frequency

This method of application of the high frequency current uses glass electrodes which are placed in direct contact with the client's skin. The current is dispersed at the point of contact with the client and as the effects are concentrated around the electrode, they are superficial.

Effects of direct high frequency

- Increases metabolism.
- Warms and relaxes the tissues under the electrode.
- Improves the skin texture.
- Improves the moisture balance of the skin.
- Calms the sensory nerve endings.
- Produces ozone which has an anti-bacterial, germicidal effect on the surface of the skin. This effect can be intensified with sparking.

Reasons for using direct high frequency

- To improve the condition of seborrhoeic or oily skins.
- To improve the condition of oily areas, e.g. T-zone, blemished skin on any area of the body.
- To aid the healing of pustule-prone skins by using sparking on the skin.
- To destroy bacteria through the creation of ozone through sparking.
- To stimulate secretion in a dry skin by treating the skin for a few minutes, e.g. 3–4 minutes.

Preparation for direct high frequency treatment

1 Observe general safety precautions for using electrical equipment.

2 The machine is placed on a stable trolley.

3 The machine is checked and tested by the therapist to ensure it is working correctly.

4 The products required for treatment are selected and placed on the trolley.

Direct high frequency treatment

1 The client is greeted at reception and escorted to the treatment area.

2 A consultation is carried out to check for contraindications and to explain the effects of the treatment.

3 The client removes their jewellery, which is kept safely by the therapist until the end of the treatment.

4 The client is helped onto the couch and their clothing and hair protected accordingly.

5 The therapist ensures the client is warm and comfortable.

6 The skin is cleansed with the appropriate products.

7 A suitable medium is selected and applied to the client's face and neck, e.g. oxygenating cream and gauze.

Method

1 Ensure the mains lead is plugged into the mains supply and that all switches are off and all dials are at zero.

2 The therapist tests the machine in front of the client and reassures them where necessary about the buzzing noise it makes.

3 The selected electrodes are wiped with disinfectant and stored safely for use.

4 The electrode is placed firmly in the holder.

5 The therapist either places the electrode in contact with the client's skin and moves it around using small circular movements whilst turning the mains control switch on and the intensity dial up to suit the client's tolerance, or places their finger in contact with the electrode before turning the machine on, then the intensity dial up, and placing both finger and electrode in contact with the client's skin before removing the finger.

---

information point

The application of the direct high frequency electrode creates warmth on the skin and converts the stable oxygen molecules in the oxygenating cream to unstable ozone molecules (which have a germicidal effect).

---

6 The treatment time will vary depending upon the client's skin condition, e.g. oily skin 8–15 minutes, dehydrated skin 3–4 minutes.

7 At the end of the treatment, or between changing electrodes, the therapist must keep the electrode in contact with the client's skin whilst turning the intensity dial to zero and switching the machine off before removing the electrode from the skin, or place their finger on the electrode before lifting it off the client's skin and turning the intensity dial to zero and switching the machine off. Some units have a secondary on/off switch directly on the handle to assist with an easier change over of electrodes, etc.

Note: When sparking to create a germicidal effect which may destroy bacteria, the electrode is lifted off the skin. The distance created between the electrode and the skin should only be a few millimetres, causing the current to 'jump' from the electrode to the client's skin thus creating a spark which in turn produces ultraviolet rays which destroy bacteria. The germicidal effect is created by the ionisation of the oxygen in the air which creates ozone. Controlled quantities of ozone help promote the healing of pustules and papules. Pores are constricted when the sparks stimulate the skins nerve endings.

8 The selected medium is removed and either further treatment such as a face mask may be given or the skin is toned and moisturised with appropriate products.

9 The client is helped from the couch, the record card completed, appropriate home-care and further salon treatment advice is given along with samples of the skin-care products used and the client's next appointment is confirmed.

10 The therapist tidies the treatment area and cleans the electrodes used by carefully wiping with hot water and then disinfectant. Special care must be taken not to wet the metal end connector of the saturator. The electrodes are stored dry for later use.

information point

- To produce a high frequency current the equipment requires a capacitor and an inductor of a special type to increase the output voltage.
- Older style circuits used a spark gap inductor called a Tesla coil.
- The special transformer contained in the handle of the machine (which holds the electrodes selected for treatment) is known as the oudin coil or resonator.
- The actual flow of current from a high frequency unit is small although the voltage is very high. The overall power is quite low.
- With high frequency the current disperses into the client's body at the point of contact.
- As the effects are concentrated around the electrode they are superficial, but care must be taken when sparking not to over-treat as this can lead to over-desquamation and drying of the skin during subsequent days.

SELF-CHECKS

1 Give four examples of vacuum applicators and in each case briefly outline their purpose.

2 List ten contraindications to vacuum suction.

3 State four reasons for giving a vacuum suction treatment.

4 Describe a high frequency current.

5 Name and describe the two different treatments that can be given using the high frequency machine.

Neuro-muscular electrical stimulation (NMES)

This treatment is referred to by many different names, such as electrical muscle stimulation (EMS), faradic (after the original type of current used for muscle stimulation), or by manufacturers' trade names, e.g. Slendertone™ and Ultratone™. It is used to improve and maintain muscular tone and is a passive form of exercise, as the client lies and relaxes whilst the machine emits electrical impulses to stimulate the muscles' motor nerves to bring about muscle contraction. To be more effective the treatment has to be part of a course to develop the full effect within the muscles. It is extremely beneficial for clients who do not enjoy physical exercise or who are contraindicated to strenuous exercise or for those wishing to tone particular muscle groups, e.g. abdominals for postnatal mothers.

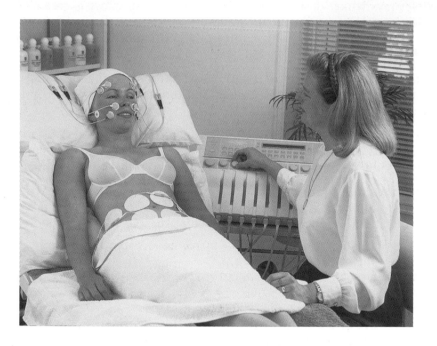

Neuro-muscular electrical
stimulation

NMES machines use an interrupted direct current of a low frequency and relatively very small pulse width which is released into the body via a conductive electrode which is connected to the faradic unit via electrical leads. The majority of machines offer the therapist the facility to use the equipment on both face and body by using different electrodes and by varying the parameters of the current. Machines, however, are available for just face or body. Faradic treatments have been extremely popular for figure improvement programmes particularly when combined with other salon treatments such as gyratory massage and galvanic along with home-care advice on diet and exercise. In recent years there has been great technological advancement by equipment manufacturers who have developed and adapted faradic currents to develop more specialised salon treatments for figure improvement (see Chapter 6).

NMES units generally have the following controls:

- A mains switch for turning the unit on or off. This is often combined with a timer.
- A safety aspect on most modern machines is a re-set feature which prevents the machine working if any of the electrode outlet dials are not at zero.
- Intensity dials for each electrode outlet. As these dials are increased, so is the intensity of the current flowing through the electrodes.

- Contraction (surge or stimulation period) and relaxation dials which enable the therapist to select the appropriate times to suit the area of the body being treated and the existing condition of the client's muscle.
- A pulse sequence, wave form or phasic control. On the majority of equipment only two types are found: mono-phasic and bi-phasic. Mono-phasic emits pulses flowing in one direction only. Bi-phasic emits pulses flowing in both directions; back and forth or negative to positive then positive to negative. The other selections available either on this dial or as a separate mode dial are:

  a Mono-phasic on a regular basis. Pulses are emitted as per the machine setting, e.g. contracting for 2 seconds and relaxing for 2.5 seconds.

  b Bi-phasic on a regular basis. Pulses are emitted as per the machine setting.

  c Mono-phasic and bi-phasic on an irregular basis. With this setting the machine is programmed to alter the pattern of the set contraction and relaxation time. This is particularly useful when a client is a little apprehensive of the treatment and tends to automatically tighten their muscles when they expect the contraction to occur. It is also useful to add variety to the treatment for a regular client.

- A frequency dial. This enables the therapist to select the number of pulses per second emitted from the machine to stimulate the motor points. Traditionally for superficial muscles, such as those of the face, 120 is used, whereas for work on larger muscles between 60 and 90 is used. However, the most recent research has shown a wider application of frequency is beneficial, especially when recreating passive exercise most closely similar to physical activity.

- A pulse width. This changes the actual width (i.e. the length of time it stays in the muscle) of each pulse emitted. The higher the setting of this dial the longer the time and therefore the greater is the effect to the muscle. For facial muscles a lower setting is usually used, e.g. 80 ms, whereas on the large body muscles a higher setting is required, e.g. from 160 ms upwards, and if the client has a lot of adipose tissue the dial may be started at a higher setting still, such as 240 ms (m is the abbreviation for millionth or micro, hence here this means a time base in microseconds, which is very quick).

- Some machines have master output control which can increase the percentage intensity of current to all the electrodes in use without turning them up individually.

- Pulse ramp envelope control. Usually only available on more specialised units, this controls the configuration of pulses in the contraction time. It is adjusted to enable more comfortable, effective contractions.

- Sequential programming. Some specialist units offer the facility to create your own sequential treatment where frequency, contraction, relaxation and pulse width can be pre-programmed and altered at regular intervals and stored in the memory.

Electrodes

There is a wide variety of electrodes available for use with faradic-type machines. To enable the current to flow to stimulate the muscles, a positive electrode (anode) and negative electrode (cathode) are needed.

The most widely used modern faradic electrodes for application of the current to the body are rubber pads which are impregnated with an electrical conductor, such as carbon, on one side. These pads can vary in shape and size but are used in pairs to enable the current to flow from one to the other.

For facial treatments there are three types of electrode available for use:

- Facial block electrode (dual head). The most popular type manufactured and used houses the anode and cathode in its insulated holder. They vary in form and in use, e.g. some have an in-built intensity control to adapt the current easily, the distance between the anode and cathode may be fixed or if the electrode has

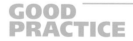

GOOD PRACTICE

Care must be taken not to over-work the muscles.

information point

- The mushroom electrode is not particularly used in salons but has traditionally been used by colleges.
- Facial faradic treatment is an extremely beneficial treatment for tightening the contours of the face, but is widely under-used by therapists.

a stylus the therapist can alter the distance between these. They are ideal for stimulating a number of motor points which are situated closely together on the face.

- Mushroom electrode (disc electrode). A metal disc in the electrode must be covered in several layers of lint to protect the client. The indifferent electrode is protected with a foam pouch and is placed in contact with the client's body by either lying it under the shoulder or, as with some machines, by using a wrist clip. The mushroom head is placed on the motor point of the muscle, acting as the active electrode and completing the electrical circuit.
- Mask electrode. This houses a variety of electrodes inside to stimulate all the muscles of the face at the same time. This would not be used on claustrophobic clients.

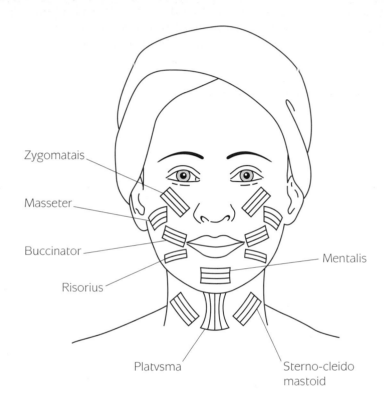

Electrode placement on muscle groups for facial faradic treatment

Types of padding

The selection of the padding method for treatment will be dependent on a number of things:

- The phase control to be used. With bi-phasic the current is even from the positive and negative electrodes whereas with mono-phasic the current is stronger from the negative electrode.
- The areas to be treated and the number of pairs of electrodes available, e.g. if there are a large number of muscles to stimulate there may be insufficient electrodes to use the longitudinal method and therefore split padding may have to be used.
- Manufacturers' instructions. These should always be followed carefully as the manufacturers will recommend the most suitable type of padding to gain maximum benefit from their machine.

Longitudinal padding

Modern longitudinal padding involves placing the anode and cathode on to the top and bottom motor points of the same muscle, e.g. rectus abdominus, triceps, rectus femoris, etc., bringing about a smoother, even contraction. This term was used to describe the padding of the origin and insertion of a muscle whereby the current had to flow via the motor point to bring about a contraction. Modern longitudinal padding usually refers to the placing of the electrodes on to a muscle with two motor points.

Dual or duplicate padding

This type of padding involves using the anode and cathode of a pair of pads on one or two muscles on one side of the body and then placing another pair on the adjacent muscle group, e.g. the obliques, rectus abdominus, adductors, abductors, etc.

Split padding

With this type of padding a pair of pads is split and placed on the same muscle group on opposite sides of the body, e.g. gluteus maximus, pectorals, etc.

GOOD PRACTICE

- To gain maximum benefit when using duplicate padding, use mono-phasic and place the cathode on the weaker muscle.
- Where duplicate or split padding is used, a greater current intensity will be needed.

ACTIVITY

With a colleague, carry out three different body NMES treatments using the different methods of padding. Discuss the effectiveness and comfort of each method.

CONTRAINDICATIONS

to NMES
- Disorders of the nervous system.
- Disorders or injury of the muscular system.
- Loss of skin sensation.
- Recent scar tissue.
- Broken bones.
- Hypersensitive skins.
- Heart conditions.
- Pacemakers.
- High or low blood pressure.*
- Thrombosis or phlebitis.
- Highly apprehensive clients.
- Epilepsy.*
- Diabetes.*
- Migraine sufferers.
- Cuts and abrasions.
- Highly vascular conditions.
- Metal plates, pins, bridges, IUD or if the client has an excessive amount of fillings.
- Over bony areas.
- Pregnancy.**
- * Only to be carried out with medical approval.
- ** Exclude the abdomen.

Effects of NMES

- Stimulates the nerves and causes muscle contraction which acts as a passive form of exercise to strengthen and tone muscles.
- Increases blood circulation.

Reasons for using NMES

- To strengthen and tone poor muscles, e.g. abdominal and pectorals of postnatal mothers.
- To improve the contours of the face and body, e.g. platysma, abdominal, gluteals.
- To assist in tightening muscles after weight loss.
- To assist in improving a client's posture by stretching and toning shortened muscles, e.g. pectorals in kyphosis.

Preparation for NMES treatment

1 Observe general safety precautions for using electrical equipment.

2 The machine is placed on a stable trolley.

3 The machine is checked and tested by the therapist to ensure it is working correctly.

4 The products required for treatment are selected and placed on the trolley.

NMES treatment

1 The client is greeted at reception and escorted to the treatment area.

2 A consultation is carried out to check for contraindications and to explain the effects of the treatment. A skin sensitivity test is carried out on the area to be treated.

Note: If performing a body treatment, the client's measurements can be noted prior to treatment.

3 The client removes their jewellery, showers and may have a heat treatment to relax the muscles prior to treatment and/or an additional salon treatment, e.g. gyratory massage.

4 The client is helped onto the couch.

5 The therapist ensures the client is warm and comfortable.

6 The skin is free of grease as this would act as a barrier to the current and prevent a good contraction.

7 The therapist tests the machine in front of the client.

8 If treating the body, elasticated straps are wrapped and firmly secured around the area to be treated.

9 Having considered the client's needs and the machine being used, the therapist selects an appropriate method of padding, dampens the electrodes with warm water or conductive gel and places them firmly in contact with the client's skin.

Method

1 Ensure the mains lead is plugged into the mains supply and that all switches are off and all dials are at zero.

2 The therapist selects the appropriate treatment time, contraction and relaxation period, the mode, pulse sequence and width.

3 If performing a facial treatment, the therapist dampens the facial electrode and places it firmly in contact with the treatment area.

Note: If using the mushroom electrode, the therapist first places the indifferent electrode firmly in contact with the client's skin (behind the shoulder or strapped to the wrist). If using a mask electrode, it is firmly strapped around the client's face and neck and, as the electrodes are simultaneously activated by the intensity dial, the therapist would check on client sensation and comfort until contractions

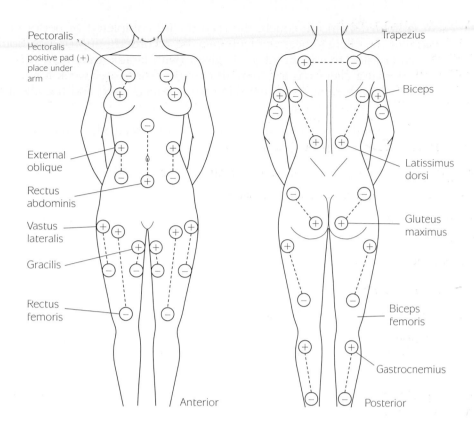

Pectoralis
Pectoralis positive pad (+) place under arm

Trapezius

Biceps

External oblique

Rectus abdominis

Latissimus dorsi

Vastus lateralis

Gluteus maximus

Gracilis

Rectus femoris

Biceps femoris

Gastrocnemius

Anterior

Posterior

Example of faradic padding on the bi-phasic mode

were achieved. The treatment time would begin at around 8 minutes and build throughout the course of treatments to 15 minutes.

4　The therapist slowly turns up the intensity dial during the contraction time only, checking with the client on how it feels.

GOOD PRACTICE

- It is very important to use a good conductive medium.
- If working on the body all electrodes need to be turned up individually until the client feels a slight tingling sensation. This allows the client time to relax and adjust to the treatment before the therapist turns the individual intensity dials to achieve a contraction.

information point

Some machines allow the therapist to increase the intensity during the treatment to all electrodes by adjusting the master output dial.

When working on the face, neck and décolleté areas, it is advisable to contract the muscle 6–8 times before switching the intensity dial off during the relaxation period and moving the electrode to the next muscle. The sequence is then repeated 2–3 times throughout the course of treatments.

When working on the body, the therapist must ensure even contractions are achieved on all the muscles being worked. If a muscle is weaker it will need a lower intensity than a stronger more toned muscle. The treatment time is usually around 20–40 minutes depending upon the treatment effects and condition.

It is important to ensure that the client is warm and comfortable throughout the treatment.

5　At the end of the treatment the therapist ensures all dials are switched off before removing the electrodes. It is advisable to turn the intensity control down during the relaxation period.

6　If recommended, further treatment may be given.

- Saline solution used to be applied to the electrodes as a conductor but most manufacturers today feel that there are sufficient mineral salts present in tap water to act as a conductor.
- Faradic pads deteriorate with use and become less conductive so will need replacing regularly.

7 The client is helped from the couch, the record card completed (if performing a body treatment the client's measurements may be recorded), appropriate home-care and further salon treatment advice is given (with faradic treatment it is recommended that a client has a minimum of 2–3 sessions per week for 6–8 weeks) along with samples of any skin-care products used and the client's next appointment is confirmed.

8 The therapist tidies the treatment area and cleans the electrodes used by carefully wiping with hot water and detergent.

GOOD PRACTICE

Poor contraction of muscles may be due to:
- Any grease left on the skin.
- The electrodes being too dry (they may need re-damping during the treatment).
- The electrodes not being firmly in contact with the skin.
- The intensity selected being too low.
- The pulse frequency and width not being set correctly.
- Trying to stimulate muscles through large quantities of adipose tissue which can act as a barrier to the current.
- Incorrect positioning of the electrodes. It is important to switch the intensity dial to zero before moving the pads.
- Faulty connections on the machine or leads. The leads need regular checking and maintenance.
- Muscle fatigue.

Galvanic treatments

Galvanic treatments have become extremely popular over the last few years. The current brings about chemical and physical reactions within the body and it is commercially used with professional products to improve the client's face and body appearance. There are a wide variety of gels and ampoules manufactured and recommended for different skin types and conditions.

The galvanic machine can be applied with the appropriate products to offer two treatments to the client:

- Desincrustation – this is given to deep cleanse the skin.
- Iontophoresis – this is used to introduce beneficial ingredients into the skin for particular skin types or conditions, e.g. oily, dry or couperose skins.

Galvanic treatment is used on the body to assist in the dispersal of cellulite.

The principles of the galvanic treatment for face and body is the same but the application, products used, treatment time, further salon treatment and home care advice are different. The machines use a direct current of a low voltage. They can be purchased for face or body work individually or combined in a face and body unit or in a combined unit with another electrical treatment such as high frequency. This last combination is commonly found in salons as these two treatments are popularly used with professional products for improved skin care (see Chapter 6).

Galvanic units consist of:

- A mains control switch which may be connected to a timer.
- Outlets for connecting the electrodes, which are used in pairs (anode and cathode).
- Intensity dial and milliamp meter for registering the amount of current applied (and directly to indicate the level of the client's skin resistance).
- Polarity switch which is often referred to as 'normal' or 'reverse' where 'normal' indicates that the internationally accepted law of colour coding applies (red = positive, black = negative).

information point

The range of products available include gel and ampoule preparations and specially formulated solutions.

It is extremely important that the therapist reads and follows the manufacturer's instructions as although there is a standard understanding that the red wire of an electrode is positive and the black lead is negative, most manufacturers have adapted their machines to enable the therapist to reverse the polarity of the leads at the flick of a switch which could easily cause confusion if the manufacturer's instructions are not read.

The therapist must fully understand their unit and if terms such as 'normal' and 'reverse' are indicated, know accurately how this refers to the polarity of the leads and outlets. Usually this is a simple point to clarify, but it should not be assumed as manufacturers vary in the use of terminology and presentation, i.e. some units have separate outlets for the anode and cathode and others are coupled.

The intensity of the output is measured in milliamps (mA) and can be registered on either:

- a moving coil meter, i.e. a gauge with an arm
- a LED (light emitting diode)
- a LCD (liquid crystal display).

For facial therapy treatment, intensity settings are low and indicated by the product directive and the type of skin being treated. Ranges between 0.2–0.6 mA are common, but individual sensory responses are an important factor to be considered along with manufacturer's instructions.

For body therapy the following calculation can be used to work out the maximum milliamps current setting for a pad size:

Manufacturer's recommended maximum = 0.05 mA per square centimetre

Pad size = 11 × 11 cm = 121 cm²

Maximum current setting = 121 × 0.05 = 6.05 mA

Terminology referred to in galvanic treatments

- Anode – positive electrode.
- Cathode – negative electrode.
- Active electrode – the electrode in contact with the client's face during facial treatment.
- Indifferent electrode – the electrode held by the client to complete the electrical circuit.
- Anions – negatively charged ions, used in professional products which determine the polarity of the active electrode.
- Cations – positively charged ions.
- Anaphoresis – the flow of anions to the anode.
- Cataphoresis – the flow of cations to the cathode.

The galvanic treatment operates on the basic principle that like poles repel and opposite poles attract (see the figure below). The products selected are repelled into the skin by the active electrode which must be of the same polarity as the product.

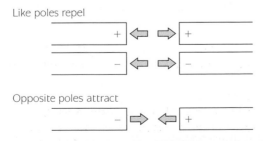

Like poles repel

Opposite poles attract

Like poles repel, opposites attract

information point

- The type of product, its viscosity, etc., will determine the most appropriate method of application.
- Each product will list the most active ingredients for a specific purpose, i.e. products for couperose skins tend to contain a vasoconstrictor such as horse chestnut.

information point

Galvanic machines contain:
- A rectifier – changes the alternating current to a direct current.
- A capacitor – smoothes out any irregularities in the direct current.
- A transformer – reduces the voltage of the alternating current given out at the mains supply.

GOOD PRACTICE

The polarity of the active electrode is determined by the product used, so care should be taken to read the manufacturer's instructions. The majority of products tend to be 'negative to positive' but the actual time for which the negative or positive poles are used will once again vary depending on the type of treatment being given and the manufacturer's instructions.

During desincrustation treatment a process called saponification takes place. This occurs due to the sodium within the skin reacting with water to make sodium hydroxide and hydrogen which is an alkali and causes emulsification and removal of excess sebum and grease.
- Some conductive electrodes are conductive on both sides. This is not recommended for safe body application. If these are to be used care must be taken to insulate the top of the pad before securing with elasticated straps.
- During a facial treatment the active cathode removes the body's sebum and in doing so lowers the skin's resistance to the current; it may therefore be necessary to reduce the intensity of the current during treatment.

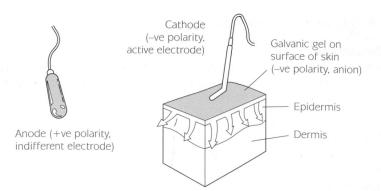

Anaphoresis

Electrodes

There is a variety of electrodes available for use on the face.

Types of active electrode:

- Metal rollers.
- Metal ball – single/double prong.
- Tweezer or flat head electrode.

Tweezers or flat head electrodes are usually covered with either dampened gauze, lint or cotton wool, according to the manufacturer's instructions or worked over a gauze masque soaked in active solution.

Types of indifferent electrodes:

- Metal bar. Some companies recommend that the electrode is covered in a dampened sponge pouch.
- Flat plate. These are generally supplied with a sponge pouch which is dampened before application.

Body electrodes

Galvanic pads come in pairs, having a positive and negative electrode, and should be supplied with sponge pouches which are designed to protect against galvanic burns. The sponges are dampened prior to use and the active side of the galvanic pad is placed face down. Several layers of a lint wadding can be used instead but care must be taken to ensure an even contact is made.

Note: It is important to check that the sponge or lint layers do not dry out during treatment.

CONTRAINDICATIONS

to galvanic treatment

- Loss of skin sensation.
- Recent scar tissue.
- Infectious skin diseases or disorders.
- Broken bones.
- Hypersensitive skins.
- Heart conditions.
- Pacemakers.
- Low blood pressure.
- Epilepsy.*
- Diabetes.*
- Migraine sufferers.
- Cuts and abrasions.
- Highly vascular conditions.
- Metal plates, pins, bridges or an excessive amount of fillings.
- Pregnancy.*

* Only to be carried out with medical approval.

GOOD PRACTICE

- Sponge pouches must be thoroughly washed after use with warm water and detergent then soaked in a suitable disinfectant and thoroughly rinsed.
- Sponges will deteriorate with wear and tear and must be replaced as needed.

Effects of galvanic treatment

Effects at the cathode

The cathode produces an alkali effect on the skin by bringing about a chemical reaction between sodium ions and the hydroxyl ions of water to produce sodium hydroxide which is an alkali, thus creating the following effects:

- Breaks down the acid mantle.
- Relaxes the pores.
- Increases the blood circulation – vasodilation occurs.
- Hyperaemia.
- Warmth in the tissues.
- Brings about saponification – the emulsifying and removal of sebum.
- Creates a softening and drying effect on the skin.
- Stimulates nerve endings.
- Moisture is temporarily drawn to the cathode.

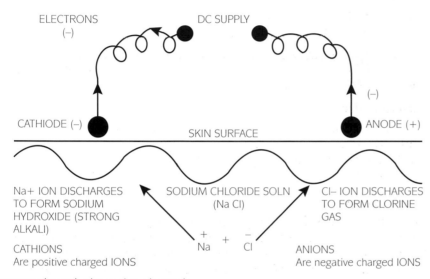

Flow of current through the active electrode

Effects at the anode

The anode produces an acidic effect on the skin by bringing about a chemical reaction between the chloride ions and hydrogen ions present in tap water to produce hydrochloric acid and oxygen, thus creating the following effects:

- Restores the acid mantle.
- Tightens the pores.
- Hardening of the skin.
- Creates warmth in the tissues.
- Reduces circulation.
- Soothing effect on the nerve endings, if used for a short time.

ACTIVITY

Research the variety of products available for use with galvanic equipment. Consider their size, cost, ingredients and usage.

Reasons for using galvanic treatment

- To deep cleanse the skin.
- To introduce active ingredients to benefit the client's skin condition.
- To assist in dispersing cellulite.

Preparation for galvanic treatment

1 Observe general safety precautions for using electrical equipment.

2 The machine is placed on a stable trolley.

3 The machine is checked and tested by the therapist to ensure it is working correctly.

4 The products required for treatment are selected and placed on the trolley.

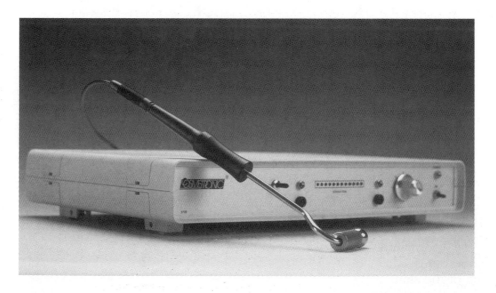

Galvanic unit and attachments

Galvanic treatment to the face and neck

1 The client is greeted at reception and escorted to the treatment area.

2 A consultation is carried out to check for contraindications and to explain the effects of the treatment. A skin sensitivity test is carried out on the area to be treated.

3 The client removes their jewellery.

4 The client is helped onto the couch and their clothing and hair protected.

5   The therapist ensures the client is warm and comfortable.

6   The skin is cleansed with suitable products and if using a cream-based product the therapist must ensure that there is no residue left on the skin which would act as a barrier to the current.

Note: A vapouriser can be used to soften the skin and lower the client's skin resistance. There is also a variety of conductive lotions available that may be used.

7   A suitable medium is selected and applied to the client's face and neck, e.g. desincrustation gel or active ampoule. It is usually recommended that ampoules are applied with a gauze masque rather than directly onto the skin.

Note: The type of product selected for facial work will influence the type of electrode used, e.g. metal roller and ball electrodes tend to be used with gels whereas the other electrodes tend to be used with ampoules.

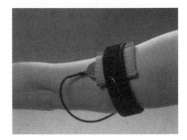

information point

Galvanic equipment tends to include the arm clip indifferent electrode.

Method

1   Ensure the mains lead is plugged into the mains supply and that all switches are off and all dials are at zero.

2   The therapist tests the machine in front of the client and explains its use.

3   The selected electrodes are wiped with disinfectant and prepared for use according to the manufacturer's instructions.

4   The therapist ensures the electrodes are correctly fitted and that the correct polarity for the product being used is selected.

5   Depending on the type of indifferent electrode being used, it is either given to the client to hold firmly or is placed under the client's shoulder or clipped to the client's arm.

6   The therapist places the selected active electrode in contact with the client's skin and moves it around using small movements whilst turning the mains control switch on and the intensity dial up according to the manufacturer's instructions. Do not begin treatment on the forehead or around the eyes.

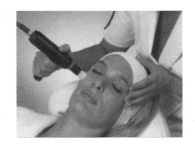

Note: The client is advised that they may get a metallic taste in the mouth if they have fillings whilst working around the mouth and nose area. Some clients feel a slight warmth in the tissues, others don't feel any reaction, but do not be tempted to increase the milliamp intensity beyond recommended levels as blood vessels can dilate and if there is insufficient product on the skin a galvanic (chemical) burn could result. Ensure that the machine is working correctly and any manufacturer's instructions for equipment/product are being followed.

7   The therapist moves the active electrode slowly over the client's face and neck in a methodical pattern. The treatment time will vary according to the type of treatment being given, the skin condition and the manufacturer's instructions, so it is essential that the therapist studies these carefully. Carlton Professional recommend the following for use with their products and equipment:

   Desincrustation – 15–20 minutes negative to positive.
   Iontophoresis – 5–7 minutes negative to positive.

The positive polarity is generally used for the final 2–3 minutes.

It is important that the therapist keeps the active electrode moving and in contact with the skin whilst turning the intensity dial to zero before removing the electrode from the skin to reverse the polarity.

8   At the end of the treatment the therapist ensures all dials are set to zero and switched off before removing the electrodes.

9 The selected medium is removed and further treatment, such as facial massage or direct high frequency, may be given or the skin is toned and moisturised.

10 The client is helped from the couch, the record card completed, appropriate home-care and further salon treatment advice is given, along with samples of the skin-care products used and the client's next appointment is confirmed.

11 The therapist tidies the treatment area and cleans the electrodes used by carefully wiping with hot water and disinfectant.

Galvanic treatment to the body

1 The client is greeted at reception and escorted to the treatment area.

2 A consultation is carried out to check for contraindications and to explain the effects of the treatment. A skin sensitivity test is carried out on the area to be treated.

3 The client removes their jewellery, showers and may have a mild heat treatment to relax the tissues prior to treatment and/or an additional salon treatment such as gyratory massage.

4 The client is helped onto the couch.

5 The therapist ensures the client is warm and comfortable.

6 The therapist ensures the skin is free of grease as this would act as a barrier to the current.

7 The therapist tests the machine in front of the client and checks all leads are providing a working circuit.

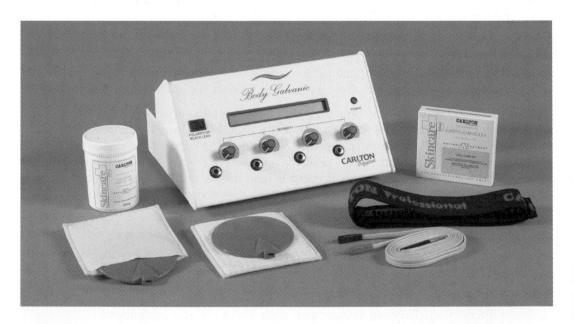

Super galvanic equipment

Method

1 Ensure the mains lead is plugged into the mains supply and that all switches are off and all dials are at zero.

2 Elasticated body straps are wrapped firmly around the area to be treated. The therapist applies the selected product, e.g. cellulite gel or ampoule, to the skin/sponge pouch and places the insulated electrodes according to manufacturer's instructions. (If the electrodes are conductive on both sides, ensure the top surface is insulated before fixing with elasticated strapping.)

In treatment for cellulite the stronger, active, cathode pads are placed on the main cellulite areas whilst the anode is generally placed parallel or opposite.

3   The therapist ensures the electrodes are correctly fitted and that the correct polarity for the product being used is selected.

4   The intensity dials are turned up individually until either the client feels a slight tingling sensation, or until the maximum output recommended is reached.

5   The treatment time may take up to approximately 20 minutes according to the client's tolerance. The polarity is generally reversed for the last 3–5 minutes of the treatment.

6   At the end of the treatment, or in between changing polarity, the therapist must turn the intensity dial to zero before switching off the machine and removing the insulated electrodes from the skin.

7   The selected medium is removed and further treatment such as NMES may be given. Care should be taken in any subsequent pad and product placement to avoid over-irritation or stimulation.

8   The client is helped from the couch, the record card completed, appropriate home-care and further salon treatment advice is given and the client's next appointment is confirmed.

Note: For treatment of cellulite it is recommended that the client has a minimum of 2–3 sessions per week with a total number of 12 treatments before a significant difference can be seen.

9   The therapist tidies the treatment area and cleans the electrodes used by carefully wiping with hot water and then disinfectant.

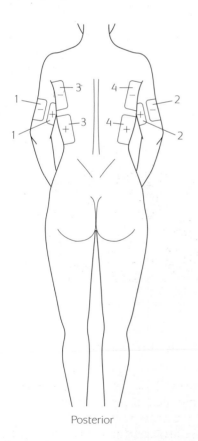

Posterior

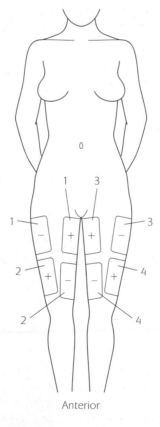

Anterior

Example of galvanic padding

- For treatment of cellulite, diet and exercise should be combined with body galvanic treatments.
- The client's cellulite condition can often appear worse before improvement is seen due to the redistribution of fatty fluids in the area.
- Body galvanic treatment helps to relax and loosen the adipose tissues and waste elements that bring about cellulite. It is not effective as a treatment on its own.

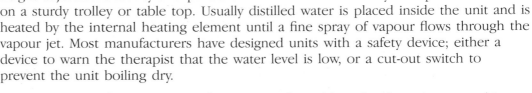

ACTIVITY

1 Identify three clients with differing skin conditions and design individual treatment programmes for them using electrical equipment. Carry out the treatments keeping a record of the products and equipment used, duration of each treatment, home-care and clients' views and evaluate the effectiveness of the programmes.
2 With a colleague, design and carry out a programme, including the use of electrical equipment, to assist with figure improvement. Keep a record of the treatments and home-care and evaluate the effectiveness of the programme.

Vapourisers

For years vapourisers have been used to prepare a client's skin for further treatment, such as prior to a cleansing face mask or galvanic treatments. The warmth of the vapour relaxes the tissues and softens the skin. It may also induce slight perspiration which has a cleansing action on the skin and the warmth will stimulate the sudoriferous glands thus assisting in the elimination of waste.

There are a variety of vapourisers available including mobile free-standing units with a height adjustment facility and portable machines that are easily transported and sit on a sturdy trolley or table top. Usually distilled water is placed inside the unit and is heated by the internal heating element until a fine spray of vapour flows through the vapour jet. Most manufacturers have designed units with a safety device; either a device to warn the therapist that the water level is low, or a cut-out switch to prevent the unit boiling dry.

Most vapourisers have an optional ozone switch enabling the therapist to combine vapour with ozone which has an anti-bacterial effect on the skin and is therefore

information point

Ozone is produced when the vapour passes over the high pressure mercury lamp which turns the available oxygen to ozone.

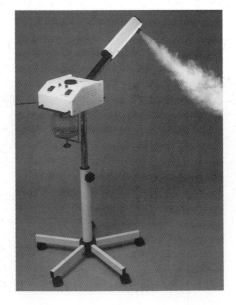

Vapouriser

particularly beneficial for congested skins or after extraction work has been carried out. Vapourisers are used for differing lengths of time and from different distances from the skin according to the desired effect and overall treatment programme.

CONTRAINDICATIONS

to using a vapouriser
- Highly vascular conditions.
- Sunburn.
- Acne rosacea.

information point

- Health and Safety legislation recommends that the maximum safety level for ozone released from vapouriser units should not exceed 0.1 p.p.m. (part per million) calculated as an 8-hour time-weighted average. If, for example, the quantity of ozone produced at a distance of 30 cm from the steamer head over an 8-hour period is 0.1 p.p.m., which, if divided by 8, gives a reading for continual use of the vapouriser for 1 hour of 0.0125 p.p.m., this would indicate that the steamer is operating well within the recommended safety level.
- A traditional vapouriser has a deliberate warmth to the vapour as well as a stimulating action. Another system known as a pulveriser (favoured in France) could be confused with a vapouriser, but in this instance the vapour jet is very fast and furious and designed to apply a cool, wet product to the skin.

GOOD PRACTICE

- To maintain vapourisers in good working order they will occasionally need to be de-scaled according to the manufacturer's instructions.
- Do not use if the vapouriser is spitting hot water: check that the kettle is not overfilled or that there is not a blockage in the jet outlet (refer to the maintenance manual).
- Some vapourisers are designed to enable the therapist to infuse essential oils to suit the individual client.

Brush cleansing

Brush cleansing machines are used to aid the desquamation of the skin and to aid cellular regeneration by stimulating the skin's blood circulation. They can be used to give a deep cleansing of the skin, to aid in the removal of peels or masks or to give a stimulating massage. The units are supplied with a variety of massage heads allowing the therapist to select the appropriate head according to the client's skin type and the desired effects of the treatment. The machines have a mains on/off switch and a variable speed control and some incorporate a directional control to enable the therapist at a turn of a dial to ensure the skin is being lifted rather than pulled down. If the machine is being used for cleansing or massage, suitable

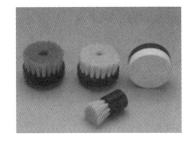

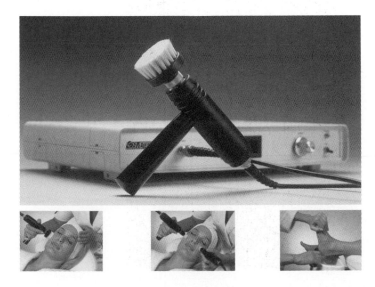

Brush peeling machine

water-based foaming products should be used to facilitate the action of the massage heads. The circular, rotating heads should be applied to the skin dampened and flat to the skin, i.e. making a right angle between skin and handle.

CONTRAINDICATIONS

to brush cleansing
- Skin diseases or disorders.
- Hypersensitive skin.
- Extremely loose skin tissue.
- Cuts or abrasions.
- Diabetes.*
- Highly vascular conditions.
- Any skin inflammation.
- Recent scar tissue.
- Sunburn

* Only to be carried out with medical approval.

information point

- Brushing can be used for lymph stimulation massage. The direction of the massage head should be 'lifting' the skin.
- Treatment time is on average 5–7 minutes.

KEY TERMS

You need to know what these words and phrases mean. Go back through the chapter to find out.

Brush cleansing

Care of electrical equipment

Galvanic

High frequency

Mechanical massagers

Micro-electrotherapy

Micro-dermabrasion

Neuro-muscular electrical stimulation (NMES)

Safety precautions

Skin sensitivity test

Vacuum suction massage

Vapourisers

SELF-CHECKS

1 State the different types of electrical treatments for:
   a the face
   b the body.

2 Describe the general effects of the following treatments:
   a neuro-muscular electrical stimulation
   b desincrustation
   c iontophoresis
   d vapourisers
   e brush cleansing.

3 List four contraindications for each of the following treatments:
   a neuro-muscular electrical stimulation
   b facial galvanic treatments
   c vapourisers
   d brush cleansing.

4 Describe the electrical currents used in the following treatments:
   a neuro-muscular electrical stimulation
   b galvanic.

5 Explain the following terms:
   a anode
   b cathode
   c anion
   d cation.

Chapter 6 Spa and specialised treatments

After working through this chapter you will be able to:

- identify the different types of spas
- name the different types of spa and specialised salon treatments
- describe the effects of spa treatments
- identify the different specialised treatments available.

Introduction

The profile of the spa industry has been raised globally by the tremendous investment made by the leisure and tourism sector. The hotel industry has seen a huge demand for luxury and short hotel breaks and few quality hotels now being built do not include spa facilities. Consumer awareness has also greatly increased via the extensive media coverage that has been afforded to health awareness and the acceptance of relaxation time without the 'guilt'. The growth of the spa market has mushroomed in the past 40 years. It has moved away from the strict traditionalist perspective to a wider market. Client expectations have been raised, excellent service and attention to detail, space, comfort and luxurious surroundings are expected.

There is a demand for high quality therapists who can treat guests as individuals and deliver unique, innovative and a comprehensive range of therapies.

Water is the heart of a spa experience. Water treatments are therapies as well as social activities. The benefits of water have been advocated by many ancient civilisations such as the Egyptians, Babylonians, Chinese and Persians. One of the cultures we associate with water is the Romans; they believed in *Salus per aquae* ('health through water'). Spa treatments are associated not just with indulgence but health maintenance, and incorporate holistic and spiritual elements. Spa areas and treatments are often designed around bathing traditions from earlier times such as Greek, Roman and Turkish to name but a few. Treatments are designed to stimulate the body senses – hearing, touch, smell – and usually have extended treatment times to balance the pace and pressure of modern life.

Types of spas

- **Destination spa**. These were commonly known as health farms but they no longer target the market of those wishing to slim but have moved with the times to the luxury, pamper, health living, de-stress market. Some destination spas are in magnificent locations with a wealth of services and they focus on improving the individual's lifestyle. Guests will stay at the facility where fitness, diet and the environment of the spa location will play an integral role in their general wellbeing. To view an international destination spa, visit www.chivasom.com.
- **Medical spa**. These centres or institutions tend to focus primarily on preventative care, diagnostic testing, healthcare programmes, complimentary therapies and medical services. On-site doctors and other related medical professionals are normally available.
- **Medispa**. In the USA these facilities link the day spa experience to other medical services such as cosmetic surgery and cosmetic dermatology, an extension to a doctors' surgery. Facilities that were only once available within a hospital setting can now be found in the tranquil calm setting of the spa environment.
- **Day spas**. These focus on wellbeing, relaxation, personal service, offering a comprehensive range of body and facial treatments, therapeutic massage and a range of water therapy-based experiences. They may offer nutritional advice, spa cuisine, weight management and fitness facilities. They are usually located in urban or city locations for people with a limited amount of time. To view an example of a UK day spa, visit www.elemis.com.
- **Hotel/Resort spas**. These spa facilities are an integral part of the hotel/resort. They form part of the services found within the hotel or leisure complex and the facilities enhance the guests' experience at the hotel and provide the business traveller with the opportunity for some peace within their busy schedule. The location and setting of these spas are an important aspect of the client experience in a resort spa.
- **Mineral spring spa**. These spas can overlap with medical spas in that the water is known for its restorative or curative properties, for example thermal springs. Town names are good indicators of places with natural springs. The focus is on relaxation as well as on health and wellbeing. They will have their own on-site source of thermal/spring or seawater. For an example of this type of spa, visit www.thermaebthspa.com.

Spa design

Key factors to consider are the location and style of the property, the company philosophy and its target market. The choice of colour and materials need to be carefully selected to enhance the experience rather than assault the senses. Some spas are themed, incorporating historical references such as Roman or Italian frescoes or Greek mythology. Influences of Asian cultures are popular not only in the design but also in the treatments, whether it is Indian, Indonesian or Japanese. Design has moved away from the basic and clinical to contemporary, minimalist and luxurious. In the treatment and wet areas, careful consideration needs to be given to wall and floor surfaces for hygiene and safety reasons and particular attention given to the effects that humidity can have on building materials.

As with all spa and specialised salon treatments, it is essential to research the companies' products and equipment, the effects, potential market and growth of the treatments. It is important to note that with these specialised salon treatments the therapist must undertake all necessary training from the manufacturer/agent concerned.

Water

Water can be used in a variety of states as liquid, in steam or as a solid. It is an excellent medium for conductive heating or cooling. No spa is complete without it.

Water testing

Clean water is critical in a spa pool. With higher temperatures and increased bathing loads, water testing and clean water maintenance is essential to ensure health and safety of clients and staff and to prevent the spread of waterborne infections such as Legionella and e-coli that can proliferate in all water systems of the spa. It is critical that staff operating the spa have detailed knowledge and understanding of water safety.

The water should be clear; any cloudiness indicates a problem, whether it is improper pH levels, an inefficient filter or that the water is too hard. Most spa installation companies will give guidance on staff training. Testing must be completed on a regular basis; frequency will depend on pool type and chemicals used. An average is a two-hourly check on such things as chemical levels of the disinfectant, ATP (adenosine triphosphate) and pH levels. The pH test is a critical test and must be maintained regardless of the types of disinfectants used.

Some spa operators use ozone as a powerful disinfection system, others use a dosing system of chemicals to prevent bacteria and fungal growth, such as chlorine and bromine. Chlorine is not only a disinfectant but it is an oxidiser in that it also burns up small particles of debris from the water. There will also be a non-chemical or mechanical filtration process to remove debris from the pool, such as strainers or sand filters. These will have to be replaced regularly. Daily cleaning of the surface of the pool as well as back washing and weekly cleaning of the drainage system must also be carried out.

> **GOOD PRACTICE**
>
> Never collect water for testing in glass and never allow any glass in the spa area. Glass in water becomes completely invisible!

Spa facilities

- **Tepidarium**: a Roman thermal bath. The tepidarium is a lukewarm room positioned between a cool room and hot room or bath, with a constant radiant heat of between 37 and 39 °C.
- **Laconium**: a dry heat room for resting and relaxing; it uses a radiant heat of 60–65 °C and 15–20% humidity. Cooler than a sauna, its aim is to aid the elimination and detoxification process of the body. Laconiums will usually contain heated ceramic couches and they are usually part of a sequence of treatment linked to other heat or water therapies. The client should shower before entering and after 15 minutes in the laconium the body will start to perspire; after 20 minutes the client can shower to help detoxification and refresh (using a Kneipp hose). It is important to rest for a 20-minute period after use or before returning to the laconium, and rehydrate with several glasses of water.
- **Caldarium/Aroma bath**: a mild steam room that is infused with aromatic herbs such as lavender, rose, jasmine, eucalyptus. It has high humidity and radiant heat of about 42–45 °C. Its purpose is to aid elimination and detoxification. The room will usually contain heated seating and a Kneipp hose for showering down. A client's stay in the caldarium is usually for 20 minutes. Client should shower before entering. Just like the laconium it is usually part of a sequence of treatments linked to other heat or water therapies. Shower at the end of the treatment. Then rest for 20 minutes after treatment and rehydrate and apply a good body lotion or link to a Cleopatra nourishing bath of oil, honey and milk or nourishing soft pack treatment on the dry float bed.
- **Sanarium**: similar to sauna but higher humidity levels and lower temperature.
- **Hamman**: Turkish or Middle Eastern communal bath house or steam room for sweat bathing. Hamman means 'spreader of warmth' in Arabic. The room has a radiant heat of 60–80 °C and high humidity. Clients should shower before and after use.
  The central element of Hamman is 'Hot stone', a polished granite table of stone on which therapists can perform a wet massage. After treatment clients should rest for 20 minutes and rehydrate and apply a good body lotion or link to a Cleopatra nourishing bath or nourishing soft pack treatment on the dry float bed.

to laconium/caldarium/hamman
- High or low blood pressure.
- Skin disease.
- Infections.
- Respiratory disorders, particularly severe asthma.
- Pregnancy.
- Raised body temperature or fever.
- Cardiovascular disease.
- Uncontrolled epilepsy.
- Diabetes.

GOOD PRACTICE

All heated rooms should contain an emergency button.

Hygiene and maintenance

- Encourage the client to clean seating after use with the Kneipp hose.
- Disinfect and clean all ceramic or wood walls and floors and surfaces daily.
- Check with manufacturers for suitable products.
- Ensure essence bottles are filled or elements and fibre optic lighting is working correctly.

Dry heat treatments

The general effects of heat treatments

information point

- Hyperaemia is the term given to describe the increase in the flow of blood brought about by vasodilation.
- The effects of heat treatments will vary according to the length, temperature and type of treatment given, for example electrically heated under- and over-blankets create a heated environment which can be a very gentle sudation, or that of a personal sauna cocoon.

- Increase body temperature.
- Metabolism is increased as heating of the body accelerates the natural chemical reactions that occur within the body, e.g. burning of energy, production of carbon dioxide. This in turn will increase the demand for oxygen and nutrients within the tissues, therefore increasing the amount of waste produced.
- Circulation is increased. As the temperature in the body is increased, the blood vessels dilate to allow the blood to flow more quickly to the surface thus reducing the body temperature. Other factors which trigger this process, known as vasodilation, are the stimulation of the sensory nerve endings and an increase in the body's metabolism.
- Blood pressure is lowered as the pulse rate increases, causing the superficial blood vessels to dilate, which automatically lowers the blood pressure due to the reduced resistance to the flow of blood through the blood vessels.
- The heart rate increases to meet the demands of the body on the circulatory system.
- Perspiration is induced to help cool the body. This aids removal of waste from the body and has a cleansing and softening effect on the skin.
- The activity of the sudoriferous and sebaceous glands is increased.
- Muscle fibres are relaxed in preparation for further salon treatment, e.g. massage.
- Sensory nerve endings are soothed by mild heat.
- A sense of general relaxation is achieved.

General safety precautions to be observed in the spa area

- Ensure all equipment is serviced regularly.
- Always follow manufacturers' instructions.
- Hygiene is of the utmost importance, so ensure all equipment is maintained and cleaned according to the manufacturer's recommendations.
- Floors in the spa area should be non-slip.
- Spillages should be cleared up immediately.

- Clean towels and gowns must be regularly replenished.
- Dirty laundry baskets should be emptied regularly.
- Soaps, shampoos and body lotions should be replenished.
- Clients must always be checked for contraindications.

Sauna

In Scandinavian countries, pine log cabins were built by the side of lakes to enable people to take a cool dip between sessions in the sauna. Today they are commonly found both indoors and outdoors. Saunas produce dry hot air and the pine logs absorb the condensation produced in the sauna.

A sauna resembles a wooden cabin. Saunas are usually made from pine logs or panels which are packed together with insulating material (fibreglass) to prevent heat loss and ensure the heated air remains dry. They contain pine shelving at different heights for resting on. Pine slats (duck boards) on the floor protect clients' feet from heated flooring which could burn them. A thermostatically controlled electric stove, on top of which is a tray of non-splintering stones (coals), is used to heat the sauna. Manufacturers should ensure that the heating capacity of the electric stoves have the correct power rating for the size of the sauna.

When installing saunas the contractors should check that there is sufficient space around the cabin to enable air to circulate. An air inlet is found at floor level and an outlet is found near the top of the cabin.

As the power rating for sauna stoves is much higher than for normal household electrical appliances, the sauna stove is fitted directly to the consumer's mains electrical supply. (They cannot be run from a plug socket!) A thermometer should be placed as near as possible to the roof of the sauna to accurately measure the temperature inside the sauna.

It is important to have some way for a client to measure time whilst in a sauna so either an egg timer or clock should be in the sauna or a clock on a wall outside which can be seen through the window of the sauna door.

Note: Remember to make sure timers are working correctly.

information point

- The stones used in a sauna are igneous dolerite rock, a type of rock that withstands rapid heating and cooling without splintering.
- Birchwood twigs used to be used in Scandinavian countries by sauna users for their suppleness to stimulate the blood circulation by tapping them on the skin.

information point

- If the air is too dry the body's natural perspiration evaporates quickly, which has a cooling effect on the skin, and signs of dehydration such as tiredness and dry throats can occur.
- If the humidity of the air is too high, perspiration produced to assist in the cooling of the body does not evaporate leaving people feeling hot and clammy.
- A hygrometer is used to measure humidity.

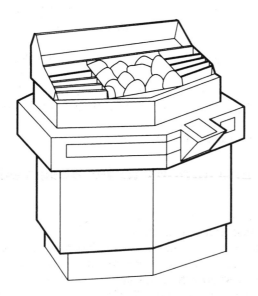

Sauna stove

Water can be ladled onto the coals of the sauna stove. This creates steam and increases the humidity in the sauna, which in turn reduces the rate of the evaporation of sweat from the client's skin making the sauna feel hotter. Hot air does not have the same heat capacity as hot water, therefore the temperature of a sauna does not feel as hot on the skin as water would. The temperature of a sauna can vary between 50 and 120 °C (the boiling point of water is 100 °C).

GOOD PRACTICE

- A comfortable sauna temperature for a new client unaccustomed to a sauna treatment is 60–80 °C.
- A comfortable sauna humidity is approximately 50–60%.
- As hot air rises, a thermometer should be placed near the top of the sauna.

Care of the sauna

- Hygiene is of utmost importance as although the air in the sauna is too hot for growth of micro-organisms, bacterial infection could be housed and grow in the wooden walls and furnishings of the sauna due to the warm, moist conditions.
- The sauna should be regularly disinfected by scrubbing the benches and floor with disinfectant products recommended by the manufacturer.
- Disposable client footwear can be used to reduce the risk of passing contagious foot conditions such as verrucas.
- At the end of the day, the sauna doors should be left open to allow for a change of air. This prevents stale odours from lingering.

CONTRAINDICATIONS

to a sauna
- Low and high blood pressure.
- Heat conditions.
- Thrombosis or phlebitis.
- Bronchitis.
- Asthma.
- Epilepsy.
- Dysfunction of the nervous system.
- Oedema.
- Recent scar tissue.
- Severe bruising.
- Diabetes.*
- Early stages of menstruation.
- Pregnancy.*
- Heavy colds/fever.
- Infectious skin diseases.
- Athlete's foot.
- Verrucas.
- Sunburn.
- Claustrophobia.
- After alcohol consumption.
- After a heavy meal.
* Only to be carried out with medical approval.

- The moisture content of the air is referred to as humidity. Relative humidity is the measurement of moisture content as a percentage of the maximum it can hold at that temperature. 100% is the maximum capacity of moisture content in air.
- 60–70% relative humidity is a comfortable humidity for working conditions.
- As the temperature of air increases, so does its capacity for holding moisture, e.g. if the temperature of a salon was 20 °C and the relative humidity measurement was 70%, then raising the room temperature to 100 °C would decrease the relative humidity to approximately 20%.
- The relative humidity in a sauna can be as low as 10%. This causes perspiration to evaporate very quickly, thus causing a cooling effect on the skin so that the sauna does not feel as hot as the actual temperature recorded in the sauna. Water loss is from the whole of the body and it should be remembered that if the temperature is high and the relative humidity is low then there is a danger of dehydration, breathing difficulties and scorching of the lungs.

Effects of a sauna

- Increases body temperature.
- Metabolism is increased.
- Blood pressure is lowered.
- Pulse rate increases.
- Circulation increases.
- Perspiration is induced which aids removal of waste from the body and has a cleansing and softening effect on the skin.
- The activity of the sudoriferous and sebaceous glands is increased.
- Muscle fibres are relaxed in preparation for further salon treatment, e.g. massage.
- A sense of wellbeing is achieved.

Preparation of the sauna

1 Observe general safety precautions.

2 The sauna stove is switched on to allow the temperature of the sauna to build up prior to use. A large sauna will take approximately 1 hour to heat up whereas a smaller sauna will take approximately 30 minutes.

3 The air vents should be open to allow the air to circulate.

4 A pine bucket filled with water is placed in the sauna with a ladle. Pine fragrance can be added to the water to produce a pleasant fresh smell when used on the coals.

5 Paper towels may be placed on the floor.

6 Showers are checked and appropriate products are made available for clients, e.g. shower gels and caps.

7 Towels are replenished.

8 Throughout the day the laundry basket is emptied and towels, etc. replenished.

Note: Different establishments will offer different services to clients and will outline these to therapists in their induction programme, e.g. towels may be placed in the sauna for clients to rest on, clean bath robes may be placed in the sauna area.

Sauna treatment

1 The client is greeted at reception and taken to a changing area.

2 A consultation is carried out to check for contraindications and to explain the effects of treatment.

Note: In spas a detailed consultation is undertaken on the guest's arrival by a member of their medical staff. The therapists would still explain the effects of the treatment to a new guest.

3 The client removes items such as contact lenses, spectacles and jewellery before showering to remove deodorants, body lotions, fragrances, etc.

4 The client is taken to the sauna and advised if it is their first treatment to spend approximately 5–8 minutes on a lower shelf, allowing them time to adjust to the temperature of the sauna. It must be stressed to the client that if at any time they feel light-headed they must come out of the sauna.

5 The therapist informs client of the time and asks them to take a cool shower or use the plunge pool for a short time to cool the body, stop perspiration and tighten the pores which have dilated due to the heat of the sauna and through perspiration. The temperature of the plunge pool/shower should be approximately 15–21 °C.

6 The client can return to the sauna for 10–20 minute periods in between taking cool showers or using the plunge pool for up to a total treatment time of approximately 30 minutes.

7 The client should relax after a sauna either in a rest area or by having a further treatment such as a massage, and drink plenty of fluids to prevent dehydration.

information point

Male clients tend to prefer a higher sauna temperature to females.

ACTIVITY

Research the different size saunas available, noting their client capacity, initial setting up and running costs. Evaluate which would prove to be the most cost-effective for a large salon, hotel and health spa.

Vibratory sauna

The vibratory sauna machine looks like an elongated steam cabinet as it allows a client to lie flat inside it. It is manufactured from moulded plastic with a vibrating couch which has a built-in head rest. Control panels on the outside allow the therapist to set the temperature, duration, vibration along with the stereo and fan control for cooling the sauna. There are control panels situated at a convenient location inside the chamber to enable the client to alter the temperature, music and to operate the fan. During treatment heat is introduced into the sauna whilst the couch vibrates gently, to relax the client's muscles and help reduce stress. The built-in stereo system allows the therapist to play therapeutic tapes and aromatic oils can be used to further enhance the client's relaxation.

REMEMBER

Skin can tolerate much higher air temperatures than water temperatures.

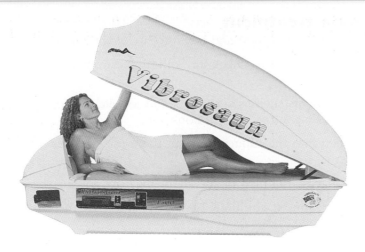

A vibratory sauna

to vibratory saunas
- Thrombosis or phlebitis.
- Circulatory conditions.
- Infectious skin conditions.
- Sunburn.
- Pregnancy.*
- Menstruation.
- Heavy colds or fevers.
- After alcohol or a heavy meal.
- Low and high blood pressure.
- Epilepsy.
- Diabetes.*
- Dysfunction of the nervous system.
- Oedema.
- Recent scar tissue.
- Athlete's foot.
- Verrucas.

* Only to be carried out with medical approval.

information point

The vibratory sauna is a personal treatment – the temperature can be set to suit the individual client.

Effects of a vibratory sauna
- Increases body temperature.
- Increases circulation.
- Heart rate increases.
- Pulse rate increases.
- Blood pressure is lowered.
- Increases metabolism.
- Induces perspiration.
- Relaxes muscle fibres.

Care of the vibratory sauna
The sauna should be cleaned between clients according to the manufacturer's instructions.

Preparation of the vibratory sauna
1. General safety precautions should be observed.
2. Fresh paper towels are placed over the vibratory couch.
3. The sauna should be switched on at the mains. (There is no need to preheat the chamber.)

Vibratory sauna treatment

1 The client is greeted at reception and taken to a changing area.

2 A consultation is carried out to check for contraindications and to explain the effects of the treatment.

3 The client removes items such as spectacles and jewellery prior to showering to remove deodorants, fragrances, body lotions, etc.

4 The client is helped into the cabinet and the therapist switches on the vibratory couch and music.

5 The room lights may be dimmed or the client may opt to wear eye shields.

6 At the end of the treatment, the body is cooled slightly by the fans which automatically cut in.

7 The client is helped out of the cabinet and may take a cool shower prior to resting. The drinking of suitable fluids is recommended.

GOOD PRACTICE

- Some clients are irritated by music so therapeutic tapes should only be used with the client's agreement.
- As clients are all individuals, it is important to establish what types of fragrance they like before selecting aromatic oils.

SELF-CHECKS

1 List the ten general effects of heat treatments.

2 Explain the term 'relative humidity' and its relevance to a sauna treatment.

3 Give four points that should be considered when taking care of the sauna.

4 Describe in detail the preparation, client consultation, treatment and after-care advice given for a sauna treatment.

5 State the effects of a vibratory sauna treatment. Also state four contraindications to treatment.

Bath therapy (balneotherapy)

Balneum is the Latin word for bath.

There are a variety of bath experiences that can be individual or shared. They can be for the whole body or for immersion of one part of the body such as feet. Baths are the simplest form of hydrotherapy. New inventions in baths now incorporate chromatherapy and light technology.

Temperatures can vary depending on the effects to be achieved, from cold baths 10–21 °C, neutral baths 32–36 °C through to hot 36–40 °C. The head is not normally immersed.

Hot baths

There is an increase in body temperature due to heat conduction from the hot water and this induces an artificial fever. It is because of this that hot baths should only be used for short periods from 2 to 15 minutes. Heat loss will only be via the parts of the body that are not immersed. Hot baths are used for muscles aches and spasms. Hot baths:

- relieve pain
- induce perspiration
- have a cleansing effect
- increase temperature.

Cold baths

This type of bath is only used for short periods from a few seconds to 3 minutes. Temperature ranges from 10–21 °C. It is used as a metabolic stimulant and general exhilarant. They should not be given to children, older people or people who are contraindicated. Cold baths:

- relieve pain
- have a stimulating effect
- have a diuretic effect
- reduce temperature.

Cold baths used to be very popular, particularly after a sauna. However, clients today tend to prefer cool baths. Perhaps tolerance of different temperatures has altered with the advances in technology which brought about such development as central heating and air conditioning.

Contrast baths

Contrast baths describe the situation where two different temperature baths are found next to each other so that the client can move from one to the other. It is designed to stimulate the peripheral circulation. The treatment time may vary slightly dependent on the temperature of the baths, but generally the client would spend between 1–5 minutes in the hot water (38–44 °C) and 15–60 seconds in the cold water (10–16 °C). The total treatment time would last approximately 10–30 minutes. They are not suitable for anyone with obstructive vascular conditions. An example of a contrast bath is a *Sitz bath*.

Sitz bath

The Sitz bath treatment from Germany is an example of a contrast bath; it uses the effects of contrast bathing. Two baths are used, one containing hot water, the other cold. For the first 5–10 minutes the client sits in the hot bath with their feet immersed in cold water. The client then changes and sits in the cold bath with their feet immersed in the hot water. The cold water causes the blood vessels to constrict, which in turn will force the blood supply to the area of the body immersed in hot water. The overall effect of this treatment is to flush the blood into the pelvic area bringing nourishment to it, then to flush it out taking away waste. This type of bath was recommended for any illness which affects the lower part of the body.

Scotch douche

The Scotch douche treatment utilises hot and cold water, which is alternatively run up and down the client's spine to stimulate the spinal nerves by sluicing blood in and out of the spinal area. This treatment is believed to help sufferers of migraines and other ailments such as aches and pains in the back.

Another treatment using the effects of differing temperatures is the Spanish mantle treatment. Cold, damp, cotton sheets are wrapped around the client and hot water bottles are placed around the body or a radiant heat lamp is used to induce perspiration. The client would be left to perspire for up to 3 hours. It was claimed that when the sheets were finally removed the elimination of toxins from the body changed the colouring of the sheets.

Artificial brine baths

These baths can be made by adding 5–8 lb of sodium chloride to 40 gallons of water. Treatment time is for 10–15 minutes. The temperature of the water should be 32–40 °C. The more salt added, the bigger the increase in the buoyancy of the water.

Cleopatra's bath

This provides exclusive individual bathing in an ergonomically designed bath, filled with water to shoulder level and set at a temperature of 36 °C. Ideally the client should exfoliate and shower before entering the bath The bath contains air jets to give a water massage. The client should be supported into the bath so they are correctly aligned with the jets. They should also be supported out of the bath. Always ensure the client rests for 20 minutes after bathing, and if not having a massage the client should apply a hydrating body lotion and rehydrate with several glasses of water. Products in the bath will vary depending on manufacturer's instructions and the aim of the treatment, but usually involve combined aromatic herbs or seaweed extracts.

Reflexology foot baths

These tiled foot baths provide a seated communal area within the spa and incorporate air jets for foot massage. The temperature is usually set between 33 and 38 °C.

Seaweed bath

Specially treated seaweed is placed in a bath of hot sea water. The heat releases iodine-rich oils into the water. It is used for sufferers of arthritis and rheumatism.

Roman bath (Celtic bath)

Named after ancient Roman practices, a Roman bath was a group of pools and heated or steam rooms varying in temperature. The modern version of a Roman bath includes a whirlpool with built in seating and air and water jets.

Precautions with specialised baths

- Assist clients in and out of the bath.
- If the client feels unwell, turn off any air jets. Bring the water temperature down if the bath is heated, by running cold water in while the bath is emptying. Once the temperature has dropped slightly, empty the bath and help the client out.
- Always ensure the client rests for 20 minutes.

CONTRAINDICATIONS

to specialised baths
- High or low blood pressure.
- Skin disease.
- Infections.
- Respiratory disorders, particularly severe asthma.
- Pregnancy (not in the first 4 months).
- Raised body temperature or fever.
- Cardiovascular disease.
- Uncontrolled epilepsy.
- Diabetes.

Hygiene and maintenance

- Clean the bath according to manufacturer's instructions. Normal cleaning agents can affect the pH level of water or induce foaming in the bath. Baths should be cleaned and disinfected after each use.
- Daily clean at the end of the working day so they are left clean and dry overnight.
- Do not use abrasives on the bath surface.
- The bath jets should be rinsed and cleaned every morning before first use by a client.

REMEMBER

Hydrotherapy means treatment with water in any physical state (i.e. liquid, water vapour, steam, ice).

Showers

There are a wide variety of showers now available in spas. Water is applied via a shower apparatus – it can be directional, vary in pressure and temperature, and deliver varying quantities of water to all the body or various parts of the body.

Scotch hose/jet blitz

The aim is to improve general circulation and re-energise the client. With the client standing, they receive a powerful water massage delivered by a therapist with a high-pressure hose (it can have interchangeable head attachments) of alternating hot (38–40 °C) and cold water (13–22 °C) or sea water to stimulate the circulation. The therapist is positioned approximately 3 metres away. The duration will vary depending on the client response.

Vichy shower (affusion)

The Vichy shower originated from the thermal spa town in France. It is a horizontal shower bar containing 5–7 shower heads. Clients lie face down on a wet table (place face guard to protect face) whilst above them is a multi-jet shower that sprays them with water of varying temperatures from 37–40 °C. The temperature of the water is controlled by a thermostat. The pressure is variable from a light rain sensation to a needle shower, similar to percussive massage. A Vichy shower is very energising and it stimulates the circulation. It can be combined with exfoliation, removal of wrap products or mud and be part of a lymphatic massage sequence.

Affusion

With affusion, water is poured from a pail or a hose or is thrown or falls on a client seated or standing. It is the forerunner of the shower and water temperatures are usually 13–22 °C. Affusions are used in Kneipp hydrotherapy procedures. Vichy showers are also known as rain showers or affusion showers.

Monsoon shower

This is a hot or cold invigorating shower that delivers approximately 50 or more litres of water a minute.

CONTRAINDICATIONS

to various showers
- Pregnancy.
- Skin disease.
- High or low blood pressure.
- Uncontrolled epilepsy.
- Fever or raised body temperature.
- Infections.
- The colon area.
- Severe varicose veins.
- Cardiovascular disease.
- Respiratory disease: severe asthma.
- Menstruation and coil – avoid abdomen.

SELF-CHECKS

1 List the types of baths.
2 What care should be taken of the different types of baths?
3 List the different types of showers.
4 State five contraindications to showers.

Rasul

This is an Arabian/ancient Egyptian cleansing ceremony that takes place in a specially designed ceramic steam chamber that infuses the air with aromatic herbs. The ceremony uses four different types of bolus medicinal earth – *terra sigillata* – which can be self-applied to different areas of the body. The Rasul chamber is warm with low humidity, which causes the mud to dry. Then after 20 minutes steam is released to help liquefy the mud on the skin helping absorption and the person can then massage the mud against the skin to aid exfoliation. The minerals in the mud are slowly absorbed as the heat increases and the person perspires. After a further 20 minutes, a tropical rain shower is automatically released from the ceiling of the Rasul to wash away the mud. After treatment clients can visit a tepidarium and relax for 20 minutes. Encourage the client to drink several glasses of water to rehydrate and apply a good body lotion or link to a Cleopatra nourishing bath of oil, honey and milk or nourishing soft pack treatment on the dry float bed.

Serial chamber

This provides a gentle steam environment with a radiant heat of 35–40 °C, combined with peloid treatments. Lighting and sound therapy can also enhance the serial chamber. The treatment consists of two stages. The application of a body pack such as mud, salt or chalk applied all over the body with hands or a brush; then on entering the chamber the temperature will climb to 45 °C for 15 minutes. The pack is then allowed to dry and is massaged against the skin in the warm chamber. The second stage is a warm shower or individual body jets, which removes all the pack from the body. After treatment clients can visit a tepidarium and relax for 20 minutes. Encourage the client to drink several glasses of water to rehydrate and apply a good body lotion or link to a Cleopatra nourishing bath of oil, honey and milk or nourishing soft pack treatment on the dry float bed.

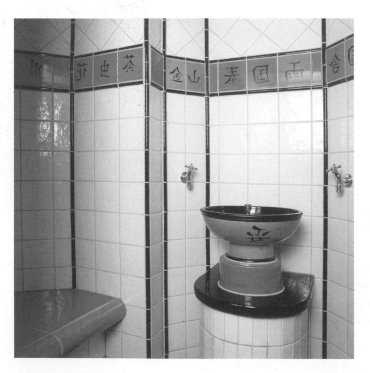
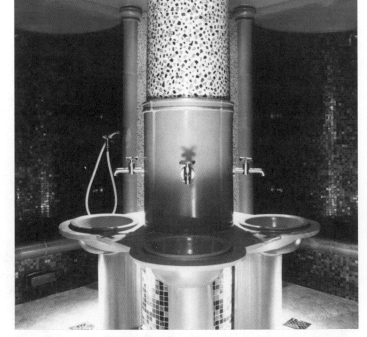

Serial chambers

to Rasul/Serial chamber
- High or low blood pressure.
- Skin disease.
- Infections.
- Respiratory disorders, particularly severe asthma.
- Pregnancy.
- Raised body temperature or fever.
- Cardiovascular disease.
- Uncontrolled epilepsy.

Hygiene and maintenance
- Encourage the client to clean seating after use with Kneipp hose.
- Daily disinfecting and cleaning of all ceramic or wood walls and floors and surfaces. Check with manufacturers for suitable products.
- Ensure essence bottles are filled or elements and fibre optic lighting is working correctly.

REMEMBER
All heated rooms should contain an emergency button.

Steam treatments

Steam treatments were first used by the Turks and Romans and are sometimes referred to as Turkish baths. The original Turkish and Roman baths were found in large buildings which contained steam baths of various temperatures, where people met socially for a relaxing bath.

Today there are a variety of steam treatments available.

Steam cabinets

Steam cabinets are designed for individual treatment enabling clients to sit in the cabinet with their heads outside so that they can breathe in the normal air of the room.

A modern steam cabinet can be constructed from either metal or moulded fibreglass. The fibreglass model is more expensive but is easier to clean, and as fewer towels are needed to protect the client from the heat of the metal they tend to be more popular.

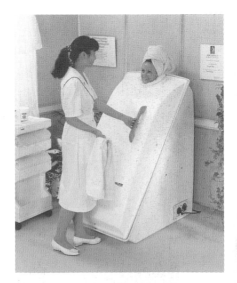

Steam cabinet

Steam cabinets have an opening for the client's head and a hinged door for easy access to and from the cabinet, making them more suitable than saunas for clients who have a tendency to suffer from claustrophobia. Inside there is an adjustable seat which is raised or lowered according to the client's height. Beneath the seat at floor level is a water tank, made from cast iron or aluminium, which is heated by an electrical element. The size of the water tank varies and should be considered when purchasing a steam cabinet. The larger the capacity of the tank the longer it can be used before the therapist needs to refill it. Therefore in a spa where the steam cabinets receive more use, a cabinet with a large water tank would be more beneficial.

To operate the steam cabinet the therapist will find a:

- Mains switch on the wall. The cabinet must be fitted directly to the mains electrical supply due to the power rating of the heating element.
- Timer switch to set the time for prior heating of the cabinet and the actual treatment time.
- Temperature gauge to set the cabinet to the appropriate temperature.
- The timer and the temperature gauge are generally found adjacent to each other on the outside of the cabinet often at floor level near the heating element.

Steam cabinets produce wet heat as the thermostatically controlled water tank heats the water until it boils, producing wet steam which mixes with the air inside the cabinet or room creating water vapour (at a lower temperature than the 100 °C required to boil water) at a temperature tolerable to the skin. The highest temperature advised for use in a steam treatment for the body is 45 °C.

The relative humidity of the air inside the steam cabinet or bath is generally around 92–97%. As the air is virtually saturated, the sweat produced by the sudoriferous glands, due to the heating of the body by the water vapour, is unable to evaporate and cool the body and therefore it trickles off the body.

Steam rooms

Steam rooms accommodate a number of clients who may take a treatment at the same time.

The length of time for a steam room to heat up ready for use will depend upon its size. Some are designed for individual use whilst others can accommodate up to eight people. Individual steam 'tubes' provide a mini steam room environment, which takes up a small amount of space and is easily affordable for salons.

Advantages of using a steam cabinet

For the client:

- Steam cabinets are a more private treatment than the communal steam room.
- The temperature can be adjusted to suit the individual client.
- Clients are able to keep their head out and keep their hair dry.
- It is far more suitable for claustrophobic clients as their head is out of the steam.
- The client is able to breathe in the air in the room rather than steam.

For the salon:

- The running costs are much lower than with a steam room as the heating element in a steam cabinet uses far less power.
- The initial financial outlay is much lower.
- The space required to accommodate the cabinet in the salon is much smaller.

Care of steam cabinets and rooms

- Hygiene is extremely important as moist heat provides an ideal breeding environment for micro-organisms.
- The steam baths and rooms must be cleaned down with suitable disinfectants recommended by the manufacturers before and after treatment.
- The doors of the steam bath and room should be left open at the end of the day to allow for an interchange of fresh air, preventing stale odours.
- Disposable footwear can be used to prevent the risk of cross-infection of contagious foot conditions.

to steam treatments for the body
- Thrombosis or phlebitis.
- Asthma and other respiratory conditions.
- Low or high blood pressure.
- Heart conditions.
- Epilepsy.
- Diabetes.*
- Athlete's foot.
- Verrucas.
- Infectious skin diseases.
- Sunburn.
- Pregnancy.*
- Menstruation.
- Clients on restricted diets who may have a tendency to become light-headed.
- Heavy colds/fevers.
- After a heavy meal or alcohol.
- Claustrophobia.**
- Dysfunction of the nervous system.
- Severe bruising.
- Recent scar tissue.

* Only to be carried out with medical approval.
** Some clients find the steam cabinet less claustrophobic.

> **information point**
>
> If given approval by a medical practitioner, clients with skin conditions such as psoriasis and eczema may receive wet heat treatments which may help these conditions.

Effects of a steam treatment for the body
- Body temperature rises.
- Metabolism is increased.
- Circulation is increased.
- Heart rate increases.
- Pulse rate increases.
- Blood pressure is lowered.
- Perspiration is induced.
- Cleansing and softening of the skin takes place.
- Superficial muscles are relaxed.

Preparation of the steam cabinet

1 Observe general safety precautions.

2 The cabinet is cleaned with sterilising liquid.

3 The metal heating trough is filled with water.

4 A towel is placed over seat to protect the client and if using a metal bath, towels must be placed inside to protect the client. Place a towel over the opening in the bath to prevent heat loss.

5 The water tank guard must be in place to protect the client from burning themselves.

6 Turn on the mains switch and set the temperature gauge to maximum to heat the bath. Set the timer to allow sufficient time for the bath to heat. (This will vary depending on the capacity of the water tank. Note the manufacturer's recommendations for heating time. A general guide for the time taken for a small tank to heat is approximately 15 minutes.)

7 Once heated, adjust the temperature gauge to 50–55 °C and check the timer switch does not click off allowing the temperature to fall.

Steam cabinet treatment

1 Greet the client at reception and take them to the changing facilities.

2 A consultation is carried out to check for contraindications and to explain the treatment and its effects.

3 The client removes items such as jewellery, spectacles and contact lenses and showers to remove deodorants, fragrances, body lotions, etc.

4 The client is helped into the bath. A fresh towel is placed around the client's neck for protection and to prevent heat loss.

5 The timer is set to the appropriate time, generally 15–20 minutes.

6 The therapist should reassure the client throughout the treatment and be at hand should they need them.

7 At the end of the treatment, help the client from the bath and direct them into a cool shower.

8 The use of an exfoliating product is recommended to speed up cellular regeneration and general skin texture.

9 The client should relax after the steam treatment and drink plenty of liquids.

information point

Steam cabinets can be purchased with aromatherapy atomising systems to enable the therapist to infuse the cabinet with selected essential oils to suit the individual client.

GOOD PRACTICE

It is important to look directly at the client's face and not at the client's body when helping them in and out of baths and showers. Imagine how you would feel if a fully clothed person stared at your naked body!

Steam capsules

These are ergonomically designed steam units where the client reclines in a single capsule. They can incorporate a range of treatments such as aromatics, steam, infra-red, rain showers and colour therapy. They can be utilised with mud or seaweed wraps.

ACTIVITY

With a colleague, design and carry out a survey to establish the percentage of people in your local area who have undertaken a heat treatment in the last 12 months. Note the type of treatment, the age ranges, gender and reasons for treatment.

Mud treatments (pelotherapy)

Mud treatments are not new and have been used since 400 BC. Hippocrates used medicinal mud for healing wounds and cold treatments. *Peloid* comes from the Greek work *Pelos* for mud. Peloids vary in composition and there are four main varieties:

- peat
- moor
- earth moor
- muds.

Peat is composed of organic matter found at above ground water level. Moors contain vegetable and inorganic components and usually contain a lot of lime. Muds are mainly inorganic (disintegrated rock) with only a small amount of organic debris.

Peloids have different physical properties from being able to retain water, thermal conductivity, convection and radiation.

- Terra sigillata: a medicinal mud produced on the island of Lemnos Greece. It became as valuable as gold.
- Moor: Mud rich Neydharting Moor is in Upper Austria and dates back to the Ice Age. Moor mud is nutrient-rich as a result of the decomposition of over 1000 plants and herbs. It was first discovered by the Celts in 800 BC. In 1945 an Austrian biochemist, Professor Otto Stober, pioneered the field of moor therapy. After research the moor mud is now available on the national medical schemes of Austria, Germany, France, Italy and Switzerland due to its healing properties and as a natural remedy for arthritis and rheumatism.
- Fango: the Italian word for mud. Fango therapy includes treatments that use a highly mineralised nutrient rich mud used for cleansing and revitalising the skin.
- Parafango battagilia: developed in 1952 by Professor Hesse in Germany. It is a mixture of fango mud and paraffin wax. The warm paste can be moulded to the body for the treatment of sports injuries and rheumatism.
- Dead sea black mineral mud: this is particularly good for skin diseases such as eczema and psoriasis.
- Hungarian wellness mud: this mud comes from Kolop, south-east of Budapest. It is used in medicinal spas in Hungary.

Herbal rituals

Indonesian rituals acknowledge beauty from within and the importance of inner health. The most famous of these are:

- Mandi Lulur: a traditional ritual from the royal palaces of Java, Indonesia, also known as Javanese Lulur. It is a skin sweetening, lightening and softening treatment that was originally a royal bridal treatment to prepare women for their wedding day and night. Historically, for 40 days prior to the marriage the lulur would be used on the skin; now it is usually for a week prior to the wedding. Lulur recipes vary according to royal family traditions. Most lulur bases would be made of various flowers, herbs and spices such as rice, sandalwood, ginger, cumin and turmeric. The paste is applied to the body and allowed to dry, then buffed and rinsed off with yoghurt. Usually applied after massage and before soaking in a rose petal and jasmine bath.
- Boreh: an Indonesian tradition remedy used by rice farmers at the end of a working day. Boreh is made by hand using a variety of ingredients depending on botanical availability and family recipes but it usually contains crushed ginger root, cloves, turmeric and nutmeg. It is recognised as traditional medicine believed to help warm the body and relieve aching joints and sore muscles. A warm paste is applied to the body and allowed to dry traditionally overnight, then rinsed off and massage performed.

Thalassotherapy

The word originates from the Greek *Thalassa* meaning sea.

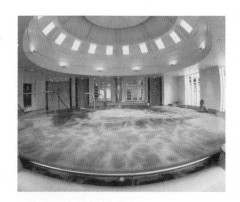

In 400 BC Euripides wrote 'The sea heals man's illness'. In 1791 Dr John Lafthn opened the first marine hospital in Margate. Then in 1822 the first marine therapy centre opened in Dieppe in France and in 1899 Dr Louis Bagot founded the first thalassotherapy centre at Roscoff. Purified seawater is almost identical to blood plasma and contains all 92 trace elements essential for life. Seaweed treatments were also popular at the turn of the twentieth century in Ireland in County Clare, Galway and Cork. The basic principle of thalassotherapy is that through treatment, immersion or exposure to sea air, sea water and marine extracts, minerals will be absorbed into the body system and have restorative effect that can help remineralise and detoxify the body.

Thalassotherapy

Thalassotherapy is a salt water hydrojet massage used to ease aches and pains, and to trim and tone tissues. It is renowned for its healing properties. The treatment will also restore balance and energy to the body.

Thalassotherapy consists of a large pool which can hold up to 15 people at a time and consists of different areas with pressure jets situated underneath. The treatment takes 30 minutes during which time a person progresses around the pool to the different areas. The treatment can also be combined with an algae wrap.

The pool contains 1 ton of salt which consists of three main elements:

- magnesium, a natural sedative to make the client feel relaxed and sleepy
- zinc, which has healing properties and is especially good for sufferers of eczema and psoriasis
- sodium, which has a firming and toning effect, particularly when used in conjunction with the side jets in the pool.

Main benefits of thalassotherapy treatment

- Relieves stress.
- Regulates blood pressure.
- Purifies the body of toxins.
- Regulates hormonal activities.
- Strengthens the cardiovascular system.
- Increases body metabolism.
- Cleanses the sinuses and respiratory passages.
- Improves the quality of skin and hair.

Marine/Algotherapy

This is the use of seaweed or seaweed extracts and algae-based treatments. Seaweed/algae extracts can be incorporated into wraps or baths and body products. There are over 25,000 varieties of seaweed recorded and many more thousands waiting to be discovered. Seaweed has been used for many years as a detoxification treatment. Kelp contained in seaweed is known for its ability to increase metabolism and aid elimination through the lymphatic system. Seaweeds are high in trace elements, minerals and amino acids. Enzymes in seaweed are called algaenic acids; they work on the lymphatic system by engulfing waste and toxins. When seaweed extracts are added to water treatments their trace elements are absorbed into the body through osmosis, as in a seaweed wrap or bath.

Seaweed is grouped by its colour.

- Blue: *Cyanophyta* – contains organic iodines which aids in detoxification
- Green: *Chlorophyta* – high in vitamin content such as B12
- Red: *Rhodophyta*
- Brown: *Phaeophyta*.

The algae most used in health and beauty are *Fucus*, *Ascophyllum* and *Laminaria* varieties. They are rich in iodine and have antibacterial properties.

SELF-CHECKS

1 Name the different types of muds and their effects.
2 List the different types of steam treatments.
3 Name and describe two rituals.
4 What is thalassotherapy?

Body wraps

Body wraps have been used in the professional beauty market for a number of years in varying forms. Most are marketed as a 'slimming treatment' as body tissues are compressed and slight fluid loss will result in inch loss together with a slight weight decrease. Body wraps offer other benefits such as cleansing the skin, tightening loose tissue, detoxifying the body, revitalising and helping improve cellulite and stretch marks.

Body wraps normally consist of three principles:

- Specialised products that contain active ingredients designed to be absorbed by the skin and aid in the elimination process. Examples of key ingredients most commonly used are seaweed, used for its diuretic effect; mineral extracts, used to nourish the skin; and oceanic clay, which acts as a poultice to draw toxins from the body.
- A wrapping medium – these can be almost like elastic bandages or even be some form of plastic or rubber sheeting.
- Thermal activity. This can be in the form of a heat treatment – infrared lamps or a thermal blanket – and is designed to keep the client warm as the wrapping medium and products cool. Some manufacturers suggest exercises to keep warm and to help with toning the body at the same time.

Most body wrap treatments are designed to be taken in courses attended regularly together with home-care products and diet and exercise advice.

Example of a body wrap treatment

1 A detailed consultation is carried out with the client checking for any contraindications, and the client is weighed and measured.

2 Specific measurements are marked to show the client exactly where the tape measure was placed.

3 The wrapping medium is prepared, in particular bandages are normally soaked in a special 'clay' solution. (This should be done before the client arrives.)

4 The client is then wrapped in the bandages/wrapping medium and most manufacturers suggest that the bandages are applied upwards in line with venous return. Particular attention should be observed to wrapping the back so as to offer lumbar support.

5 Extra amounts of the product are sometimes added for specific areas.

6 Once all the bandages/wrapping medium are in place, check with the client that they feel comfortable.

7 A thermal device is used to keep the client warm while the bandages cool. During treatment time it also induces relaxation. Some manufacturers recommend gentle exercise or the use of a toning table. (In this case the client will normally wear some form of protective tracksuit.)

8 After approximately 1 hour the bandages/wrapping medium are removed and the client is remeasured. Whereas some manufacturers recommend taking a shower to remove traces of product left on the skin, some products will have been completely absorbed and a shower is not necessary.

9 Finally, recommend home-care and retail products necessary for the maintenance of the treatment and confirm the next treatment.

Envelopment treatments/wraps

Prior to most wraps the client will first exfoliate using dry body brushing or a *dulse scrub* (seaweed) or salt scrub first, then shower.

Salt glow, also known as body glow or Turkish scrub, is exfoliation with coarse salt, essential oils and water, followed by a shower and application of massage or body lotion. However, it will depend on the product company or effects to be achieved. Some wraps do not require pre- or post-showering and some are used in conjunction with dry floatation.

Materials used for wraps

Clients can be wrapped in a variety of materials depending on the effects to be achieved. The wrap can be pre-soaked in cool or hot infusions of herbs or essential oils. The wrap may have a coating of fango on it before applying to the client. Types of materials used for wrapping are linen sheets, thermic film, soft foil, elasticised or plastic bandages, sand and towels. Compression wraps are used for cellulite and as part of a slimming package.

Products used with wraps

- Muds: which are used to help to remineralise the body.
- Algae/seaweeds: to help to detoxify the body.
- Flowers: rose petal and jasmine.
- Baltic chalk: chalk is used from the Baltic island of Ruegen and has a detoxification affect.
- Wine and clay mixed together: exfoliation and vineotherapy combined. The wine helps to combat free radicals responsible for ageing. It also uses grape extracts from the seed and wine yeast.
- Aloe vera: for moisturising and conditioning the skin.
- Essential oils are used for their warming, cooling or elimination effects with wraps. Cooling would be camphor or menthol. Warming would be cinnamon or eucalyptus or clove.
- Hay bath: the client lies on a bed of hay whilst the top of the body is covered with a thick layer of wet hay flowers and wrapped and covered with a heat blanket or used in conjunction with dry float. The main ingredient in the hay is cumarin. The process purifies and detoxifies.

Example of a hot herbal linen wrap from Dermalogica

This is used for muscle aches or detoxification. Unbleached linen is steeped in hot herbal 'tea' inside a special moist heating unit. The massage couch is prepared with a metallic spa sheet with a thick wool insulation blanket underneath. The hot sheets are then taken out of the water, wrung out and quickly laid flat on the massage table. The client lies on the sheet and it is wrapped around them. The smell of the warm herbs will provide an inhalation treatment. A cool compress is placed on the forehead or thyroid area. Treatment time is usually 30 minutes and scalp massage can be included whilst the client is wrapped. (Dermal Institute)

Floatation treatments

There are two types of floatation treatment – wet floatation and dry floatation.

Wet floatation tank

These are made from moulded fibreglass and can vary in size. They are generally rectangular, shaped like a small room, with a door opening outwards on the side of the tank. Inside the interior colour is usually blue and there is approximately 30 cm (12 inches) of warm, saturated salt water heated to body temperature on the floor surface, which will allow everyone to float. A small interior light illuminates the

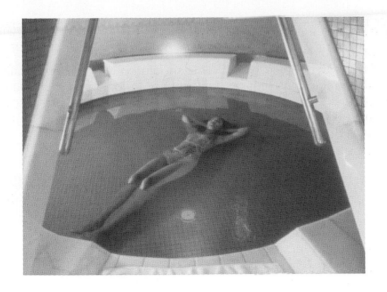

Wet floatation

tank enabling the client time to climb in and settle before switching it off. The switch control is in easy reach on the side wall.

The tanks are often found in spas and leisure centres and are situated in a separate room with access to a shower. Clients are advised to shower to remove any body creams, etc., and to apply petroleum jelly to any cuts preventing the brine (salt water) from entering any abrasions and causing a stinging sensation. It is suggested that no clothing is worn in the tank. Ear plugs are provided and often a neck cushion, which can be very reassuring to the weak or non-swimmer who believes they cannot float. A small step at the side of the tank allows the client to climb easily into the illuminated tank and a pull bar allows easy closure of the door. The client can take their time to adjust to the warm, slightly restrictive environment before switching off the interior light. There is usually an intercom system which enables the therapist to check the client is comfortable, play therapeutic music and reassure the apprehensive client that someone is at hand should they need them.

The tanks generally have a small, round ventilation hole which also allows the client to be phased into total darkness by first switching off the interior light and using a delay switch to turn the lighting off in the outer room (light can still enter the tank from the outer room through the door frame and the ventilation hole). This is extremely beneficial for apprehensive clients. The client lies on their back, the neck supported if they wish by a neck cushion, allowing the brine water to support their body thus relaxing all superficial muscles and releasing tension in the body. If the client wishes, therapeutic background music is played and after the client has had sufficient time to drift off, the music quietly ends allowing a peaceful and tranquil period before the music is quietly reintroduced, slowly bringing the treatment to an end.

Afterwards the client needs to shower to remove the brine from their skin and hair using professional products that could also be sold to them by the therapist. Spas book an hour treatment. Out of this the client would spend 40–45 minutes in the floatation tank. After a beneficial treatment the exhilarating, uplifting experience of 'walking on air' brought about by the total relaxation of mind and body can make this an almost addictive treatment.

Care of the floatation tank

- The tank must be free of debris such as oils, scum, loose hairs, etc.
- The inside of the tank, above the water line, must be cleaned a minimum of once a week or as necessary.

- The water in the tank must be filtered between uses and the temperature checked.
- The level of the water has to be checked between clients.
- The pH of the water should be 7.6. This should be checked on a daily basis.
- The level of bromine must not be higher than 2 p.p.m. and must be checked at least once a week.
- The tank must be tested either by an independent laboratory or by the Environmental Health Department.

CONTRAINDICATIONS

to wet floatation
- Claustrophobia.
- Highly nervous clients.
- Severe cuts/abrasions.
- Recent scar tissue.
- Infectious skin diseases.
- Severe eczema/psoriasis.
- Plantar wart (verruca).
- Tinea pedis (athlete's foot).
- After alcohol consumption.
- Heart conditions.*
- Epilepsy.*
- After a heavy meal.

* Only to be carried out with medical approval.

Effects of a wet floatation treatment
- Warms the body tissues aiding relaxation.
- Relaxes muscles through the buoyancy of the water.
- Eases aches and pains.
- A general feeling of wellbeing is achieved.

Preparation of the wet floatation tank

1 Observe general safety precautions.

2 Check the tank and shower areas are clean.

3 Ensure the level and temperature of the water are correct.

Wet floatation treatment

1 Greet the client at reception and take them to the changing facilities.

2 A consultation is carried out to check for contraindications and to explain the effects of the treatment.

3 The client removes items such as jewellery, spectacles and contact lenses, and may shower.

4 The client protects any minor skin abrasions with petroleum jelly and inserts ear plugs.

5 The client enters floatation tank, closes the door and in their own time switches off the interior light.

6 If the client wishes, the therapist can play piped music during the floatation time.

7 At the end of the treatment the therapist would advise the client to shower to remove the salt from skin and hair.

8 The client should rest in a relaxation room and drink fluids as required.

Dry floatation tank

Dry floatation tanks were originally developed in Austria and have been extremely popular there for many years. They are made of a stainless steel frame containing a tank of water which can be thermostatically controlled, into which a duck board is set which can be lowered to suspend the client in water with no pressure points.

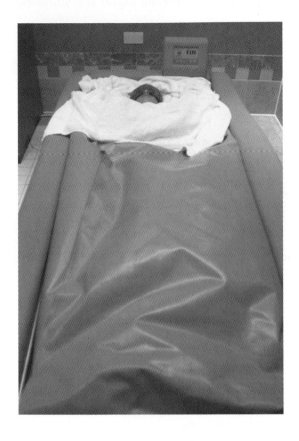

Dry floatation

The water tank is sealed by a flexible membrane, the tank is clad in upholstered panels which make it appear rectangular in shape, similar to a bath tub. The client lies on the raised bench which is protected by paper roll. Protective paper sheeting may be placed over the client. The therapist pushes a control button to lower the board thus suspending the client's body weight, protected by vinyl, in warm water, the temperature of which remains constant.

The dry tanks are mainly found in health spas in treatment rooms with easy access to a shower. The dry floatation method can be used in a number of treatments some of which involve coating the body in various ingredients for different effects, e.g. mud can be used for its exfoliating and softening effects, a mixture of hay softened with its own juices and eucalyptus essential oil is said to be beneficial for sluggish lymph circulation and respiratory conditions, and milk and essential oils can be used for softening the skin and has therapeutic benefits. The floatation can be given on its own for the therapeutic benefit of releasing tension in the body and for relaxation.

Once the client is suspended in the dry floatation tank the therapist switches on gentle therapeutic music, dims the lights and places an alert button within easy reach of the client. The client is then left to relax for approximately 40 minutes.

The therapist will check on the client's comfort after 5–8 minutes, remaining close at hand outside the door throughout the duration of the treatment and returning to the room at the end. The control button is pressed, which slowly raises the board under the client's back and brings them back to the top of the tank, the vinyl cover is removed and the client is helped off. If a specific treatment such as mud has been used the therapist will have to place protective covering on the floor between the tank and the shower.

Care of the dry floatation tank

The tank should be cleaned with a sterilising liquid recommended by the manufacturer.

CONTRAINDICATIONS

to dry floatation
- Infectious skin conditions.
- Severe respiratory conditions.
- Heavy colds/fevers.
- Heart conditions.*
- Diabetes.*
- Epilepsy.*

* Only to be carried out with medical approval.

Effects of a dry floatation treatment

- Aids relaxation.
- Relaxes muscles through the buoyancy effect of the water.
- Eases aches and pains.
- A general sense of wellbeing is achieved.

Note: If specific treatments are used in conjunction with dry floatation then the specific benefits from these can be added to the above list.

Preparation for a dry floatation treatment

1 Observe general safety precautions.

2 The vinyl sheeting must be clean, dry and protected as necessary.

3 The board is raised to the top of the tank and the temperature control switch is turned to pre-heat the water.

Dry floatation treatment

1 Greet the client at reception and take them to the changing facilities.

2 A consultation is carried out to check for contraindications and to explain the effects of the treatment.

3 The client removes items such as jewellery, spectacles and contact lenses, etc., and may shower.

4 The client lies on top of the tank and the therapist covers them.

5 The therapist presses a switch which lowers the board.

6 The lights are dimmed and music played to suit the individual client.

7 At the end of the floatation time the therapist raises the board and helps the client up.

8 If specific treatments such as mud baths have been given, the client showers to remove the products from their body.

9 The client should relax in a rest room and drink fluids as needed.

Foam baths

Foam baths are far more likely to be found in a day or destination spa offering a variety of water treatments than in a beauty salon where the costs of purchase, installation and running could prove too high an expense. However, modifications to a general household bath can transform it for use as a foam bath.

Foam baths found in health hydros are found in the spa area and resemble a household bath in appearance. A perforated, plastic duck board is found at the bottom of the bath which will allow compressed air to be forced through the hundreds of tiny holes into the bath water. Only a small quantity of water is needed, approximately 10–15 cm to cover the duck board. The water is heated to between 37–43 °C depending on the individual client. Concentrated foam essence such as seaweed is added to the water prior to the compressor being switched on. The compressor pumps air to beneath the duck board where it will force its way through the perforated holes to aerate the water. The compressor is left on until the foam created by the aeration of the water and foam essence reaches the top of the bath. The client lies in the foam in a semi-reclined position with their head resting on the back of the bath, outside of the foam.

Care of the foam bath

The bath should be cleaned between client use with a sterilising fluid recommended by the manufacturer.

CONTRAINDICATIONS

to foam baths
- Infectious skin conditions.
- Verrucas.
- Athlete's foot.
- Sunburn.
- After consuming alcohol.
- Diabetes.*
- Epilepsy.*
- Respiratory conditions.*
- Circulatory conditions.*

* Only to be carried out with medical approval.

Effects of a foam bath

- Induces perspiration.
- Raises body temperature.
- Induces circulation.
- Muscle fibres are relaxed.

Preparation of the foam bath

1   The bath is cleaned and filled with sufficient warm water to cover the duck board.

2   A selected concentrated foam essence is added to the water, e.g. seaweed.

3   The compressor is switched on to aerate the water.

4   Once the foam reaches the top of the bath the compressor is switched off. The foam bath is now ready for use.

Foam bath treatment

1   The client is greeted at reception and taken to the changing facilities.

2   A consultation is carried out to check for contraindications and to explain the effects of the treatment.

3   The client removes items such as contact lenses, spectacles and jewellery prior to showering to remove fragrances, deodorants, body lotions, etc.

4   The client is helped into the bath.

5   Treatment time is generally around 15 minutes.

6   The client is helped from the bath.

7   A warm shower may be taken using exfoliating products for cellular regeneration.

8   The client should relax in rest area and drink fluids as required.

Aerated baths

There are many types of aerated bath to be found in health spas, hydros and clubs, and they can also be found in hotels and individual homes. They vary in size, shape and price. The simplest form is a normal household bath with an air pump outside which pumps air into the water.

Aerated baths were developed in France. They are filled with water and air is forced into the water either through a hose or through holes in a duck board in the bath. Essence may be added to aerated baths for their individual properties. Treatment time would last approximately 15 minutes.

Hydrotherapy baths

Aerated baths are used as a hydrotherapy treatment in the majority of health spas, using a hose to direct air over the body. The hydrotherapy unit is shaped like a bath with grab handles to assist the client to get in and out. The inside of the hydrotherapy unit is fitted to the shape of the client's body more so than an ordinary household bath. The unit is filled with warm water, the selected essence is added and the compressor is switched on allowing air to aerate the bath gently through the duck board. The client is helped into the bath and the therapist switches on the hose which is worked methodically over the muscle groups. The treatment time is generally around 20 minutes.

ACTIVITY

Research the range of hydrotherapy units available and compare their benefits and cost.

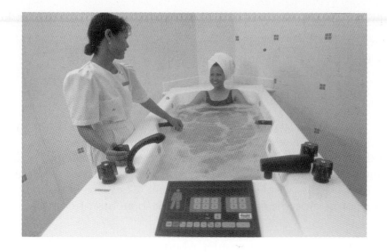

Hydrotherapy bath

to hydrotherapy baths
- Heart conditions.
- Infections skin conditions.
- Circulatory conditions.
- After a heavy meal or after consuming alcohol.
- Athlete's foot.
- Verrucas.
- Pregnancy.
- Diabetes.*
- Epilepsy.*

* Only to be carried out with medical approval.

Effects of a hydrotherapy bath
- Body temperature is raised.
- Perspiration is induced.
- Circulation is increased.
- Muscle fibres are relaxed.
- Metabolism is increased.

Preparation of the hydrotherapy bath
1 Observe general safety precautions.

2 Fill bath with warm water.

3 Add essence required.

Hydrotherapy treatment
1 The client is greeted at reception and taken to the changing facilities.

2 A consultation is carried out and the effects of the treatment are explained.

3 The client removes items such as contact lenses, spectacles and jewellery, etc., and showers to remove deodorants, fragrances, body lotions, etc.

4 The compressor is switched on for gentle aeration of the water.

5 The client is helped into the unit, where they rest in a semi-reclined position.

6 The hose is switched on and the therapist guides it over the client's body for approximately 15–20 minutes before the hose is switched off.

7 The compressor is switched off and after a few minutes the client is helped from the bath.

8 The client is taken to a relaxation area to rest.

Whirlpools

Whirlpools are sometimes called spa baths and are commonly known by the name of the American manufacturer who brought them to commercial success – Jacuzzi™. They are found in the majority of health spas, hydros, clubs and hotels and even in individual homes. They vary in size, shape and price. The larger ones can accommodate up to eight people at the same time. They are commonly found near the swimming pool in most health spas where the benefits of contrast baths can be achieved.

There are a number of factors to consider when fitting a whirlpool:

1 The floor must be:
   ● reinforced to take the large weight of the filled pool
   ● tanked and drained.

2 The plant room which houses the controls must:
   ● have a suitable power supply
   ● be within five metres of the pool
   ● be well ventilated.

3 The pool should have:
   ● a filtration system
   ● a heavy duty control panel to withstand constant wear and tear.

Effects of the whirlpool
● Increases circulation.
● Stimulates the skin and aids desquamation.
● Increases metabolism.
● Relaxes muscles.
● Relieves aches and pains (whilst in pool).
● Produces a sense of wellbeing.

The whirlpool generally has two massage effects – a gentle effect and a strong one. The gentle massage effect is created by compressed air flowing through small holes at the base of the pool. The strong whirlpool massage effect is created by jets of air pummelling the skin along with the action of the fast moving water of the pool. When these two effects are combined they create a fast stream of bubbling water.

ACTIVITY

With a colleague, select three different spa treatments that would benefit each of you. Taking the roles of client and therapist undertake the treatments selected and evaluate their physiological and psychological effects on you. Discuss and compare your findings with your colleague.

Hydro-oxygen baths

This treatment involves the client reclining in a bath-type cabinet that contains jets which are used to blast the client's body with hot water and to diffuse oxygen into the cabinet. The treatment is extremely stimulating and makes the skin more sensitive. An infrared treatment would not follow due to skin sensitivity.

information point

● The pH in whirlpools should be maintained between 7.2 and 8.0.
● The water temperature in whirlpools should be maintained between 30 and 40 °C.
● Hygiene and maintenance of whirlpools is extremely important to prevent Legionnaires' disease which is a form of pneumonia caused by the inhalation of water droplets contaminated with the *Legionella pneumophila* bacterium.

Research the different spa treatments offered by three different day and destination spas.

SELF-CHECKS

1 State the different treatments you might find in a spa area.

2 List four contraindications to each of the following treatments:

   a foam bath

   b hydrotherapy bath.

3 State two effects for each of the following treatments:

   a foam bath

   b hydrotherapy bath

   c whirlpool.

4 Explain the preparation of the foam bath.

5 State the effects of hydrotherapy treatments.

6 Briefly describe the following treatments:

   a hydro-oxygen baths

   b contrast baths.

Other therapies

Kneipp

The principles of the Kneipp Cure can be found in many spas today but it was originally developed by a German priest from Bavaria called Sebastian Kneipp who studied medicine and became involved with hydrotherapy in the 1850s. He opened a centre in 1889 and used cold baths and wet wraps as part of his treatment therapy. Alongside these treatments he also advocated exercise, dietary changes and plant therapy. The five pillars of Kneipp Cure are phytotherapy/herbology (use of plants), kinesiology (movement), dietetic (nutritional therapy), hydro (water) therapy and regulative.

Sound therapy

Sound therapy is not new and has been used in many ancient societies, for example in the form of chanting. Sound is a universal language that touches us on a deeper level. It was used during the Second World War as part of a rehabilitation programme for soldiers. Sound therapy is now being incorporated into spa treatments and spa equipments. British Osteopath Peter Manners developed cymatics or cymatic medicine. He created a sound wave machine for treatments with healing vibrations. The machine uses frequencies that are similar to the frequency of healthy cells, and it has been used in the treatment of cancer. Further research created a computerised system with 800 frequencies. This system is sometimes known as vibration therapy or bio-resonance. Liquid sound is the use of light and sound under and above water.

Transpersonal sound therapy was created by Dr Wolfgang Kölbl and his wife Dr Ruth Kölbl. It uses a variety of instruments and sound tools to increase neural networks and improve brain performance. The therapy aims to activate chakras.

Colour therapy

Colour therapy is based on the ancient art of using colour to treat disease. The human body absorbs light made up from the colour spectrum. Each colour has a

- The temperature of the surface of the skin is 33 °C or below.
- Water of a temperature above the skin's surface temperature has a hyperthermal effect as it adds heat to the body.
- Water of a temperature below the skin's surface temperature has a hypothermal effect as it draws heat away from the body.
- When water is used to cool or warm the body, it is referred to as hydrothermal therapy.
- When the mechanical properties of water, such as buoyancy, are used, it is referred to as hydrokinetic therapy.
- The temperature of the surface of hands and feet is generally much lower than the temperature of the surface of the skin of the body (i.e. below 20 °C).

frequency, a wavelength and energy. By using colour through a variety of mediums it helps restore physical and psychological balance. In spas colour therapy is being incorporated into the interior design of the spa as well as into saunas, pools, showers and types of chambers through fibre optic lighting and other colour therapy lamps. Another general example is the use of colour in the treatment of dyslexia, with the use of tinted lenses to improve reading.

Ayurveda

In Sanskrit Ayurveda means the 'science of daily living'. It is the original holistic health system and has been around since approximately 10,000 BC and contains wisdom on the maintenance of the physical, psychological and spiritual wellbeing. Ayurveda advocates that the human spirit consists of five basic elements – earth, fire, water, air and space. In an ideal situation these elements exist in balance. This theory is then refined to three tridoshas (commonly know as doshas – energies or humours) which are the governing forces of human life. They are Vata or Air, Pitta or Fire, Kapha or Earth – one or two will be dominant in an individual. The aim of the therapy is to keep these in balance. Disease occurs when these are imbalanced, therefore healing can occur when the harmony between the three doshas is restored. Ayurvedic treatments found in spas are purification (basti), synchronised body massages (Anhinga: a light, surface caress performed), Shirodhana head and face massages, herbal and steam inhalations, use of herbal pastes and elixirs, acupuncture, yoga and meditation. Ayurvedic massage is a deep massage that aims to open the chakras. It is yoga-based in its movements; the massage will incorporate breathing as well as muscle stretching as the muscle is being warmed and relaxed.

- Shirodhana: An Ayurvedic treatment involving the slow pouring of warm oil over the third eye (centre of the forehead). Switches off the chattering mind and induces a deep sense of relaxation.
- Siddha Vaidya: an Ayurvedic massage incorporating the use of a pouch of herbs and oils such as coconut.

Shiatsu

There are different forms of acupressure. The best known one is Shiatsu. Shiatsu has its base in oriental medicine and originated in Japan. It is a form of finger pressure carried out on the body. Shiatsu principles join the principles behind acupuncture (that energy flows through meridians of the body) and the ancient hands-on therapy 'anma' helps stimulate the bodies in-built healing powers. Shiatsu is particularly good for musculo-skeletal problems. For further information, log on to www.shiatsu.org.

Watsu

Watsu means underwater shiatsu. It is nurturing and intimate aquatic body work and was pioneered in Harbin Springs in California by Harold Dull in 1980. The client lies in the water fully supported by the therapist. The buoyancy of the water helps relieve stress on the joints and allows greater relaxation. There is a focus on breathing. The movements in Watsu are slow, rhythmical and continual.

Lomilomi

This is a traditional form of native healthcare in Hawaii passed down through generations of families. It arrived in Hawaii with the Polynesian voyagers. The kahuna lomilomi priests believed that physical discomfort and disease were the results of suppressed emotions, mental disturbances and spiritual disharmony. The kahuna, amongst their many skills, were masters of healing manipulation. A traditional lomilomi healing session began with investigation as to the cause of the problem, prayer and fasting, several sessions in the steam hut, then treatment with hot stones, herbal poultices and then massage – which doesn't sound too dissimilar to a stress relieving spa therapy week. Lomilomi massage is deep and uses rhythmical rocking and long stroking techniques. The favoured oil is kukui nut and coconut. It also incorporates breath work (ha).

Rolfing

Rolfing was founded by Swiss-born biochemist Dr Ida Rolf in the 1940s. Her search for solutions to family health led her to study the effect of the body structure and function. Hence 'Rolfing' or *structural integration* was born. The aim was to re-order the body segments using deep tissue massage to bring the body back into better alignment, ensuring less energy was used and the muscles worked more efficiently. A person will attend ten sessions, each session building on the previous, where work is carried out on realigning the posture. An off-shoot of Rolfing is *postural intergration* created by Jack Painter Ph.D. in the US. It combines deep body work, acupressure, breath work and Gestalt psychology.

Hellerwork

Hellerwork was started by Joseph Heller in the USA in the late 1970s after originally training with Ida Rolf. It is the exploration of the mind and body connection. It has three basic principles: body work – deep tissue to educate muscle and nervous systems; movement education – to realign posture; and verbal dialogue – to assess emotional patterns. Hellerworkers believe that memory is not just held in the brain but in the muscles and tissues of the body. Therefore by changing someone on a structural level you will affect them on an emotional level. Hellerwork has a rigid structure of 11 sessions lasting 90 minutes each. After which home-care advice on exercise and any further work needed on an emotional level is given.

Oxygen therapy

Good health requires high levels of oxygen. Oxygen is a colourless odourless gas. Oxygen therapy is based on the premise that all harmful bacteria, viruses and fungi, e.g. cold, flu, HIV, candida and cancer cells, are anaerobic and thrive in low oxygen environments. Dr Otto Warburg, twice Nobel laureate, was able to prove that cancer cannot grow in high oxygen environments. Although there are many secondary causes for cancer the primary cause is lack of oxygen for aerobic cell respiration and its replacement with anaerobic respiration. Oxygen therapy is divided into two main areas: ozone therapy and the use of hydrogen peroxide.

Oxygen bars, popularised in Japan due to poor air quality, enable an individual to breathe in oxygen-enriched air. These are not the same as hyperbaric units, which are used for the critically ill. Oxygen therapy is used in the medical arena for the treatment of many diseases. Many beauty companies are now incorporating oxygen delivery into their products, treatments and equipment. In facial treatments oxygen is being delivered to the skin via a pressurised jetting system. This is usually combined with micro-dermabrasion.

SELF-CHECKS

Describe three 'other' therapies.

ACTIVITY

Research the variety of companies retailing spa treatments, and draw together a comparison on cost, service and back up provided.

Manual cellulite treatments

A number of professional skin-care companies offer specialised manual treatments that aim to reduce and improve the appearance of cellulite. They normally work in two ways, either by the action of the product itself or the massage techniques used.

Products

There are certain ingredients, in particular plant extracts and essential oils, that are known to have an effect on cellulite. Examples of these include:

- Essential oil of rosemary – this has a tonic effect and is anti-toxic.
- Essential oil of sandalwood – eliminates toxins and decongests.
- Essential oil of patchouli – this has a regenerative effect and is healing.
- Essential oil of lavender – this has a healing and diuretic effect.
- Seaweed – acts as a diuretic.
- Horsetail extract – tonic action on the tissues.

Massage techniques

These often incorporate specialised movements that help in lymphatic drainage and compression-type movements as the circulation is reduced in these areas and needs improving if the effective elimination is going to take place.

For any of the cellulite treatments to be successful they need to be given in courses with proper home-care advice. The client should be encouraged to look at their diet and eliminate convenience-type foods – too much salt, sugar, tea, coffee, etc. – and to look at their lifestyle; in particular smoking, alcohol consumption and exercise.

The client must be able to attend the clinic at least 2–3 times a week for a course of treatments lasting from 20–30 minutes on average. The client must also be prepared to invest in products to be used at home in between salon visits and to use them daily.

Example of a cellulite treatment

1 Perform a detailed consultation, checking the area for any contraindications.

2 Prepare the client for treatment ensuring comfort throughout.

3 Uncover the area and clean with specialised toning product.

4 Apply exfoliating cream evenly to the treatment area, remove when dry using circular movements. Support the skin as required.

5 Wipe area with toner to remove any residual cream.

6 Apply cellulite treatment oil and massage the area using lymphatic drainage movements and compression techniques.

7 Apply specialised cellulite gel/serum and work into the area.

8 Often some form of heat is next applied to the area to help the absorption of the products; it may be in the form of cellophane sheeting, a warm poultice or a thermal blanket.

9 Remove the thermal medium and any traces of residual product.

10 Apply cellulite cream and massage into area.

11 Recommend home care advice and book the next treatment.

Products for home-care

Home-care normally consists of using some kind of cellulite serum/gel and cream which needs to be applied daily, preferably morning and at night, and usually following a brisk circulatory massage.

Stretch marks

These treatments aim to reactivate the dermis and increase the localised circulation. Success of the treatment will depend on regular salon treatment (2–3 times per week) over a course of 12–20 on average. The client will also need to purchase home-care products to be used in between salon visits.

Common ingredients used in stretch mark treatments include plant extracts and essential oils. For example:

- Hops – have a firming and tightening effect.
- Ginseng – aids cellular stimulation and has an anti-ageing effect.
- Horsetail – restores elasticity in fibres and collagen of the skin.
- Essential oil of mint – tones, firms and increases circulation.

Example of a stretch mark treatment

1 Perform a thorough consultation, checking the area for any contraindications and make sure that the stretch marks are at a stage where they will respond to treatment.

2 Wipe over the area with toner and exfoliate to remove dead skin cells to allow easier absorption of products.

3 Next, stimulate the area to be treated with either a body brush, body mitten, specific equipment or even brisk effleurage-type movements.

4 Apply a specialised stretch mark gel/solution and work it into the area briskly.

5 A stimulating product is applied and massaged into the area. The massage sequence should be quite brisk and include pinching-type movements.

6 Thermal equipment/product can be applied to allow the active solutions to penetrate more thoroughly.

7 Remove any residue of products.

8 Finally, prescribe the most appropriate products for the upkeep of the skin at home and book the next treatment.

Skin improvement treatments

One of the latest advances in skin improvement has been the development of skin renewal treatments. On the surface it may seem that nothing is new, peeling products have been used for a long time – even as far back as Egyptian times. As recently as 1927 chemical peels were used to dissolve dead skin tissue. However, in the last few years two substances have been generating media interest. They are retinoic acid and alpha hydroxy acid (AHA).

Retinoic acid

Retinoic acid is Vitamin A and was originally developed as a formulation for the treatment of acne vulgaris. It was found to speed up the natural shedding of the epidermis and recent trials have shown it to be very effective (if used in low concentrations) on sun damage, ageing, fine lines and wrinkles and pigmentation. It needs to be used for six months and once discontinued, stops working. There can be side effects, however, and a lot of people develop residual inflammation as the treatment reduces the thickness of the stratum corneum.

This is not performed as a salon treatment, clients usually obtain the retinoic acid on prescription. Beauty therapists need to take great care with any client using retinoic acid products. In particular avoid waxing, peeling or extracting in areas being treated.

Alpha hydroxy acids (AHA)

These are also sometimes referred to as fruit acids and were developed following the interest in retinoic acid.

They work by causing micro-exfoliation which speeds up the natural exfoliation process of the skin. Some of the ingredients literally digest the surface cells, therefore revealing new skin. This is a very important concept in the treatment of the skin as many problems that occur are the result of a build-up of dead skin cells, or hyperkeritinisation as it is technically known.

Great care should be taken with the use and administration of these products, however, as they can be extremely harsh if not used in the correct quantity.

Some key ingredients used in AHA creams are:

- **Lactic acid**. This alpha hydroxy acid occurs naturally in sour milk and dissolves the intercellular cement holding the skin cells together. It also works on follicular skin cells helping dislodge blockages and therefore helping prevent congestion.
- **Glycolic acid**. This is used for its small molecular structure as it is able to penetrate quickly and deeply and dissolves the natural moisturising factor of the skin. It can cause more irritation than lactic acid.
- **Salicylic acid**. This stimulates the formation of new epidermal skin cells in the stratum germinativum and has antiseptic properties.
- **Bromelain**. This is a pineapple derivative and is a fruit enzyme that digests surface skin cells.
- **Papain**. This comes from the papaya fruit and is an enzyme. It again digests the surface skin cells.
- **Citric acid**. This is derived from citrus fruits and is also a fruit enzyme that digests the surface skin cells.
- **Plant and flower extracts**. Examples include orange flower, aloe vera and cornflower. They are added for their soothing and hydrating properties.

Buffers

Alpha hydroxy acid treatments have a buffer added to make them less aggressive in reaction on the skin. Plant extracts and enzymes are used as buffers and they have the effect of altering the pH of the reaction.

AHA treatments exist in two forms: a concentrated strength for use by the therapist in the clinic and a lower concentration for the client to use at home daily between salon visits. The combination of the professional and the home-care products will achieve the most rapid improvement in the appearance of the skin and as a general guide most manufacturers recommend a course of at least six salon treatments to be taken once a week initially with the daily use of home care products.

Example of an AHA facial treatment

1 Perform a detailed consultation checking the area for any contraindications.

2 Remove the eye and lip make-up with a suitable product making sure there is no residue left on the skin.

3 Next, cleanse the face and neck with an appropriate cleanser at least twice and again thoroughly remove.

4 The special fruit acid solution is applied to the skin and left on according to individual manufacturer's instructions.

5 After the correct time the product is removed very thoroughly, usually with sponges and copious amounts of warm water, making sure no residue is left.

6 Extractions can now be performed where necessary.

7 The skin is massaged with a special soothing product to help calm the skin and reduce irritation.

8 A soothing mask is applied.

9 A special toner is applied often by means of a 'spray' action.

10 Finally a protective cream is applied to filter ultraviolet rays and nourish the skin.

11 To conclude the treatment the therapist explains the relevant home-care and retail advice and confirms the date of the next appointment.

SELF-CHECKS

1 Give an example of a manual cellulite treatment.

2 What is the main purpose of a stretch mark treatment?

3 Give three factors that should be considered when performing an AHA treatment.

4 What are the main benefits of a body wrap treatment and how often should it be performed?

Toning tables

Toning tables have existed since the 1930s when they were produced for physiotherapy and rehabilitation purposes. Modern tables have quickly established themselves in the professional beauty market. They normally consist of a motorised bed-type unit with various movable sections. It is possible to purchase them in two forms; either as individual units or as a multi-function unit.

Individual units are tables designed to work on one specific area of the body and would normally be part of a group of approximately six or seven units which the client uses in a treatment session lasting approximately 1 hour. The obvious advantage of having individual units is that more than one client can be using the tables simultaneously. The main drawback is that a lot of space is needed because each unit measures approximately 8 × 1.1 m (6.5 × 3.5 ft). This normally means that if the salon is going to purchase individual units either it is very large, or is going to specialise in toning tables and figure correction treatments generally. This type of toning table is very popular with health spas.

Multi-function units are beds with all the features of the individual units incorporated into them so the client does not have to move once treatment commences. This type of unit is ideal if space is a problem, but it does restrict the number of clients that can use it in any one day.

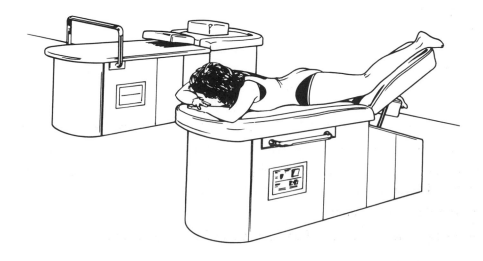

Toning tables

The main benefits of toning tables

Toning tables are designed to improve muscle tone, mobility and reduce inches without the use of any kind of weight. They work on the principles of both isotonic and isometric exercise.

Different tables or parts of the multi-function table produce varying movement, rhythm and speed which produces progressive resistance. This in turn strengthens muscle fibres as each fibre is shortened in length improving elasticity. Toning tables also increase body temperature by increasing blood circulation; this also helps in the removal of waste products and toxins.

Types of toning table

- **Circulation table** (warm-up and cool-down). This produces a gentle vibration which is designed to increase the circulation and relax tense muscles. It should be used at the start and the end of a treatment session. There is normally an arm bar present on this table to help in toning of the upper arms, back and chest.
- **Leg table**. This concentrates on the inner and outer thighs and gluteals, but has a toning effect on the entire leg area.
- **Sit-up table**. This works the abdominal area and it is suggested that 10 minutes on this table is the equivalent of around 80 sit-ups.
- **Stomach/hip table**. This table stretches and lifts the gluteals and works the abdomen at the same time. It will also help to improve overall posture.
- **Twister table**. This table alternately lifts and raises the lower legs.
- **Stretching table**. This table affects the upper body, lifting the rib cage and bust and easing tension in the upper back.

A normal treatment session will last approximately 1 hour with roughly 10 minutes being spent on each table/function. Most beds have a control panel which allows the therapist to adjust the speed of the table according to the health and general fitness of the client.

SELF-CHECKS

1 List the six classifications of toning table and explain the main purpose of each.

2 List the contraindication to specialised salon treatments.

3 What safety precautions should be observed when carrying out specialised treatments?

Electrical treatments

Specialised galvanic, high frequency and NMES treatments

Over the last decade the choice of specialised treatments has made the beauty profession one of the most innovative in existence. Modern therapy treatments have been adapted from straightforward galvanic, faradic and high frequency principles to incorporate advances in technology. Some of these treatments are designed specifically for use on the face but many are for body application. Not all are 'new' however, as some are adaptions of old ideas.

Slimming treatments incorporating iontophoresis, faradic and thermal clay

This treatment is a mixture of faradic muscle stimulation and galvanic current applied in the iontophoresis mode to allow ingredients designed to help with the removal of cellulite penetrate more deeply. The treatment stimulates the circulation, aids lymphatic drainage and increases cellular activity all at the same time as toning the muscles.

A special current-conducting clay is applied as this allows the treatment area to be larger and ensures even distribution of the current.

It is recommended that treatment is taken in intensive courses with products used at home in between salon visits.

Facial treatments incorporating galvanic and high frequency treatments

These treatments are not so new and have been used in salons now for well over 20 years. They work on the principle of combining the beneficial effects of galvanic, normally the iontophoresis mode, with direct high frequency and specialised products to produce a complete treatment that is deeply cleansing, rehydrating and increases cellular regeneration. The treatment normally lasts about 1¼ hours and is suitable for most skin types. Cosmetic houses produce specialised products to work with the equipment and an intensive training course is usually necessary to ensure therapists adhere to correct procedures to gain maximum effect. Some manufacturers have taken the treatment a stage further and developed specialised adaptations for the eyes, neck, bust and back areas offering excellent results.

Sequential body toning systems

This is the term used to describe a new range of more sophisticated toning machines that are controlled by micro-processors.

Many combine iontophoresis, infrared and programmed electro-stimulation over a frequency range of 100–800 Hz. Session times will vary according to individual manufacturers and specific programmes, but on average treatment times are approximately 30–40 minutes. Infrared is used to warm the area and thus improve the effectiveness of the treatment as current transmission will be maximised. Specialised products are applied to the area together with electrodes to release trapped fatty deposits while at the same time sequential electro-stimulation of the muscles, commencing at the ankles and gradually progressing upwards, increases the lymphatic and circulatory system to help in the dispersal of the accumulated waste products and the mobilised fat. Another key feature of such systems is that the programme can be adapted to meet the individual client's needs.

Treatments should be given in courses of approximately 12 sessions over a 1-month period for optimum results with a regular maintenance programme thereafter.

Ultrasound treatments

Treatment with ultrasound has been in existence for a long time and is traditionally used by physiotherapists. It incorporates wave-type sound energy of a frequency that is just about audible, which is transmitted via a flat, disk-shaped applicator to the tissues. It is able to penetrate to a depth of approximately 6 cm depending on the type of tissue. It agitates the cells, releasing toxins and fatty accumulations.

It is an effective treatment not only for muscular tensions, but also for cellulite and related disorders. A specialised coupling cream is normally used in conjunction with the treatment.

Interferential therapy

Interferential current is an alternative type of muscle stimulation to faradic that produces practically no sensation during treatment. The reason for this is that two medium frequency currents are delivered to the treatment area by separate circuits.

Where the two currents meet, a third frequency is produced. This is equivalent to the difference between the two original frequencies. There is no surge or interruption during treatment.

information point

Wet, elasticated bandages can replace the use of the clay masque and specially made flexible, conductive, black strapping can be used instead of traditional static electrodes.

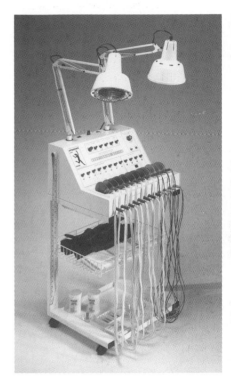

Sequential body toning equipment

information point

Specific sequencing EMS units are specially designed to closely emulate exercise by varied passive stimulation and the range of frequency, 5–70 Hz, is controlled to stimulate most effectively the range of muscle fibre activity. These units use advanced micro-processor control and offer a constantly changing parameter of stimulation. They follow the latest research into electrical muscular stimulation.

Interferential currents are used in therapy treatments for a number of reasons:

- A constant 'third frequency' will have an analgesic action which will help to reduce pain.
- A variable 'third frequency' will improve localised circulation, lymph drainage and cell metabolism which will help to reduce toxins and waste accumulations.

SELF-CHECKS

1 What conditions are treated with specialised galvanic, high frequency and faradic treatments?

2 Give the main benefits of galvanic and high frequency facial treatments.

3 What systems of the body will be affected by a sequential body toning treatment?

4 Describe interferential current.

Specialised slimming programmes

Over the last few years manufacturers have been researching and developing slimming programmes incorporating a variety of heat, vibration, galvanic, faradic and specialised products. A typical treatment can involve:

- Detailed consultation with measurements being taken.
- Pressure massage.
- Heat therapy, such as sauna, with the use of products that contain ingredients such as seaweed.
- Interrupted direct current on accupressure points (which may help to reduce appetite).
- The client is wrapped in polythene-type sheeting which induces perspiration.
- Vibration and heat from the bed form the next stage of the treatment. The heat is normally derived from infrared lamps.
- Finally the treatment finishes with a shower and measurements being checked and home-care and retail advice given.

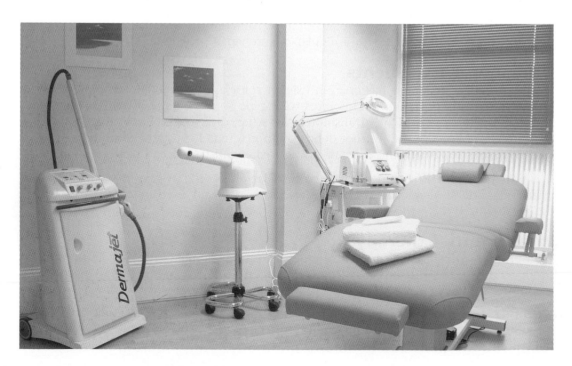

Treatment room

Lifting treatments

With advances in micro-current a number of electrotherapy companies have launched new combined units and, in some cases, support products to gain maximum effects. The following are some of the latest on the market.

- Body Sculpture by CACI™ with the Quantum™ system is an all-in-one computerised body care and slimming system incorporating micro-current for lifting and shaping, cellulite body treatments and synchronised lymphatic drainage. The computerised micro-current with pre-set programmes tightens skin and facial muscles, softens fine lines and wrinkles, increases collagen production and improves circulation. Complementing the treatment is the Body Sculpture™ range of products, which includes active collagen ampoules and aloe vera gel.
- Technique Infusion by Silhouette™ incorporates its micro-current systems to infuse a range of concentrated actives such as collagen (anti-wrinkle mask) to plump up fine lines, replenishing tired tissues; anti-acne mask (containing orris root) to purify and tighten open pores and stabilise the skin's pH whilst reducing the excessive production of sebum; Skin-lite™ mask (containing grape extract) to treat uneven skin tones and pigmentation; vitamin C eye-and-lip pads to improve the skin's elasticity, rehydrating and protecting against free radicals (pollution), softening fine lines and wrinkles and lightening dark shadows.
- Sports Compact 20™ and Super Pro 20™ by Ultratone™ are units for all sports training and beauty therapy applications. Sports 20™ features computerised physio-sequential rotating programmes for body building, strength stamina, speed, flexibility, rehabilitation, oedema reduction, TENS pain reduction and endorphin release. Super Pro 20™ features 41 sequencing programmes, 30 of which are 'multi-area' – delivering different rotating programmes to individual areas during the one treatment – and also includes a hands-free facial micro-current programme for lifting, tightening and toning.
- Ultrasound Sonocare by Ella Bache™ incorporates ultrasonic vacuotherapy and ultrasonic vascular drainage. It has an ultrasound transducer with a frequency of 0.6 MHz to optimise penetration of the active ingredients in their gels. The hand-held vacuolyser head has a suction head with an ultrasonic ceramic flange which, through a frequency of 3 MHz, vibrates. The head combines ultrasound waves with suction. Each programme involves six steps: cleansing, exfoliation, Sonocare system (cellular stimulation, muscular toning, and drainage); pulverisation; mask application and application of a day-care product.
- The VIP Body System by Scanda Sol™ combines the latest in light therapy with acupuncture to combat cellulite. Infrared light is applied to break down adipose tissue, then faradic waves are applied to acupuncture points in the treatment area to elongate and contract the muscle.
- In Cellular Electrotherapy by Biogénie beaute Concept™, alternating current signals of a harmonious electrical frequency to the dermal tissues permit direct current and sinusoidal signals to pass through the skin without irritation and enable micro-currents to effect specific results at cellular level. Biogénie Visage™, for example, is an 'anti-gravity' massage, using four sinusoidal signals delivered to the skin via sponges soaked with a conductive product and inserted into round electrodes (4 cm diameter). The sculpting massage action lifts, tones and re-energises facial tissues.

Endermologie™

Endermologie™ is a treatment developed in the early 1980s by a French engineer, Louis-Paul Guitay, who had suffered muscle and skin damage in a car accident. This treatment was for burns, to prevent skin contraction and to loosen scar tissues. While conducting these initial treatments, it was discovered that the treatment unexpectedly improved cellulite on patients suffering the condition and this is how it came to be used for aesthetic purposes.

> **information point**
>
> Cellulite is a hormonal condition exacerbated by factors such as pregnancy and the menopause. It is caused by fat stored in the adipocytes, which are fat cells in the hypodermis, swelling and distorting connective fibres and creating the orange peel effect associated with cellulite. This is turn causes the circulation to become sluggish leading to a build-up of toxins, along with congestion, leading to the dimpled effect.

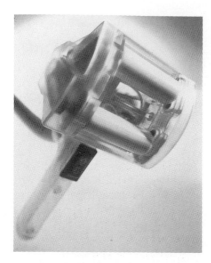

Endermologie Cellu-M6™

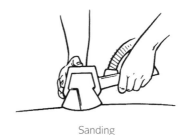

Sanding

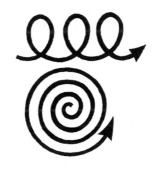

Endermologie™ treatment consists of the Cellu M6™, a hand-held massaging unit that delivers intermittent suction and rolling via two motorised heads to the area being treated as well as the surrounding soft tissues. This patented action of rollers, gentle suctionary stretch and deep massage is applied to the affected areas in a unique way. The fibrous tissues are thus stretched and weakened and this has the effect of minimising the dimpled effect.

Benefits of treatment

It is now thought that during this process of stimulation, collagen is also increased, helping to give the skin a smoother and more contoured appearance. It is worth noting that during the treatment there will be deep stimulation of the blood and lymphatic circulation which will also help in sending oxygen to the affected areas and carrying away stagnant toxic waste.

The treatment programme

The treatment works best if taken in courses, with an initial 14 treatments recommended, each lasting approximately 35 minutes. These should be taken twice a week followed by a maintenance schedule of one or two per month. A very precise 'before' and 'after' photographic record is made, with clients standing in a specific photograph measuring station which has built-in foot markers to ensure consistent positioning of the body and feet on every photograph. This gives totally measurable results to the effectiveness of the programme and is not liable to therapist error with a tape measure or different angle of camera and so on. During treatment, the client wears a special protective body stocking to prevent skin friction and to afford a degree of modesty.

Endermologie™ have developed two machines: the Cellu M6 IP™ is the larger and recommended for medical and sports applications, whilst the Cellu M6™ is the smaller and developed specifically for the beauty industry.

Example of an Endermologie™ treatment

1   First, a thorough consultation is carried out detailing all medical history and contraindications and so on. During the consultation a photographic measuring session is performed with the client being led into a special photographic measuring station. The feet are placed on specific foot markers and then the cellulite can be photographed from all angles and at an exact distance.

2   Next, the therapist helps the client into a one-size body stocking and on to the couch for treatment.

3   Treatment commences and the motorised main head is worked over the body in rhythmic patterns from the upper back, down the tops of the arms, across the back over the gluteals and all the way down to the ankles and on the front of the body. A variety of techniques are employed including:

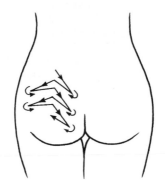

Kneading

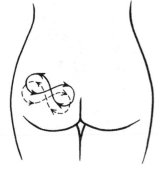

Figure of eight

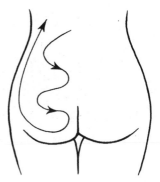

Winding

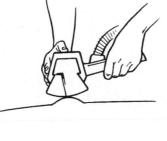

Bouncing

Endermologie™ techniques

- sanding, which is used to revitalise while stimulating the dermis to achieve tissue resurfacing following weight loss or pregnancy or as part of an anti-ageing treatment
- kneading, which is designed for areas with a high concentration of cellulite especially where it is long established
- figure-of-eight, which is specific to cellulite-ridden areas and designed to smooth tissue
- winding for the beginning and end of a treatment of a particular area which is a smoothing manoeuvre designed to control the newly regained smoothness of the skin
- bouncing, a technique that can be incorporated into all other movements except for sanding, which is especially recommended on thick and fatty areas.

4   Once the treatment is finished the client is helped off the couch and to get dressed after any more photographic evidence is recorded.

5   After-care advice and follow-up sessions are booked in.

information point

The latest development in aspiration systems is Celluloss™, by Biogénie beaute Concept™, which includes simultaneous electrical stimulation – cellular electrotherapy – to revitalise skin tissue. The patented round head utilises the design of the electrical contacts or 'feet' to direct skin tissue into central aspiration duct, avoiding surface skin tissue trauma and, therefore, is applied directly to the skin over conductive refirming cream.

Dermajet

The Dermajet is a technique similar to Endermologie in the sense that it uses a combination of vacuum and a rolling action with the added benefit of ultrasound, which produces even better results on cellulite and body contouring. It is the first patented technology to combine simultaneously a mechanical and non-invasive massage therapy technique called Endomassage with the use of external ultrasound therapy. Dermajet offers ten different programmes that allow treatments of numerous body conditions including cellulite and body contouring.

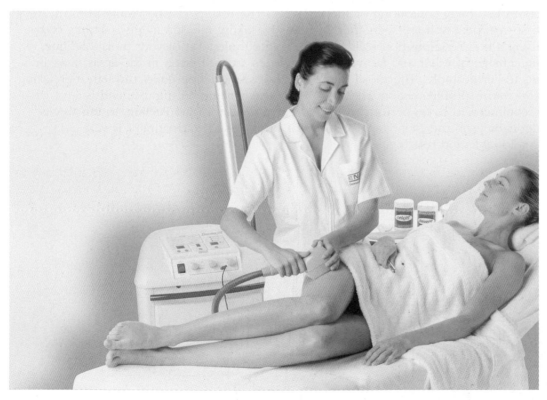

Dermajet

Endomassage

Endomassage allows a stretching of both tissue layers of the skin – the dermis and the hypodermis – and the connective tissue layer is exercised and stretched through the action of the main treatment head while the vacuum suction gently restores micro-circulation and stimulates the subcutaneous fluid exchange over the whole body. The vibratory alternating pressure/non-pressure of the ultrasound causes a micro-massage at cellular level. The friction created among molecules produces local heat and vasodilatation, increasing the effect of lipid elimination. The ultrasound can penetrate deeper into the fat layers by ultrasonic peeling to 8 cm.

This double action can be used simultaneously or separately allowing minimum trauma to the tissues with more effective results.

Thermojet

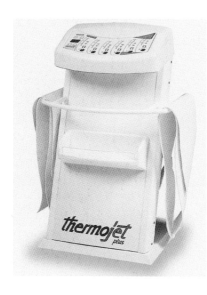

The Thermojet is an infrared technique that works on weight loss. The system uses short and long infrared waves, penetrating the dermis, hypodermis and the deeper fat layers. This stimulates the adipocyte metabolism which in turn improves circulation. The system has six independently controlled silicone bands housed in the infrared filaments. The bands are placed around the hips, thighs, waist and arms. Specific gels are applied according to the individuals needs. The client is wrapped with thermofilm and bathed evenly with the infrared rays, stimulating the metabolism and circulation and further enhancing the penetration of the active ingredients of the gels. The process creates thermolipolysis and offers a rapid treatment giving spectacular results in weight and inch loss. The treatment acts on all the different skin layers including the dermis and hypodermis where cellulite is located. Water retention problems causing swelling of the adypocytes are improved through thermotherapy and blood and lymphatic circulation is increased. The treatment works well with other non-invasive mechanical body contouring techniques and more superficial techniques such as Endomassage or deeper contouring techniques such as liposuction. The treatment gives spectacular results in weight and inch loss and controlled body contouring of specific areas. The results can be visible from the very first treatment and are seen after 24 hours by taking measurements, pictures or by using a body composition scale giving accurate evaluation of your metabolic rate, percentage of water and fat mass. The changes are produced in the areas most in need. Furthermore, Thermojet has a great stress-reduction effect through its relaxing and warm soothing action. Each treatment lasts around 45 minutes and is recommended to be performed twice weekly for Ultrasonic Peeling, to ten weeks depending on the client's expectations or problems. The treatment is very comfortable and relaxing.

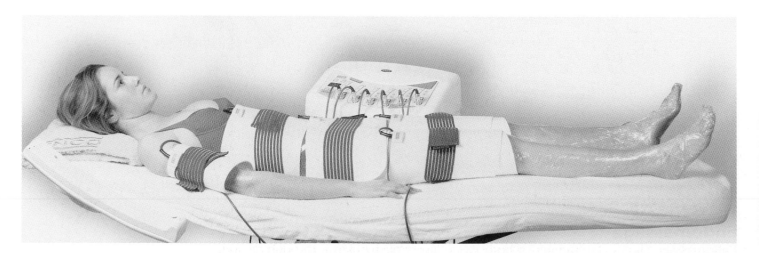

Thermojet

Thermolipolysis

Thermolipolysis is the fat burning process, which is activated by the increased body temperature and metabolic rate. The increased thermolipolytic action of the infrared works from the deep fat layers to the superficial tissue layers (dermis).

Ultrasonic Peeling

Ultrasonic Peeling is a non-invasive and non-abrasive peeling process. The treatment removes dead skin cells from the epidermis and painlessly removes comedones and pimples. The process assists the removal of discolouration and dark patches and the penetration of products like no other treatment. It also helps to hydrate and condition the skin tissue.

The Ultrasonic Peeling is an indispensable tool for anti-ageing, firming, deep peel, purifying, pigmentation and blemishes treatments.

Ultrasonic hydro-cavitation

The Ultrasonic Peeling transmits a series of ultrasonic vibrations to the skin and underlying connective tissues via elastic waves at frequencies as high as 25,000 (0 to 25,000 Hz) cycles per second, creating both mechanical and thermal action for the peeling and cleaning programme. The process removes dead cells, comedones, sebum and make-up residues. The elastic waves are beneficial to the skin due to a 'cavitation' phenomenon during which a vacuum is created in the flowing liquid when the elastic wave is introduced. Cavitation causes no injury to any cells from deeper layers where the elastic wave performs a stimulating cellular micro-massage.

The high frequency micro-vibrations also act to reduce the presence of bacteria on the skin's surface – this is a contributory cause of blemishes – by making it sensitive to unexpected changes in pressure, which promote sterilisation.

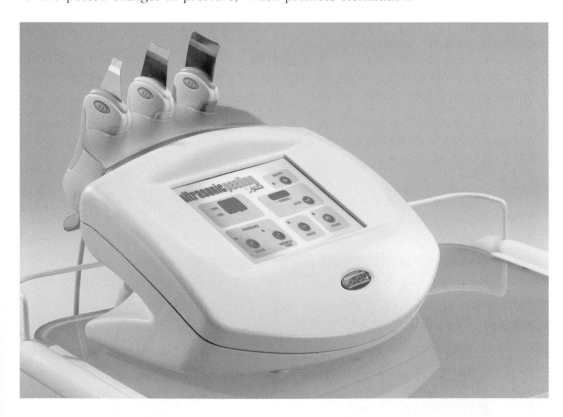

Ultrasonic hydro-cavitation

Ultrasonic elastic wave

The Ultrasonic Peeling works in conjunction with sonophoresis, causing deep internal hydration through micro-massage of the dermis and external hydration through micronisation of specific skin-care products and essential oils applied during the treatment.

Hyper oscillating vibration

The Ultrasonic Peeling increases blood circulation through the hyper oscillating vibration that is executed and transmitted deep in the skin.

The Ultrasonic Peeling treatment

Cleanse (peeling)

Using a specially designed metal spatula vibrating at a supersonic frequency, active cleaners and moisturising tonics are forced into the pores to produce remarkable results. The continuous vibrating effect in conjunction with the treatment product temporarily expands and softens the pores, allowing the thorough removal of oils, impurities, cosmetic and dead cells. The result of this supersonic frequency is a super moisturising effect, accelerated blood circulation, reinforcement of the cutaneous tissue and the increased metabolism of the cells. The ultrasonic vibration travelling down the metal spatula causes the tip of the spatula to move and vibrate so rapidly that any contact with the skin causes all particles that are not firmly attached to be lifted and removed, thus eliminating blackheads, spots, dead cells and impurities. The speed of the vibration in a confined space creates a type of aerosol effect. All impurities in the skin, emulsified by the treatment products used, are forced out of the pores and released from the skin. The Ultrasonic Peeling treatment method penetrates to a depth virtually impossible with regular facial treatment.

Regeneration (wrinkle tone)

Reversing the position of the spatula provides an intense skin micro-massage. This percussion effect aids deep penetration of the product, without affecting its ion balance.

Micro-massage (wrinkle tone and pulse)

This is performed using the Bi-action Regenerating or Whitening product, depending on the treatment decided upon. Ultrasonic Peeling is the complete solution to all physiological problems caused through ageing of the skin.

Recommended treatment time

- Peeling and purifying treatment: Treatment time is 20 minutes for the face and Ultrasonic Peeling, to 50 minutes for the face and body. For best results, the client should have a treatment once a month.
- Anti-ageing treatment: It combines the peeling, moisturising and regeneration phases, and leaves the skin hydrated, oxygenated and rejuvenated. This treatment is approximately 45 minutes and for best results, the client should have a series of 8–10 treatments once a week.

SK IV

SK IV is a combination treatment using galvanic micro-current and ultrasound currents with Matis products to improve facial skin conditions.

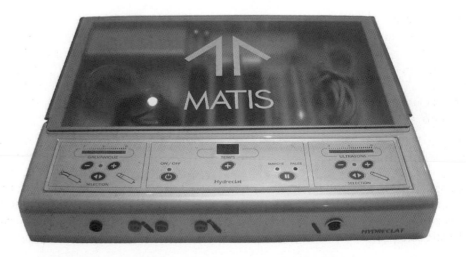

SK IV treatments are ideal for:

- Crows feet and eye bags. Your eyes are surrounded by a network of fine, narrow muscles, supporting the skin in an area which is particularly fragile. Micro-mode exercise will contract these muscles, improving the circulation in the peripheral blood vessels, thereby reducing the sagging and restoring healthier skin tone.
- Wrinkles on forehead. The vertical muscles that support the skin of the forehead are rarely used, therefore they do not adequately stimulate the blood vessels, for proper irrigation of the epidermis. Frowning will stimulate these muscles, but the creases that result will cancel out any benefits of irrigation. Using micro-mode, these muscles can be exercised in a beneficial way, improving the tone and reducing wrinkles.
- Creases around the mouth. Between the cheeks and nose, there is a long muscle called the 'joint elevator of the nasal wing and upper lip'. This muscle works in a downward direction, as a rule gradually forming a deepening, vertical crease in this area. With the use of micro-mode, you can cause this muscle to work upwards, creating better support for your skin and progressively reducing creases.
- Sagging chin line. Whenever you chew, you are using the muscles around the jaw bone, called masseters. But to correct any sagging under the chin, the muscles called the quadrate and the triangularis must be exercised. These are not used in the chewing process. The micro-mode stimulation causes these muscles to contract, tightening up any slackness under the chin.
- To improve the complexion. Beneath the facial skin, there is a complex network of muscles and elastic tissue, whose function is to support the epidermis, and stimulate the peripheral blood vessels, ensuring that the skin's foundation is well irrigated. Regular use of micro-mode improves and maintains the efficiency of this 'skin feeding system', and achieves a visible improvement of the complexion.

Lines and wrinkles – the signs of ageing

Like all organs, the skin is affected by the ageing process. In contrast to other organs, changes in the skin become visible over the years. The signs of ageing start to show as early as the end of the second or the beginning of the third decade of a person's life. At first, fine lines start to form between the nose and the mouth, around the eyes and on the forehead. As a result of facial movements that are often repeated, the first expressive wrinkles come into being: laughter creases, brow furrows and crow's feet. Over the years, the skin loses its elasticity because the dermis produces fewer and fewer collagen and elastin fibres. This results in the weakening of connective tissue causing the skin to lose its tone, the skin becomes flabby and wrinkles are formed. Due to gravity, wrinkles develop downwards, a phenomenen seen in sagging cheeks and drooping eyelids.

Cosmolight™

An exciting treatment combining holistic as well as technological advancement is Cosmolight™. The system combines a non-coherent pulsating light ranging from 600 to 1200 nm (this means that it is part of the visible and invisible light spectrum but contains no UV properties) with a 'biological resonant wave' to create a holistic therapy that heals or regenerates conditions such as acne, stretch marks, back pain, sports injuries and signs of ageing.

Cosmolight™ penetrates the skin up to a depth of 7 cm and the light is generated by a pure cold light source and gives no sensation of heat. The principal effect is to stimulate the fibroblast cells to speed up collagen and elastin production. Secondly, the biological resonant wave creates a vibratory wave which pulsates at the same rate as the body's blood and lymph systems. This has the effect of dilating the arteries to allow increased blood flow and provide greater nutrition for the newly active light-stimulated skin cells.

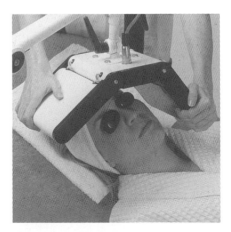

Cosmolight™

Example of a Cosmolight™ treatment

1 After a detailed consultation that checks medical history and contraindications, the client is prepared for treatment, for example for a treatment on the face, the area would be thoroughly cleansed and toned.

2 Shields are placed over the eyes to block the light and help the client relax. (The light will not damage the eyes.)

3 The therapist sets the required setting for both the light energy and the biological wave and sets the timer.

4 The three-sided Cosmolight™ light pane, each section about the size of a paperback book, is positioned over the area. The treatment commences.

5 Whilst the client relaxes under the lights, the therapists uses the Cosmolight™ pen, a needle-free acupuncture device, to stimulate meridian points, for example during an anti-ageing treatment the points relating to liver, intestines and bladder would be stimulated to improve lymphatic drainage.

6 After 10 minutes, the light panel is removed and the contents of an ampoule are applied, which will contain vitamins, minerals and anti-oxidants. The light panel is then replaced so that it can propel the active ingredients deeper into the skin.

7 After 5 minutes, the light panel is removed before a second ampoule, specific to the client's needs, is applied, followed by a further five minutes from the light panel.

8 The light pen is then used to work on deeper facial lines, scars or even cold sores.

9 The treatment panel is then placed on the soles of the feet for 10 minutes to work on the reflexology points and boost circulation. At the same time, the pen is used to stimulate additional meridian points.

10 After treatment, the client is offered a glass of water to boost detoxification and after-care and home-care advice is given.

Benefits of treatment

As a holistic treatment, Cosmolight™ has the effect of healing and regenerating a variety of conditions both inside and outside the body, including burns, cold sores, cellulite, eczema, psoriasis, fine lines and wrinkles, scars, stretch marks, spots, sports injuries and general aches and pains. It is suitable for clients of all ages and some conditions will show signs of improvement after just one session.

Skin testers

Electronic skin testers for registering the pH of the skin are widely used in the Far East, and are gaining in popularity throughout the world.

Pressure massage

This is the name given to a range of specialist equipment which causes 'pneumatic' compression of the limbs. Pressure is delivered in a rhythmical manner thus simulating the natural pumping action of muscles and aiding lymphatic flow. The treatment primarily affects the vascular system so is excellent for helping many conditions associated with inefficient blood and lymph circulation, including gravitational oedema and the early stages of cellulite.

Treatment times will vary, but an average session will last about 20–30 minutes and can be combined with other salon services such as facials and massage.

Oriental analysis

Arousing a great deal of interest over recent years, Oriental analysis has grown in popularity in recent months. It involves reading a client's face, hands, feet and body to gain a greater insight into understanding the client's wellbeing, history and personality. It is offered as a postgraduate course for therapists by Eve Taylor at her Institute of Clinical Aromatherapy and is practised worldwide by many of her past students.

Chapter 7

Tanning and light treatments

After working through this chapter you will be able to:

- describe the types of tanning treatments available to clients
- give the main benefits of the different tanning treatments
- list the pre- and after-care advice for tanning treatments
- carry out manual, air brush and automated tanning treatments
- outline the key principles of the electromagnetic spectrum
- state the differences between ultraviolet and infrared treatments
- list the three bands of ultraviolet rays and explain their main effects
- give the main benefits and uses of infrared and ultraviolet treatments.

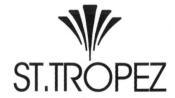

St Tropez logo

information point

Self-tan products will have specific sales benefits, e.g. St Tropez contains a slight tint of green in the formulation to prevent the colour turning orange; it has a guide colour making application easy to see and follow; and it will cover stretch marks and scars.

Social pressure to reduce the growth in skin cancer has brought about a rapid expansion in tanning products that provide the tanned look without the risk of sun exposure. Self-tanning retail products have been around for years but the gap for professional tanning treatments was seen and seized by the market leader in tanning products, St Tropez, who have been supplying UK salons since 1995. They developed their professional tanning treatment and led the way with a strong marketing and PR campaign to develop and expand the tanning treatment market we have today.

As with all markets numerous other companies saw the potential for sales and growth and quickly followed. Today there is a plethora of companies offering tanning treatments for the professional market. To provide an overview of the treatment we have decided to profile the St Tropez range of treatments to recognise the talent of a British woman, Judy Naake, in recognising a niche market and using her skills and knowledge to ensure the brand St Tropez became a household name, not just used by the 'stars', but affordable to all.

Product knowledge

With all treatments a good knowledge and understanding of all the products in the range is essential. A therapist must be able to name each product, its benefit and effects and know which are available in retail size to sell to their clients.

Remember a client is paying for your knowledge and advice so ensure you provide it at all times!

St Tropez products

There are currently seven products in their range: Body Polisher, Body Moisturiser, Tinted Self-Tanning Lotion, Factor 15 Water Resistant Sun Screen, Powder Bronzer, Whipped Bronze Mousse and Bronzing Mist.

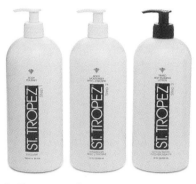

St Tropez products

Body Polisher

This is a gentle exfoliant that is used to refine and prepare the skin for the tanning treatment. The exfoliating ingredient is round beads of polystyrene that gently roll over the surface of the skin, leaving it feeling soft and even.

Body Moisturiser

This product is used professionally as a barrier cream on dry skin, problem areas and to custom blend the tan. At home the tan can be maintained by use of this rich moisturiser.

Tinted Self-Tanning Lotion

This aloe vera-based lotion contains a guide colour for easy application and an instant tan. It is non-greasy and quick drying with a pleasant scent. It is formulated to a maximum strength that can be custom blended with the moisturiser for the desired shade.

Factor 15 Water Resistant Sun Screen

This is a fast drying oil-free formula providing both UVA and UVB protection. It also contains vitamin E and aloe vera. It can be used daily as a moisturiser and protective base to reduce the damaging effects of UV. It is PABA free. PABA (para-aminobenzoic acid) is a colourless or yellowish acid found in the vitamin B complex. It is sold under a variety of names as a sunscreen lotion to prevent skin damage from the sun. It is also used as a local anaesthetic in sunburn products. However, it can cause a reaction in people with highly sensitive skins when exposed to sunlight.

Powder Bronzer

This is a fine, matt pressed powder. It can be used directly on the face or body or over the tanning lotion. It does not contain glitter or lanolin.

Whipped Bronze Mousse

This is an instant bronzing mousse that provides a tan *now*. It dries in 60 seconds and can be used on the face or body anywhere, anytime! It is based on aloe vera leaf juice, is oil-free and has a pleasant scent. The tan produced by the mousse will last 2–3 days and it is very easy to use. However, it must be noted that when wet it can stain clothes.

Bronzing Mist

This is a spray-on mist that is dispensed in a pump action bottle for a quick, simple streak-free tanning application. A weightless application drying in 60 seconds, the Bronzing Mist is perfect for those tanning emergencies and gives a deep tan lasting for days. It is also used with St Tropez Air – The Ultimate Airbrush Tan. This product can also stain clothes when wet so care must be taken.

Manual tanning treatment

Client pre-treatment advice

It is paramount that the therapist and receptionist are aware of the advice that should be given to every client prior to treatment. This includes the following:

- Each client should be issued with a treatment-advice booking slip and where a phone booking is taken this should be posted to the client.

> **information point**
>
> When the tan has developed, gentle use of the St Tropez body polisher will help to maintain the tan and ensure it wears off evenly.

> **information point**
>
> L-Tyrosine acts as a tan accelerator to enhance the body's own production of melanin.

- A patch test should be carried out.
- It is important that clients are informed as to what the treatment involves.
- Clients should be advised to exfoliate and moisturise their skin regularly prior to having the tanning treatment. This will give a smoother surface for the therapist to apply the tan and therefore a much better result will be achieved and the tan will last longer.
- Clients must be advised to stop using any other tanning products 4 days before they have the treatment. If this advice is ignored, the colour and quality of the tan cannot be guaranteed.
- Clients must be advised to wear dark, loose fitting clothing when they come to have this treatment, or bring some with them to change into afterwards. (Where possible, it is better not to wear a bra or any restrictive clothing, jewellery or shoes.
- Old underwear is preferable as the guide colour may stain some man-made fibres.
- If wearing a very tight bodice, perspiration may mark the inside of the outfit on the day.
- It is advisable for brides-to-be to have a trial run 4–6 weeks before their big day and have the treatment 2 days before their wedding, to allow them and their body to adapt to their new appearance.
- Clients should have hair removal carried out 24 hours before having the tanning treatment.

Consultation

A client consultation must be carried out prior to all tanning treatments. Existing client record cards can be adapted or specific ones purchased. This needs to fit with the customer service policy of your salon and is at the discretion of the management.

St Tropez consultation card

Preparation for manual tanning treatment

The therapist must ensure the area is appropriately prepared prior to treatment and will require the following items:

- couch
- trolley
- a large bowl
- waste bin

- couch cover
- a large bath sheet
- 2–3 small hand towels
- 2 body sponges
- 3 mitts
- tissues
- head band
- cotton buds
- cleanser (that does not contain mineral oils)
- body polisher
- body moisturiser
- auto-bronzant
- disposable gloves (tight fitting)
- disposable couch roll which may be used during the exfoliation stage if required
- disposable pants, for the client to wear.

Method

Having prepared the working area the therapist is ready to greet their client from reception and carry out the consultation process. Once the client has undressed and put on the disposable pants they are asked to lie on their back ready for treatment.

Step 1. Preparation for tanning treatment – exfoliation

1 Prepare a large bowl of hand hot water.

2 Cleanse the face using a creamy cleanser, then remove with damp sponges.

3 Mix body polisher with a little cleanser and exfoliate the face, neck and décolleté, using gentle circular movements.

4 Remove the exfoliant with dry towelling mitts followed by damp sponges.

5 Take approximately 1 large pump of body polisher and mix with the water in a cupped hand. Apply to the legs using circular movements, concentrating on the areas prone to dryness such as knees, ankles and feet.

6 Remove with two dry towelling mitts and follow with damp sponges.

7 Pat area dry.

8 Repeat the exfoliation process on the arms and take extra care on the elbows. Ensure any deodorant has been removed.

9 Continue onto the mid section, exfoliating any area where the client wishes to be tanned. Concentrate under the bust.

10 Turn the client over and repeat the process on the back of the legs and the back.

11 Return the client to the original position removing any couch roll that has been used. Brush with a dry towel if necessary to remove final traces of exfoliator.

12 At the end of this stage it is important that the therapist washes their hands.

Step 2. Tanning treatment – application to the face

1 Always start on the face. It is the first area the client will want to touch, so the drier it is at the end of the treatment the better the result will be.

2 Mix 2 pumps each of auto-bronzant and body moisturiser and blend together in your hand.

3 Apply evenly to the face and neck, avoiding the eyes and hairline.

4 Add one small pump of moisturiser to the residue on your hands; blend together for the eyelids, under eyes, ears and into the hairline.

5 Be aware that the more peroxide the client has, the more porous the hair will be, therefore on bleached or grey hair use more moisturiser.

6 Remove the tan from the eyebrows using a cotton bud, carefully.

7 Wash you hands.

8 Put on tight-fitting disposable gloves.

Step 3. Tanning treatment – moisturising the body

Generously moisturise hands, elbows, knees and feet with St Tropez body moisturiser. The product should be left on the surface and not massaged in. Take care to apply the moisturiser exactly where you want it. Moisturiser on other areas may cause a problem result, e.g. lighter marks or patches.

Step 4. Tanning treatment – application to the body
The legs

1 The legs take longer to dry than any other area of the body so it is advisable to tan the legs immediately after the face.

2 Expose one leg at a time. Use approximately 7 pumps of tan and apply using a flat hand, starting at the thigh working towards the knee. Work on the lower leg area stopping short at the ankle. You will see the aloe vera start to emulsify, changing to a creamy colour. At this point stop, and slide the residue/remainder over the knee area, ensuring that it is covered.

3 **Do not massage in; over rubbing causes the aloe vera gel to ball and this will make the tan patchy.**

4 Do not be alarmed if the guide colour is not absolutely even at this stage, remember *brown* streaks are not a problem, the *white* ones are; if there is no product there is no tan.

5 By this stage there should be a minimal amount of tan on the gloves. Take off any excess as required.

6 Add to this 1 pump of moisturiser, blend together and apply to the feet, ensuring you are applying the product between the toes.

7 Wipe the toe nail plates and the soles with a tissue and blend the tan down over the foot and ankle, ensuring you do not take moisturiser up the leg.

8 Cover the leg, even though it may still be wet, this will not affect the tan.

9 Repeat on the other leg.

The arms

1 Position the client's arm so it is lying flat at their side.

2 Starting at the shoulder apply approximately 3 pumps of tan to the outer arm working to the wrist, avoiding the elbow joint and the hand.

3 Taking 1 pump of tan and 1 of moisturiser, blend in your hands, lift the client's arm, hold at the wrist and apply to the inner arm including the under arm area and over the elbow.

4 Check your gloves and remove any excess, add 1 pump of moisturiser to the residue, blend thoroughly to cover the hand.

5 Tissue the palms, nail plates and wrist creases.

6 When using a fake tan the wrists are always difficult, therefore take a tiny spot of moisturiser into the creases, blending carefully upwards to create a subtle wrist.

7 Blend the colour carefully over the back of the wrist.

8 Repeat on the other arm.

The bust and abdomen

1 Using full strength tan, apply approximately 7 pumps, using the same technique, from the bikini line to the clavicle.

2 Do not be alarmed if this area of the body looks streaky, as you are working in different directions, providing there is ample coverage the final result will be perfect.

3 Apply a small amount of moisturiser to your gloves and blend up the clavicle.

The back of the legs

1 Use 7 pumps of tan for the back of the leg. When applying the tan to the back of the leg keep out of the heel crease and ensure you join the tan to the front of the leg.

2 Apply a small amount of moisturiser into the heel crease and blend the tan around the ankle bones.

3 Repeat on the other leg.

The back

1 Use full strength tan on the back of the body, using approximately 7 pumps. Apply up to the T-shirt line at the back of the neck then blend up into the hairline with a small amount of moisturiser.

2 Join neck at the sides and check behind the ears.

3 Leave the client lying face down, remove your gloves and tidy up your working area, allowing the tan to dry.

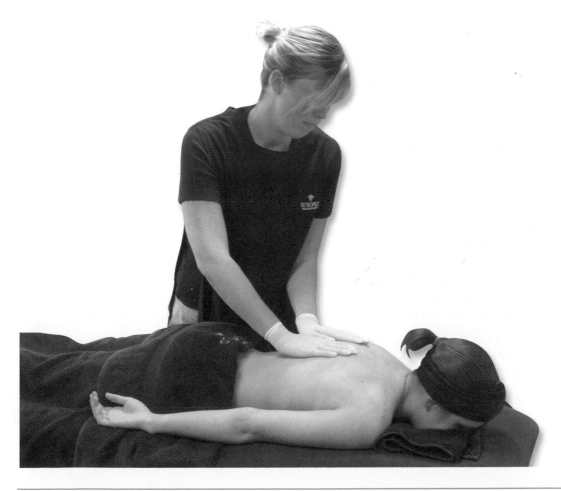

St Tropez application

Step 5. Tanning treatment – buffing the body

This is an essential part of the treatment to ensure client satisfaction and to send the client out of the salon looking perfect.

1   Turn the client over. Take one clean soft mitt, and using a flat hand gently stroke the face removing any excess guide colour.

2   Working in the same order as you applied the tan, work around the body gently lifting off the excess guide colour.

3   Start with the legs and move to the arms and mid-section.

4   Turn the client over once more and repeat the process on the legs and back.

5   Buffing essentially involves using long, soft, sweeping strokes to even out the appearances; however, be careful, as excessive rubbing will create an uneven result.

Client after treatment advice

To ensure the client receives the correct home-care and sales advice, it is important that the receptionist as well as the therapist is fully trained in the after-care service and this should include the following:

1   Remind the clients of the pre-treatment booking slips which gives after-care advice (this puts the onus on the client and legally protects you). This advice includes:

- Clients must be informed not to shower or bathe for at least 4 hours after the tanning treatment. Overnight is ideal.
- Clients must not take part in any activity that will induce perspiration during the tanning development time.
- Clients must not get their skin wet during the tanning development time.
- Clients must not apply any deodorant, perfume, body products or make-up while the guide colour is still on the skin.
- When leaving the salon, any restrictive clothing, footwear or jewellery may affect the result.
- It is not advisable to have any other treatments on the same day.
- It is recommended that clients do not swim after having had the treatment as the chlorine in swimming pools does bleach the tan.
- Clients should be advised to gently body polish, using the body polisher, every 3–4 days to prolong the tan and help it wear off evenly.
- Clients should also be advised to use moisturiser, as it will help to prolong the life of the tan.
- The tan will generally last 7–10 days depending on how the client treats her skin and her lifestyle.

2   Retail the recommended products, always ensuring that a 'Products and Application' leaflet accompanies a sale.

3   Make the client another appointment.

information point

- Dihydroxyacetone (DHA) is the tanning agent used in self-tanning lotions; it has no known toxicity. It is derived from fructose and is also used as an emulsifier, humectant and fungicide.
- The Food and Drug Administration in the USA declares that this colour additive is safe and suitable for use in cosmetics and drugs that are applied to colour the skin (self-tans).
- It is a white powder that turns colourless in liquid form.
- DHA works with the bacteria and amino acids on the surface of the skin. (Skin chemistry is unique. Therefore different results occur from person to person and even area to area.)
- It colours the skin a brown shade, giving it a sun-tanned appearance.
- It has a sweet taste and characteristic odour.
- It is currently used in most self-tans on the market, in varying quantities.

Pigmentation disorders

The therapist must give the appropriate advice to clients with pigmentation disorders wanting to use self-tanning products. As the ingredients, etc. vary from manufacturer to manufacturer it is important to seek clarification from the supplying company on what effect their tanning products will have.

Vitiligo

The St Tropez tan will cover vitiligo; however, it will not disguise this pigmentation disorder in one application.

Instructions for disguising vitiligo

1 Apply the full strength tan to the lighter areas as thickly as possible, custom blend using the moisturiser with a cotton bud to the darker edges if necessary.

2 Allow to dry. Do not worry if it looks streaky at this stage.

3 Allow to develop, ideally overnight.

4 Wash off the guide colour.

5 If the tan is not dark enough, repeat approximately every 8 hours until the vitiligo patch is disguised.

6 Finally apply the tan, either as a full strength application or mixed with the moisturiser over the whole area.

Hyperpigmentation

Using a self-tan will make areas of pigmentation darker but to even out patchy pigmentation try applying the product around the patch or custom blend the tan and moisturiser together. It is really a case of trial and error; all skin types are different, the texture, skin chemistry, hydration and colour is unique and it is impossible to say exactly what will happen.

General points on results and products

If a client is very pale, it should be explained that their skin will have a subtle colour. A second application may be required to give a more tanned look. (Often clients like the effect after one application and do not wish to appear too dark.)

If a client is already tanned or has recently come back from holiday, their tan will be enhanced.

The shelf life of the body polisher and moisturiser is approximately 2 years. Auto-bronzant will last 6–9 months once opened, 2 years unopened. It is recommend to lock the pumps between use.

St Tropez tanning products are all safe and suitable for pregnant ladies, providing there are no other contraindications, as is the treatment. (The abdomen can be omitted if the client prefers and it may be necessary to adapt the treatment position.) Leave the nipple area if breast feeding!

Clients all have unique body chemistry and the tan reacts differently on each individual. (Rather like perfume gives a unique aroma on different people.)

Trouble-shooting

If you experience a problem result, it is probably down to human error, either something that the therapist has done during application or something that the client has done after leaving the salon.

GOOD PRACTICE

With vitiligo, either perform the treatment in the salon, or retail a bottle for the client to do at home, prior to coming in for an all-over tan.

information point

An uneven sun tan e.g. watch strap marks or bikini strap marks can be disguised in the same way as vitiligo.

information point

In general tanning products do not contain sun filters so a client will tan and burn through a self-tan. A SPF (sun protection factor) product must be used if the client is going out into the sun. It is important to check with the company which SPF product is compatible with their tanning products. In the case of St Tropez a SPF 15 sunscreen is compatible with their tan.

Remember that the results of a self-tan are only as good as the skin you are applying it to. As a therapist you can only work with what you have got. If the client has dry, uneven patches of skin or uneven pigmentation it is advisable to point this out tactfully/professionally during the exfoliation stage.

If a problem arises, you have to try and establish what has gone wrong, in order that it can be avoided in the future. You also need to put right the situation for the client – this can be tricky!

Each problem needs to be treated individually as and when it arises.

The first thing you should say to the client is 'come back to the salon and show me'.

It is very difficult to trouble-shoot over the telephone, you do need to see the client in order to assess the situation. Here are a few guidelines based on experience!

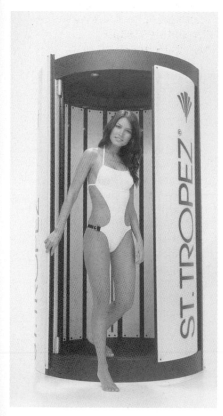

St Tropez Airport

<table>
<tr><td>REMEMBER</td></tr>
<tr><td>If a tan develops well on one part of the body and not so well on the other, it must be due either to the application technique, the skin texture before application or client actions afterwards.</td></tr>
</table>

Problem:	A streaky tan
Reason:	Something left on the skin beforehand, or
	Insufficient tan being applied, or
	Over-rubbing of the tan, or
	Client not following the after-care advice.
Action:	Exfoliate to try and even out the streaks, apply product again either full strength or 50/50 depending on the colour and situation.

Problem:	White patches
Reason:	Something left on the skin beforehand, or
	Spreading the moisturiser too far, or
	Missed patch during application, or
	Client not following the after-care advice.
Action:	Apply more tan carefully to the white patch.

Problem:	Dark patches
Reason:	Texture/colour of skin before application.
Action:	Gently exfoliate to try and even out the colour.

Problem:	No colour developed
Reason:	Client on strong medication, or
	Individual body chemistry of client, or
	Client showering too soon.
Action:	Discuss all of the above and maybe try a patch test.

Automated/air brush tanning treatments

Over the last two years tanning treatments have taken on a new dimension through the introduction of self-tanning booths and airbrushing. There are numerous companies retailing airbrush tans and electronic self-tanning booths but again after researching the market our decision is to profile the St Tropez systems, namely 'the Airport'.

When selecting an automated/manual booth system, it is essential that consideration is given to the warranty and service offered by the company.

To maintain any electrical equipment in good working order, it is essential that the owner and therapists carefully follow the maintenance guidance provided by the company.

Airport Service and Maintenance

Warranty:

All Airports are supplied with a 12-month warranty (parts and labour). An additional extended warranty may be purchased directly from Imagen, which would be renewable on a yearly basis. Imagen undertake all warranty obligations on the equipment within the UK.

Service:

The first year service agreement is purchased with all new Airports. Imagen provide the Service Agreement, which includes refurbishment of the system following six months and 12 months of operation. As with the warranty, this service can be extended on a yearly basis.

St Tropez Airport warranty and service

Maintenance of the Airport

At the end of each day:

- Switch off the Airport and ensure the booth is not left running overnight.
- Clean the inner spray chamber skins, the foot grate and the surrounding floor area with a damp cloth.

Weekly:

- Using the cleaning brush provided, gently scrub the nozzle area of the spray gun to remove any St Tropez residue.

Monthly:

- Replace the primary filter below the foot grate.

The air brush treatment

The air brush tanning treatment is carried out with the client standing inside the booth which ensures all the spray tan is drawn down away from the client restricting inhalation of the product. It also ensures a touch dry tan at the end of the treatment.

Pre-treatment advice

It is important that the client is given the following advice when booking their treatment:

- Do not wax or shave on the morning of the treatment.
- It is preferable not to apply any type of perfume, deodorant or aromatherapy oils as they may affect the treatment.
- The evening before your application you will need to exfoliate your entire body paying special attention to dry areas such as elbows and knees before moisturising.
- Wear dark, loose fitting clothes.

Method

Prior to carrying out the treatment the therapist should carry out a self-tanning consultation ensuring the client does not suffer with any respiratory problems or if they do that they have sought medical approval prior to treatment. Then they must thoroughly explain the procedure and after-care advice to the client:

information point

St Tropez is distributed in the UK by Beauty Source Ltd, they can be contacted at:
Beauty Source Ltd
Unit 4C Tissington Close,
Nottingham, NG9 6QG
Tel: 0115 9836363;
Fax: 0115 9836350

1 The client enters the Airport and, whilst standing in a warm air stream, St Tropez Bronzing Mist is applied by a trained professional using a spray gun. The treatment takes just a few minutes to cover the whole body offering a quick flawless tan. After the application the client stands in the warm air stream for a few minutes to allow the tan to dry so they can step back into their clothes straight after the treatment.

2 On leaving the salon:
- The tan will start to develop 2–3 hours after application and continue to develop for up to 24 hours. Therefore it is preferable not to shower for up to 8 hours after the application.
- Any product left on cotton bed linen will wash out.
- It is recommended that clients avoid any activity that may cause perspiration during the development time.

3 Maintaining the tan:
- With the correct after-care the tan will last longer.
- Apply St Tropez Body Moisturiser, a hydrating body lotion containing l-tyrosine. This ingredient activates the melanin in the skin ensuring the tan lasts the longest possible time.
- Avoid exfoliating the skin until the tan has naturally worn off. Do not rub but pat the skin dry after showering.
- Avoid swimming pools, as chlorine will bleach the tan.

SELF-CHECKS

1 Why is it important to moisturise the elbows and knees prior to tanning treatments?

2 Why are self-tanning treatments so popular?

3 At what stage in a tanning treatment is the client's skin exfoliated?

4 When in the manual tanning treatment is the tan applied to the face and why?

ACTIVITY

Research the different manual and automated tanning systems on the market and make up a table comparing their key benefits and after-service warranty.

GOOD PRACTICE

If the client suffers from any respiratory problems, they must consult their doctor before booking a treatment.

information point

The distance between the air gun and the skin is approximately 20 cm (8 inches) unless spraying the hands and feet. Only spray the product on the *downward* stroke and always keep the airgun *straight*, in a level position. Spray product until you see a sheen on the skin, almost as if the client was perspiring lightly.

Manual air brush application

1 The therapist should wear tight fitting disposable gloves to protect their hands.

2 Ask the client to remove their glasses, jewellery, deodorant, perfume and make-up prior to the treatment.

3 Ensure the client has exfoliated themselves prior to treatment and if they haven't ensure they shower and exfoliate in the salon (always have retail products in the shower area as this helps in selling the products afterwards).

4 Provide the client with disposable pants and a hair turban to protect their hair. A black bikini or black underwear may be worn but the mist product will come in contact with the fabric.

5 Ask the client to step onto the self-adhesive foot protectors and then enter the Airport, standing centrally and facing forward.

6 The therapist or client must apply a generous coating of moisturiser to the client's hands and tops of their feet, paying particular attention to the nails and cuticles.

7 If the client's elbows and knees are dry apply moisturiser to the tip of the elbows and knees.

8 Explain to the client the sensation they will feel as the air and mist is dispelled from the air gun.

9 Ask the client to step inside the booth facing the therapist.

10 Ask the client to take a deep breath on the count of three whilst you work down the face, repeat this if needed to ensure all of the face is equally covered.

11 Ask the client to stand upright with their head back and arms out then apply the tan working down the neck to their pants.

12 Ask the client to pull their body upright and raise their arms up in the air, this lifts the breasts up enabling the therapist to spray out under the breasts.

13 Apply the tan to the legs working down the leg ensuring full coverage.

14 With the client facing you sideways on ask them to raise their arm up in the air with their fist clenched then apply the tan stating lightly at the wrist working down under the arm and down the side of the body (remember the distance of the air brush to the skin increases around the wrist and hands). Ask the client to lower their arm down slightly out from the body then apply the tan moving down from the shoulder and off at the hand. Repeat this on the other side.

15 With the client's back facing you ask them to fold their arms across their chest then using the air brush release the tan starting at the top of the right shoulder working smoothly down the back; take your finger off the release button and move to the top of the back, continue working down the back until you have reached the other side.

16 Apply the tan to the legs following the same pattern as on the back.

17 Whilst the client stands in the warm airflow to dry, check the whole body to ensure an even application of tan.

18 The client leaves the Airport stepping onto disposable paper. The disposable shoes are removed (place the shoes in a lined waste bin).

19 Advise the client not to touch the tan until completely dry and repeat the after-care advice outlined in the Treatment Advice Slip.

20 If the client has very fair eyebrows, wipe over the eyebrows with a cotton bud.

St Tropez Auto Airport

The Auto Airport is a unit designed to evenly spray the client with atomised St Tropez Bronzing Mist to create the perfect tan. This deluxe treatment enables a salon to maximise profit through automated tanning treatments. These operate with little interaction with a therapist although it is paramount that each client is given pre and after-care advice either by a trained receptionist or therapist. Many salons operate these treatments by providing and displaying guidance on the use of the tanning booths.

To obtain the best results from the Airport treatment it is paramount that the client has followed the pre-treatment advice:

- Do not wax or shave on the morning of the treatment.
- It is preferable not to apply any type of perfume, deodorant or aromatherapy oils as they may affect the treatment.
- The evening before your application you will need to exfoliate your entire body paying special attention to dry areas such as elbows and knees before moisturising.
- Wear dark, loose fitting clothes.

GOOD PRACTICE

- Always hold the gun straight.
- Only spray product on the downward stroke.
- Always follow the same routine.

information point

- If the client is obese, it will be necessary to make them stretch in different directions to ensure even coverage of the tan, this is only possible with the air gun application.
- If a client has a hairy chest or back it is not advisable to offer these tanning treatments as the hair will restrict the tan being applied to the skin.

A consultation should be carried out and the following information given:

Before entering the booth:

- Protect hair with a turban.
- Place self-adhesive protectors on feet, ensuring that you step firmly on the pressure sensitive pads.
- Apply a generous coating of moisturiser to hands and tops of the feet. Pay particular attention to the nails and cuticles.
- Apply moisturiser to the tip of the elbows and knees if the skin is very dry.

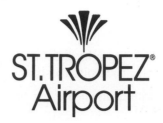

ST.TROPEZ® Airport

Treatment Advice for the Client

What is Airport?
Airport is a unit designed to evenly spray you with atomised St. Tropez Bronzing Mist in a warm and comfortable environment. Application is quick, safe and easy and enables a flawless St.Tropez tan to be achieved in a lunch break!

Preparation for Application
Do not wax or shave on the morning of the treatment.

It is preferable not to apply any type of perfume, deodorant or aromatherapy oils as they may affect the treatment.

The **evening before** your application you will need to exfoliate your entire body, using the St. Tropez Body Polish. Pay special attention to dry areas of the body such as hands elbows knees and feet before moisturising with the St. Tropez Body Moisturiser.

Wear dark, loose fitting clothes.

Application
You enter Airport and whilst standing in a warm air stream St. Tropez Bronzing Mist is applied by a trained professional using a spray gun. The treatment takes just a few minutes to cover the whole body.

Following the application you stand in the warm air stream for a few minutes to allow the tan to dry so you can step back into your clothes straight after the treatment.

Once leaving the salon
The tan will start to develop 2-3 hours after application and continue to develop for up to 24 hours. Therefore it is preferable not to shower for up to 8 hours after the application.

Any product left on cotton bed linen will wash out.

Do not take part in any activity, which may cause perspiration during development time.

Maintaining your tan
With the correct aftercare your tan will last longer

Daily apply St. Tropez Body Moisturiser, a hydrating body lotion containing l-tyrosine. This ingredient activates the melanin in the skin ensuring your tan lasts the longest possible time.

Exfoliate your skin with St.Tropez Body Polish every 2 days to ensure your tan fades evenly.

Do not rub but pat the skin dry after showering or bathing.

Avoid swimming pools, as chlorine will bleach your tan.

St Tropez advice slip

* If you suffer from respiratory problems, please consult your doctor before booking your treatment.

Within the booth:

- Before pressing the start button, carefully step into the booth, facing the spray jets and relax.
- Position your feet with the backs of your heels on the edge of the footplate.
- Hold your head upright and do not look down during the spray cycle.
- Your head will be sprayed during the four spray cycles. During the few seconds that the head is being sprayed, please keep your eyes shut and hold your breath.
- Remember to stand in the position shown by the manufacture and stay still during each spray cycle described.

Drying:

- When the spray cycle is complete stand in a relaxed pose with the hands slightly away from your sides for the duration of the dry cycle (approximately 2 minutes).
- When the green light around the start button goes out, carefully exit the booth.

After leaving the tanning booth:

- Remove foot protectors.
- Wipe the nail plates with a tissue to remove any tan.
- The tan will fully develop over the next 12 hours.
- To gain best results follow the St Tropez advice slip.

SELF-CHECKS

1   Why is an automated tanning treatment not suitable for a male with a hairy chest or an obese client?

2   What type of tanning treatment is most beneficial for an obese client?

3   What is the pre-treatment advice given to a client prior to an automated tanning treatment?

4   State the home-care advice for a manual tanning treatment.

Light treatments

There are two main forms of radiation that the therapist needs to be aware of, each forming part of the electromagnetic spectrum. *Ultraviolet* is used mainly for its skin tanning effects while *infrared* is used as a method of warming the tissues for therapeutic purposes.

The electromagnetic spectrum

The electromagnetic spectrum consists of a continuous band of radiation given off from the sun in varying frequencies and wavelengths. The radiation given off can be divided into bands according to their wavelength:

- Gamma rays (shortest wavelength).
- X-rays.
- Ultraviolet rays.
- Visible light (red, orange, yellow, green, blue, indigo, violet).
- Infrared rays.
- Radio waves (longest wavelength).

Wavelengths are typically measured in nanometres (nm). A nanometre is a millionth of a millimetre. The wavelengths of visible light are in the range between 400 and 770 nm with the lower (shorter) wavelengths being at the blue end of the visible spectrum and the higher (longer) wavelengths being at the red end of the visible spectrum. Infrared rays have wavelengths in the range of 770 to 4000 nm while ultraviolet rays have wavelengths between 200 to 400 nm.

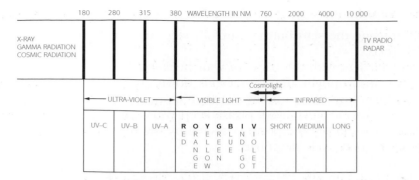

			R									

Spectrum of electromagnetic radiation

Electromagnetic rays can be uniquely defined in terms of their wavelength. The wavelength is defined as the distance from the point on one wave to the same point on the next wave. Rays also have a frequency which is defined as the number of cycles or complete waves that pass a fixed point each second. Frequency is calculated and shown as a reading of hertz, i.e. the number of cycles per second. Shorter wavelengths such as ultraviolet will have a higher frequency than longer wavelengths such as infrared because they require more cycles to cover the same distance.

The bands of radiation used in therapy treatments are ultraviolet and infrared.

Infrared radiation

As mentioned previously, infrared rays have wavelengths of the order 770 to 4000 nm, which means that they have longer wavelengths than visible light. This form of radiation can be divided into two bands:

- infrared rays which are longer wavelength rays of approximately 4000 nm
- radiant heat rays which are shorter wavelength rays of approximately 1000 nm.

An infrared lamp or non-luminous lamp type emits a gentle warmth with a barely detectable glow. The lamp operates at a fairly low temperature so the intensity of the output is also low.

A radiant heat lamp or luminous lamp type emits a more intense heat with a very visible glow. The lamp operates at a much higher temperature with an output of heat radiation and visible light.

Infrared and radiant heat lamps are used in therapy treatments to warm the tissues and the difference in the wavelengths produces varying effects. Traditionally, in beauty therapy, a warm source is used to produce the infrared energy and the bulbs are then coated red to indicate a hot surface.

Infrared rays penetrate the epidermal layer only irritating the cells to release histamine which results in the blood vessels dilating thus generating heat in the tissues. This redness is often termed hyperaemia and has a soothing effect as opposed to a stimulating one as the nerve endings are not greatly affected.

Radiant heat rays penetrate into the dermal layers causing immediate dilation of the blood and lymph vessels which forces the fluids away from the skin into the underlying structures producing a deep heat effect.

Types of infrared equipment

Infrared and radiant heat lamps normally come in the following forms:

- Fireclay lamp – this is basically a wire coil surrounding a clay support with a reflector shield.
- Filament lamp – this is like a large light bulb that also contains a built-in reflector shield and is made from red-coloured glass. Dimmer devices are added

so the intensity of the lamp can be reduced to emit infrared rays as opposed to radiant heat.

- Quartz heat lamp – this type normally contain quartz rods with a heating element inside. (Sometimes seen as old-fashioned bathroom heaters.)

There is a European recommendation that when using high wattage bulbs the cowl, the part that holds the bulb, should be double skinned to allow an outer and an inner space between the bulb and the cowl. This creates a cooling effect as air drawn into the lower ventilating holes or slits warms, rises, and flows out through the upper ventilation holes or slits.

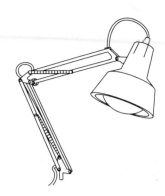

Infrared heat lamp

General effects of infrared and radiant heat on the body

Infrared and radiant heat are used in the therapy clinic as a general heat treatment to help relax the client and to relieve pain and tension. These effects are achieved as:

- Metabolism is speeded up as a result of the increased heat which will ultimately increase the demand for oxygen and nutrients and speed up the excretion of waste and toxins.
- Vasodilation occurs due to the heat on the blood vessels increasing blood circulation.
- Sudoriferous gland activity is increased due to the vasodilation effect (this will bring about further elimination of waste products).
- There is a soothing effect on sensory nerve endings.

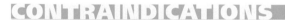

CONTRAINDICATIONS

to infrared and radiant heat treatments
- Heart and vascular conditions.
- Fever, heavy colds and influenza.
- Skin diseases and disorders.
- High or low blood pressure.
- Burns and sunburn.
- Metal pins and plates.
- Diabetes (due to impaired circulation).
- Oedema.
- Cuts, scars and skin abrasions.

Harmful effects of infrared and radiant heat treatment

If the treatment is not carried out correctly any of the following may occur:

- Burning of the skin.
- Giddiness or fainting.
- Headaches.
- Permanent eye injury.

Safety precautions for infrared and radiant heat treatment

- Always carry out a detailed consultation before treatment checking for any contraindications.
- Always follow manufacturer's instructions with regard to operating any equipment.
- Accurately time and position the lamp according to the cosine and inverse square laws (see pp. 214–15).
- Protect the client's eyes.

- Ensure skin is properly prepared and carry out a skin sensitivity test prior to treatment. (See Chapter 5.)
- Ensure lamp is secure with no trailing wires, is dust-free and is regularly serviced.
- Preheat lamp before positioning over treatment area.
- Do not leave the client unattended.

SELF-CHECKS

1 List the key principles of the electromagnetic spectrum.

2 Name the three types of infrared equipment available.

3 What is the average wattage of an infrared bulb?

4 List four effects of infrared/radiant heat.

5 List five contraindications to infrared and radiant heat treatments.

The cosine law

The cosine law shows the comparison between intensity of rays and the angle at which these rays make contact with the skin. The lamp should be placed perpendicular to the skin ensuring the rays fall at right angles to the body which will give maximum intensity.

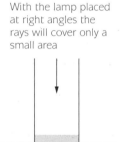

With the lamp placed at right angles the rays will cover only a small area

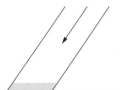

With the lamp placed at a reduced angle the rays now cover a larger area thus reducing the intensity

The cosine law

The inverse square law

With any radiation treatment distance is extremely important and in particular it is important when using ultraviolet where very little heat is generated. It goes without saying that the closer a lamp is to the body the higher the intensity of radiation will be. The inverse square law states that the intensity of radiation will differ inversely with the square of the distance from the lamp. This means that if the distance from

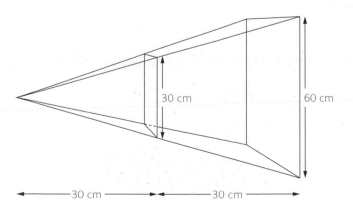

30 cm

60 cm

30 cm

30 cm

The inverse square law

the lamp is doubled the intensity of the rays will be quartered. In practical terms the intensity of radiation at a distance of 30 cm is four times that at 60 cm, i.e. 4 minutes' treatment at 60 cm will give the same effect as 1 minute's at 30 cm.

ACTIVITY

Research the uses of infrared heat treatments within a health spa.

Ultraviolet radiation

Ultraviolet rays have wavelengths within the range of 200 to 400 nm, i.e. beyond the violet end of the visible light spectrum.

They are invisible to the naked eye and are classified as follows:

- UVA rays.
- UVB rays.
- UVC rays.

UVA rays

UVA rays have wavelengths of 315–400 nm and penetrate deeply into the dermal layer of the skin. This damages the collagen and elastin fibres causing premature ageing together with increasing the risk of skin cancer. UVA rays expand melanin already present within the skin causing a short-term tanning effect.

UVB rays

UVB rays have wavelengths of 280–315 nm and will penetrate only to the basal layer of the epidermis. UVB stimulates melanocytes present in this layer to produce more melanin causing a much deeper, longer lasting colour than UVA alone. It is UVB which causes thickening of the epidermis and is also responsible for sunburn and for the development of skin cancers.

Pre-sensitisation test

This should be carried out 24 hours before the client wishes to have the UVB treatment. One way to carry out such a test is to take a sheet of paper and cut four small holes in a line about 1 cm apart. Place the sheet over the forearm and mount the UV lamp at the standard distance. Expose the area to UV rays for 1½ minutes then cover over the first hole, continue UV exposure and after a further 30 seconds cover over the second hole, after another 30 seconds cover the third hole and the final hole after another 30 seconds. The arm should be inspected the following day to see which of the areas most closely resembles a first degree erythema so the appropriate exposure time can be worked out for the client.

information point

- If a client chooses or is recommended to have a UVB treatment, a pre-sensitisation and a skin sensitivity test (see Chapter 5) must be carried out in addition to the therapist observing contraindications and safety precautions.
- It is paramount that the cosine and inverse square laws are implemented.

Ultraviolet and infrared penetration of the skin

UVC rays

UVC rays have a wavelength shorter than 280 nm and are harmful to living cells. UVC rays are absorbed by the earth's atmosphere and therefore are not found in natural sunlight or used in salon tanning treatments.

The effects of ultraviolet radiation

Current research into the effects of ultraviolet radiation have proved that it is responsible for premature ageing of the skin together with being the primary cause of skin cancer. In extreme moderation, however, there are some beneficial effects:

- Has a slightly germicidal effect on the skin.
- Causes hyperkeratinisation which is thought to help with some skin conditions such as acne vulgaris and psoriasis.
- Gives a psychological feeling of wellbeing.
- Produces a tan.

Harmful effects of ultraviolet treatment

- May cause sunburn if exposure is too long.
- Is the primary cause of skin cancer.
- Thickens the epidermis giving a 'leathery' appearance.
- Irreversibly damages collagen and elastin fibres leading to premature ageing.
- Causes dehydration of the skin tissues.
- Can cause allergic reactions.
- Can produce dark pigmentation patches.

The tanning mechanism

Ultraviolet rays are absorbed by the skin where they stimulate an enzyme called *tyrosinase*, found within the epidermis, which converts into an amino-acid known as *tyrosin* which then changes into *melanin*. This is an immediate response to exposure to ultraviolet and is followed by the increased production of new skin cells which quickly migrate to the stratum corneum layer to develop in colour. Prolonged exposure to UVB in particular will stimulate greater melanocyte production causing a deep and lasting tan.

The way in which this tanning mechanism works will depend on the individual skin type and colouring. These skin types are normally categorised as follows:

- Group 1 – very sensitive, burns easily and never develops a tan.
- Group 2 – sensitive skin which burns easily and tans with difficulty.
- Group 3 – normal skin which tans fairly slowly and may burn slightly.
- Group 4 – tans very easily without burning.
- Group 5 – genetically pigmented skin which rarely burns.

Sunburn

Sunburn is the result of damage to the skin and is the body's way of protecting itself. Sunburn presents as erythema a few hours after exposure. Erythema is the result of histamine being released in the tissues which causes dilation of the blood capillaries. In extreme cases plasma exudes from the blood vessels into the tissues causing blisters.

There are four degrees of erythema which are as follows:

- First degree – presents as slight redness with no irritation and disappears after 24 hours.
- Second degree – presents as a more marked redness with irritation lasting for 2–3 days.
- Third degree – presents as very hot skin which is sore and swollen with pigmentation and lasts for up to one week; desquamation will occur.
- Fourth degree – this is similar to a third degree with the addition of blisters and peeling. This can be quite serious and require medical treatment.

HEALTH AND BEAUTY THERAPY: A PRACTICAL APPROACH

SELF-CHECKS

1. Briefly explain the relevance of the cosine and inverse square laws.
2. Give the three bands of ultraviolet rays and explain their main effects.
3. State the purpose of the skin sensitivity and pre-sensitisation tests.
4. List the contraindications to ultraviolet treatments.
5. Give five harmful effects of ultraviolet radiation.
6. Briefly outline the stages of tanning.
7. Give a brief description of the four degrees of sunburn.

Types of ultraviolet equipment

Within the beauty salon ultraviolet radiation can be utilised in four ways:

- Mercury vapour lamps.
- Solarium.
- Sun-bed.
- Wood lamp.

Mercury vapour lamps

This type of equipment consists of a lamp surrounded by a layer of quartz, which allows UV rays to pass through. The space between contains argon gas and a small amount of mercury. Two electrodes are encased at either end. When the unit is switched on, ionisation of the argon gas occurs and electrons flow through the tube; this, together with the ionisation of the mercury, produces ultraviolet radiation. This type of equipment is rarely used in the therapy clinic but can be seen in hospitals for the treatment of certain skin conditions such as psoriasis.

Solarium

These normally consist of a lamp or a group of lamps suspended in an overhead fashion and often combining infrared bulbs with UVB emitters. Traditionally these were used for either preparing the client's skin for exposure to sunlight by using UVB rays or for preparing the client for further salon treatments, such as massage, by using the infrared lamps contained within the unit.

Modern technology has seen the development of solarium-type units which encompass a padded bed area and air conditioning together with a small, high-pressure area for the face. Some also include music facilities. Those with infrared as well as ultraviolet rays generate more heat and thus have a relaxing effect for the client. Individual manufacturer's instructions need to be followed closely to calculate treatment exposure and classify the type of UV rays emitted.

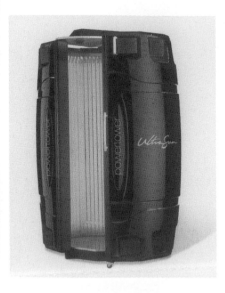

Ultrasun Powertower™

Sun-beds

These are the most popular form of UV equipment seen in the salon today and normally consist of a single or double-sided plastic covered bed containing UV tubes. Modern beds are usually contoured to ensure even tanning treatment. The tubes are often made from a product called Vita-glass™ which allows the UV rays to pass through. Vita-glass™ has a phosphorous lining which absorbs UVC and most UVB rays thereby emitting almost exclusively UVA. At the ends of the sun-bed tube the rating and specification will be stamped. Those with a built-in reflector will be marked R-UVA. Great care must be taken to ensure the correct type of replacement lamp is chosen for each sun-bed.

Note: R-UVA tubes should not be fitted into early models of sun-bed which have reflector panels between each lamp fitting position because a 'striped' tan will result! Check ratings of lamps carefully and consider the overall intensity per bed according to the number of lamps used.

GOOD PRACTICE

- Always ensure the plastic surfaces have been cleaned between clients, using a specific product for the purpose, as the wrong type of cleaner can damage them.
- Always use the manufacturer's recommended emission tubes and keep detailed records of tube use.
- Never leave a client unattended throughout the treatment.

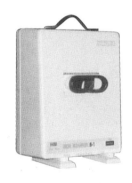

Wood lamp and skin scanner

Wood lamp

Wood lamps can be used to assist the therapist in the analysis of their client's skin. 'Black' ultraviolet tubes illuminate skin conditions in degrees of reflected light, which gives a far clearer view than the naked eye sees in normal light. A variety of lamps is available; traditionally they are designed to be used in a darkened room. Some incorporate the use of a magnifying lamp and a black-out screen; the most consumer conscious enable the client to view their skin 'illuminated' at the same time as the therapist. An accurate and very visual analysis of their skin condition is very motivating and encourages a client to follow the treatment and home care schedule recommended by their therapist.

Ultraviolet treatment

As with any salon treatment, a detailed consultation should be carried out with the client before using UV equipment. Contraindications and a skin sensitivity and/or pre-sensitisation test should be checked thoroughly.

CONTRAINDICATIONS

to ultraviolet treatments
- Any person who does not tan naturally in the sun.
- Any person prone to frequent bouts of cold sores (herpes simplex).
- Pigmentation disorders: vitiligo, chloasma.
- Vascular problems.
- Migraine and headache suffers.
- Any person prone to fainting.
- Pregnancy (as this may lead to increased pigmentation – chloasma).
- Previous history of skin cancer, problems with moles.
- Fever, colds and high temperature.
- Certain drugs may cause photosensitisation: antibiotics, tranquillisers, diuretics, contraceptive pills, anti-diabetic tablets, cold injections, quinine, blood pressure medications. (Consent from the client's GP will be required in these cases.)

- Pressure points do not tan as the blood supply is minimised to the part of the body under pressure thus preventing oxidisation of melanin.
- Controversy over the safety of sun-tanning treatments, and in particular their correct use, is likely to result in more detailed legislation being developed over the coming years.
- In certain countries such as Thailand, Malaysia, etc. tanning treatments are not popular.
- In Australia extremely high levels of natural sunlight and an outdoor way of life from an early age, together with the controversy over the depletion of the ozone layer, has resulted in the formation of cancer councils and foundations across the Australian states. These aim to promote public awareness of protection of the skin from possible skin cancers.

Safety precautions for ultraviolet treatment

If it is considered safe to give treatment the client must:

- Remove all make-up and perfume and ensure that the skin is completely dry.
- Remove watches and jewellery and contact lenses.
- Shower with an unperfumed product.
- Cover hair, especially if treated with colours or permanent wave solutions.
- Avoid applying any suntan preparations except those recommended for UV treatments by specialist manufacturers.
- Wear protective goggles at all times.

Check the client's skin type and colouring. Explain all procedures clearly to the client and supervise the treatment at all times. Ensure that high standards of hygiene are maintained in the treatment area and that the manufacturer's instructions are clearly followed. Specialist clothing which has a UV protection factor of 40 can be purchased.

GOOD PRACTICE

- Treatment should be discontinued if the client has any adverse reaction to the treatment.
- Accurate records should be kept of all treatments given.
- Ideally, perspiration during a sun-bed treatment should be minimal. Most beds contain body-cooling fans to reduce sudoriferous gland activity.
- It is essential that the sun-bed room has sufficient ventilation.

ACTIVITY

Research the variety of sun-tanning equipment available. Compare their cost, size, facilities, durability and cost-effectiveness within a salon environment.

SELF-CHECKS

1 Explain the benefits of using a wood lamp in the salon.
2 State the differences between ultraviolet and infrared treatments.
3 State the main benefits and uses of infrared and ultraviolet treatments.
4 List the safety precautions to be observed when carrying out:
   a solarium treatment
   b infrared treatment.
5 Explain why pressure marks from a sun-bed do not tan.

KEY TERMS

You need to know what these words and phrases mean. Go back through the chapter to find out.

Auto tanning treatments

Air brush tanning treatments

Manual tanning treatment

Cosine law

Electromagnetic spectrum

Infrared

Inverse square law

Pre-sensitisation

Radiant heat

Solarium

Sun-bed

Sunburn

Tanning mechanism

Ultraviolet

Wood lamp

Chapter 8 Make-up

After working through this chapter you will be able to:

- carry out specific make-up application techniques for a variety of occasions
- use corrective techniques on how to disguise minor blemishes
- understand the main principles and practice of make-up application
- enhance face shapes, noses, eye and lip shapes
- select make-up according to skin colour, type and age
- identify the different conditions that can be treated with camouflage make-up
- list the contraindications to camouflage techniques
- have knowledge of the basic principles required to carry out treatment
- carry out a basic camouflage make-up treatment
- understand the lighting effects for photographic and fashion make-up
- carry out a photographic and fashion make-up.

Introduction

Make-up is an art – it needs patience and practice in order to apply make-up effectively. Colour co-ordination is also necessary to give a flattering effect.

Consider your client as a person – the image they are trying to project, their colouring, clothes, the function they are attending and most of all their personality, e.g. you would not apply bright red lipstick on a shy, introverted client.

Make-up routine

- Make sure the couch is in a good position for light and there are no shadows on the client's face.
- Check that the client is comfortable.
- Remove hair from face.
- Wash hands.
- Cleanse, tone and moisturise. Give moisturiser time to soak into the skin and sort out colours and effect that the client wishes.
- Tidy eyebrows if necessary.
- Blot moisturiser.
- Foundation. Choose a foundation with a texture suitable for the client's skin type such as:

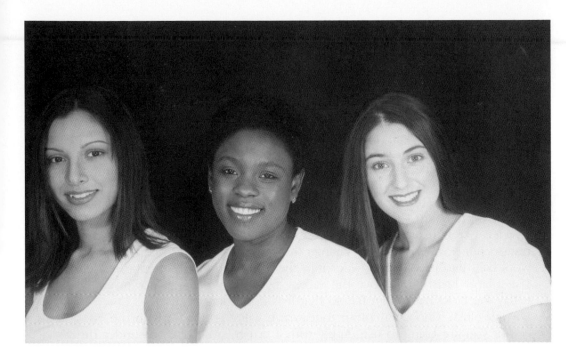

Different skin types

- Mature skin: light textured fluid foundation, light textured mousse, tinted moisturiser
- Combination skin: tinted moisturiser, matt foundation, semi-fluid foundation, colour wash
- Dry/dehydrated skin: crème foundation, mousse, semi-fluid foundation, tinted moisturiser
- Oily skin: oil-free foundation, matt foundation, gel, colour wash.

Choose a colour which matches the client's skin tone. It may be necessary to mix two foundations together to achieve this effect. One shade deeper foundation can be used on evening make-up. Apply foundation to the centre of the face with a sponge and blend outwards, make sure that there are no tidemarks.

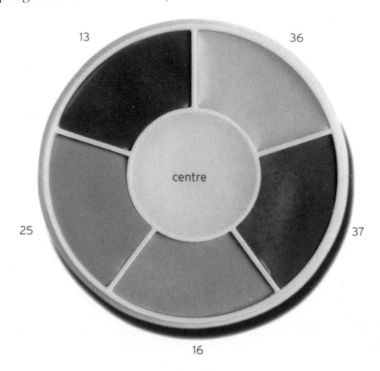

Supercover corrector wheel

Use downward movements to prevent blocking pores. Depending on the texture of the foundation, it may be easier to apply with a dampened sponge.

- Concealer. Most people require concealer around the eye area. Use a fine texture around this area as thick creams clog around the expression lines. Any spots, blemishes or red veins should be covered with a thick concealer and a brush. Apply concealer on the area and blend edges into the foundation with the brush. Check that the concealer is the same colour as foundation otherwise it will emphasise the problem.
- Contour. Use foundation a tone darker to contour and correct feature faults. Foundation is generally better to use than powder which can look artificial in daylight.
- Crème blusher. This is applied before powdering. Dot crème blusher on and blend with a damp sponge.
- Powder. Use translucent powder, it is more effective for setting make-up and translucent powder does not change the colour of the foundation. Use cotton wool balls and press the powder into the foundation with circular movements. Use a large brush to remove the excess; by using the brush downwards it helps to lay the facial hair down flat so that it is not so noticeable.
- Powder blush. Choose a colour tone which will co-ordinate with the eye and lip colour you are going to use. Apply with a brush, sweeping out under the zygomatic arch.
- Eyebrows. Brush eyebrows and use a little gel to keep the eyebrows in shape, pencil with fine feathery strokes.
- Eye make-up. Eye colour comes in various forms – gels, creams, pencils and shadows – generally speaking, eye shadow powder is most effective as it is easy to blend and longer lasting.
- Mascara. Apply from the root to the tip of the lashes.
- Water spray. Spray the make-up with fine spray of mineral water to set the make-up.
- Lipstick. Outline lips with lip pencil and fill in lipstick, blot lips with a tissue and apply lipstick again.
- Remove towel and headband before showing the make-up to the client.

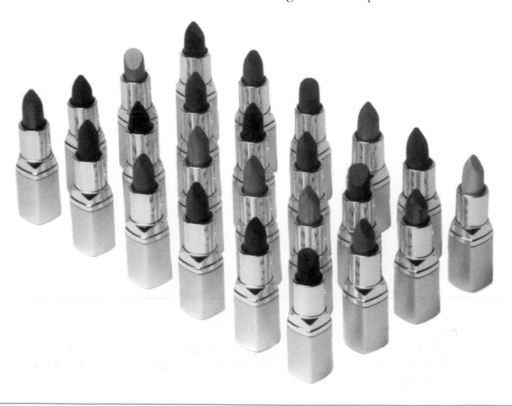

Supercover lipsticks

HEALTH AND BEAUTY THERAPY: A PRACTICAL APPROACH

Guide to foundation types

- Oily skin. Use a fluid, non-greasy astringent-based foundation.
- Dry skin. Use a cream foundation with a moisturiser.
- Congested skin. Use medicated or specialised foundations.
- Sensitive skin. Use a non-allergenic crème or fluid foundation.

These are all recommendations because make-up is an art, therefore a lot will depend on individual preference.

Make-up tools

A good make-up artist will use a selection of excellent quality sable make-up brushes in a range of different sizes for the different areas of the face. These should be hygienically washed after each client and stored in an appropriate way. Make-up sponges are most often used for the application of foundations.

Face shapes

The shape of the face is determined by the position and shape of the bones, the muscle tissue and the amount and degree of subcutaneous fat. The perfect face shape is considered to be oval, which means that the forehead and the chin area are of equal proportion. With corrective make-up the aim is to try and emulate these proportions by the clever use of shaders and highlighters.

- **Shaders.** In corrective make-up a shader which is darker than the skin colour will minimise flaws and irregularities.
- **Highlighters.** In corrective make-up a highlighter which is lighter than the skin colour will accentuate and emphasise features.

The different face shapes are:

- Diamond. This has a pointed narrow forehead and chin and is corrected by shading of the forehead and chin whilst the temples and sides of the jaw are highlighted.
- Heart. This shape has a jaw that is smaller in proportion to the forehead. It is corrected by shading the tip of the chin and forehead to reduce them whilst the jaw line is highlighted. Blusher is applied to the cheeks.
- Inverted triangle. This has a wide forehead with a pointed chin and is corrected by shading of the three corners. Blusher is used on the cheeks to enhance these features.
- Rectangle. This shape has a wide jaw and forehead and is corrected with shader to remove the four corners; highlighter and blusher are used on the cheeks to accentuate them.
- Round face. This shape has wide cheeks and shading is used at the side of the face to make it look thinner. Highlighter is used down the centre of the face. Blusher is applied to cheeks.
- Square. This shape has a wide jaw area. Shader is used to reduce the four corners; the chin is highlighted, which lengthens the face and blusher is applied to the cheeks.

Eye make-up

Eye make-up is used to correct shape faults, accentuate the eyes and to detract interest from poor features by bringing colour to the eyes.

Types and application

Eye shadows

- Cream shadows – these are used on top of foundation but must be set with powder as they tend to crease. They should not be used on older clients with wrinkled skin around the eyes.

information point

Make-up is an art that uses light and dark to enhance the natural features of a client. Imagine you are painting a picture and you want the image to appear as if it falls back away from the paper then you will use a darker shade than the paper. The same principle applies in make-up – to sink back, shade; to bring forward, highlight.

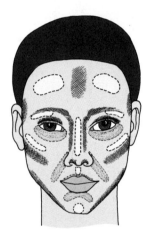

 = Highlighter

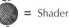 = Shader

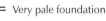 = Very pale foundation

Specialised contouring techniques for photographic work

The product	Product selection	Application	Features	Benefits
Eye shadow	Choose shades that complement the client's eye colour and skin tones. Matt colours give a more natural look, especially for mature clients. On younger clients and for a more vibrant look, use pearlised shadows to highlight.	Using a sponge applicator, apply a base colour over the central area of the upper lid. Follow this with a medium tone to create shaping and darker colours to define. Use a fine brush to blend colours after application. To use eye shadows as eyeliner, mix with a little water and apply with a fine liner brush.	Used to add colour and gives definition to the eyes.	Accentuating and correcting. More natural, especially for clients. Lifts, brightens and gives a more dramatic look. Easy to blend.
Eye pencil	Select a shade to complement eye shadow and blusher colours. Pencils give a more subtle look in comparison to liquid liners, which tend to be stronger. Select pencils that feel soft and glide easily onto the skin.	Eye pencils are applied to the upper lid following the line of the lashes. Eye shadows may be applied over the pencil to add colour and dimension. To define the lower lid, ask the client to look upwards.	Slim pencil shape. Soft texture. Wide colour range available.	Quick and easy to apply. Subtle look.
Mascara	Choose a shade that compliments the client's hair colour taking account of the eye shadows used. Use colourless mascara after eyelash tinting to thicken and define lashes.	Apply to top lashes with a downward motion, then lift lashes with the mascara brush to curl. Protect the cheeks with tissue under the lower lashes. Apply mascara with a downward stroke. Use a mascara comb to remove any excess, this will also help to separate the lashes.	Rich colour and texture. Eyelash colouring. Colourless variety.	Makes lashes darker and thicker. Gives shape and definition to eyes Enhances texture and reflects natural colour.
Lip pencil	Choose a shade to compliment the lipstick colour to be used.	Use the pencil to outline the lips. If you have difficulty in creating an even line, rest the little finger on the chin and apply the pencil with a dot-to-dot movement then go back and join up the dots.	Slim pencil shape. Soft texture. Wide colour range available.	Quick and easy to apply. Subtle look. Greater choice.
Lipstick	Select a colour that compliments the blushers, eye shadows and clothing of the client.	Following the application of the lip pencil, fill in the area outlined using lip brush. Blot well with a tissue and follow with a second application. For extra staying power apply a light dusting of translucent loose powder between applications.	Creamy texture. Full colour. Wide colour range available.	Protects and conditions lips. Enhances good shape and helps correct defects. Greater choice.
Blusher	Select a colour that compliments the skin tone, eye shadows and clothing of the client.	Following the application of the foundation, fill in the area on or under the cheek bone using a large soft brush.	Powders, creams or sticks. Wide colour range available.	Enhances cheek bones, gives shape and definition to the face. Corrects defects.

- Pressed powder – these are the most usual of eye shadows. They are used over powder and must be soft to ensure evenness of tone. Available in various textures, e.g. pearlised, matt.
- Loose powder – these are usually bright sparkly colours used mostly for evening make-up. The powder should be applied sparingly, with excess dusted off the brush.
- Powder creme – available in a wand with a sponge tipped applicator. It is applied as a cream but sets into a matt film so that powder isn't needed. It gives a soft appearance and stays on well.
- Sticks – these are cream in a stick form. They must be applied on to a spatula and softened before applying to the skin.
- Pencil – these are jumbo pencils with crème eye shadow in the centre, not to be confused with eyeliners. Use as a cream, sharpening between clients. NB. Always use a tissue to stretch the skin of the eyelid upwards so that the eyeshadow may be applied close to the lashes, application should always be in an upward and outward direction so that nothing goes into the eyes or on the cheeks.

Eyeliner

The use of these swing in and out of fashion. They are used to define and open the eyes, emphasise the lashes and help correct shape irregularities. Used incorrectly they can make the eyes seem small and sunken.

- Pencil – these must be soft or pre-softened to stop dragging of the delicate skin around the eye area. They are available in various colours and should be chosen to match the eye shadow or enhance the colour of the eyes.
- Liquid – these give a matt effect and should be applied as near to the lashes as possible with a fine brush.
- Block – these must be pre-moistened and applied with a fine brush.
- Kohl – This is a soft eyeliner that is used inside the eye. The original kohl came in little pots but now a pencil version is available. It must not be used on people with contact lenses or sensitive eyes. It is applied from the front of the client right around the inner rim of the eye and smudged through the lashes to make the lashes look thicker and give definition to the eye.

Mascara

Natural lashes are rarely long or dark enough to frame the eyes well so mascara is used for this purpose. It is now available in various colours, black and brown being the most popular.

- Wand – a plastic stick with grooves in it. This just coats the lashes without separating them.
- Spiral brush – this brushes through the lashes as well as coating them with colour.
- Block – this is the best type for salon use as it is more hygienic. The shape of the brush also enables the mascara to be applied right to the base of the lashes. It is also an ideal choice for contact lens wearers or people with sensitive eyes as there aren't any lash thickeners or filaments contained in them.
- Mascara should be applied to the bottom lashes first with the client looking up. The top lashes should then be coated from the top downwards then the brush should be brought upwards to help curl them. Several thin coats are better than one thick one, but allow each coat to dry before applying the next.
- People with sensitive eyes or who wear contact lenses should avoid all tear-proof, waterproof, and lash-builder mascaras as these are difficult to remove and may irritate the eyes and eventually cause premature ageing.

Eyebrow colour

This is used to define the brows and fill in any gaps. The effect should be very light with no hard lines apparent. As the colour always looks darker when applied, a shade lighter than the client's hair colour should be used. First, the brows must be brushed to remove any build-up of make-up, then smoothed down and coloured.

- Pencil – this must be sharpened and used in fine strokes and blended with a brush.
- Powder – this is applied with an oblique-shaped brush. It is difficult to get a definite shape but a more natural effect is achieved.

The choice of colour around the eyes

Ask the client if she has any preferences and discuss.

- Age of the client – an older client will not look very good with a high fashion effect.
- Look at the colour of the client's skin, hair and eyes.
- If the client has no preferences look at the colour of her outfit.

Guides

- If the eyes are shadowed underneath, do not use brown, grey or mauve eyeshadow.
- If the client has sallow skin, do not use olive, beige or green.
- If the client has broken capillaries or a high colour, do not use mauves or red colours.
- Do not use dark colours as they drain the face of colour (on an older client).
- Do not use bright blue on blue eyes, as this tends to disguise the true colour of the eyes instead of enhancing it. The same goes for green on green eyes, etc.

Eye shapes and corrective make-up

By finding out the shape of the eye, corrective make-up may be done. The general colour contour rule applies here; that is, deeper tones diminish or regress, while brighter and paler tones emphasise or bring into prominence. The ideal eye shape is almond shaped.

Deep-set eyes

These have the appearance of being sunk into the skull, they usually have a prominent socket bone.

- Eyes are brought forward with pale bright colours blended in an oval shape.
- Prominent socket bone may be shaded with a darker tone.
- Arch of brow and the middle of the lower lid may be highlighted.
- No eyeliner should be used.
- Fine, long false eyelashes may be used.

Round eyes

These give a wide-awake or startled look to the face. Make-up should be extended to give width to the eye.

- A pale tone is used over upper lid.
- A deeper tone should be applied to the socket bone extending at the side.
- A fine dark liner or a brighter eyeshadow may be applied to the base of both the upper and lower lashes, extending at the sides.
- Highlight under the brow.
- A medium tone of the general shade should be used to lengthen the eye shape to give a more attractive profile appearance.
- False eyelashes may be applied from the middle of the eye outwards.

Close-set eyes

The gap between the eyes should equal the width of another eye. If the gap is less than this, the eyes are too close together. Accent must be placed on the outer part of the eye.

- The entire eye area should be brought forward with a pale colour.
- A winging sweep of brighter colour shadow may be applied up to the eyebrow.

Pale matt colours to open up space between eyes

Highlighter

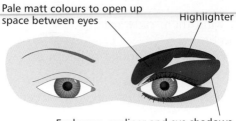

Eyebrows, eyeliner and eye shadows extended beyond outer corner of eye

a) Close-set

Eyebrows drawn slightly inside normal guidelines

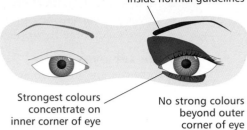

Strongest colours concentrate on inner corner of eye

No strong colours beyond outer corner of eye

b) Wide-set

Gently tapered eyebrow arch

Darkest eye shadow colour applied to centre of eyelid

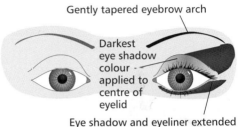

Eye shadow and eyeliner extended beyond outer corner of eye

c) Round or prominent

Highlighter

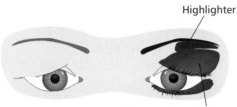

Darkest eye shadow blended over fullness of overhanging lid and blended up to the highlighter with a medium shade

d) Overhanging lids

Highlighter

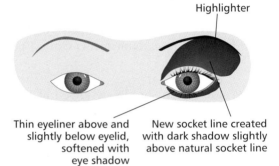

Thin eyeliner above and slightly below eyelid, softened with eye shadow

New socket line created with dark shadow slightly above natural socket line

e) Small or deep-set

Highlighter

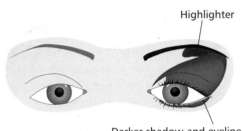

Darker shadow and eyeliner blended upwards and outwards inside outer corner of eye

f) Downward slanting

Darker socket line created above natural socket line, blended up towards highlighter

Highlighter

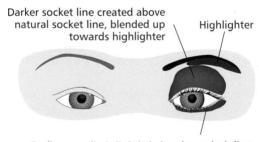

Eyeliner applied slightly below lower lash line, softened with eye shadow

g) Narrow

Socket shading above the natural socket line creates contour and depth to the eyelids

Matt neutral eye shadow blended above the middle third of eye socket produces more rounded effect

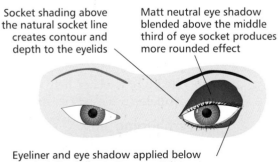

Eyeliner and eye shadow applied below lash line helps to 'open up' the eye

h) Oriental

Different eye shapes

- Highlight under extension on eyebrow.
- Pluck a little more between the brows and wing them outwards.
- Eyeliner should be applied to the outer corner.
- Concealer may be applied on the inner corners and the bridge of the nose.

Wide-set eyes

If the eyes are more than an eye's width apart they fall into this category. Accent must be on the inner corner of the eye.

- A medium shade is used over the eye area, but should not extend outwards.
- Emphasise this area with colour.
- Use eyeliner or darker shadow on inside area only.
- Highlight under mid brow.
- A shader may be used on the area between the corner of the eye and the nose.
- Keep mascara and false eyelashes to the inner corner.

Small eyes

These eyes look small in relation to the other features:

- Enlarge entire eye area with a bright but soft tone.
- Accentuate the centre of the lid with highlighter.
- Apply a darker tone above the socket bone and continue a little underneath the eye.
- A light concealer may be used at the outer corner to open the eye.
- Plenty of mascara and false eyelashes may be used but avoid eyeliner.

Droopy eyes

This is when the outer corner falls below the inner corner. Uplift is needed.

- Wing a medium tone of colour from eye to brow being careful not to extend to the outer corner of the eye.
- Use a lighter colour to contrast on the lid.
- Use a darker colour to draw in a false socket line which should be raised at the outer corner.
- Use eyeliner or a contrasting colour.
- Eyelashes should be curled up and not left to droop.
- Do not emphasise the lower outside lashes.
- No make-up should be applied to the outer corner.

Prominent or heavy-lidded eyes

This is when the eyelid appears puffy or when the eyeball seems to protrude.

- A dark matt colour should be applied near the base of the eyelashes to diminish the prominence.
- A lighter colour may be used on the rest of the eye area to bring it forward. Plenty of eyeliner may be applied to minimise the lid.
- No false eyelashes as these make the eyelid seem more prominent.

Overhanging lids

This is where the upper lid seems to rest on the eyelashes.

- Highlight the inner corner of the eye with a soft, light colour, also under the lower lashes.
- Shade the overhanging area with a darker matt shadow.
- Highlight the eyebrow bone to deflect interest.
- A stronger line of colour may be applied close to the lash roots to add vitality and definition.
- Emphasise lashes with plenty of mascara.

Eye make-up for the client who wears glasses

If the client wears glasses, check the function of the lens, as this can alter the appearance and effect of the eye make-up.

- If the client is short-sighted, the lens makes the eye appear smaller. Draw attention to the eyes by selecting brighter lighter colours. When applying eye shadow and eyeliner use the corrective techniques for small eyes. Apply mascara to emphasise the eyelashes.
- If the client is long-sighted, the lens will magnify the eye. Make-up should therefore be subtle, avoiding frosted colours and lash building mascaras. Careful blending is important, as many mistakes will be magnified!
- Curly lashes will require brushing, using a clean brush, both before mascara application and after each coat to separate the lashes.

Dark circles
- Minimise the circles by applying a concealer product.

Downward slanting eyes
- Create lift by applying the eye shadow upwards and outwards at the outer corners of the upper eyelid.
- Apply eyeliner to the upper eyelid, applying it upwards at the outer corner.
- Confine mascara to the outer lashes.

Narrow eyes
- Apply a lighter colour in the centre of the eyelid, to open up the eye.
- Apply a shader to the inner and outer portions of the eyelid.

Oriental eyes
- Divide the upper lid into two vertically. Place a lighter colour over the inner half of the eyelid and a darker colour at the outer half.
- Apply a highlighter under the eyebrow.
- White eyeliner may be applied at the base of the lash line, on the lower inner eyelid.

The eyelashes

To emphasise the eyelashes, making them appear longer temporarily, curl them using eyelash curlers.

Curling the eyelashes
- Rest the upper lashes between the upper and lower portions of the eyelash curlers.
- Bring the two portions gently together with a squeezing action.
- Hold the lashes in the curlers for approximately 10 seconds then release them.
- If the lashes are not sufficiently curled, repeat the action.

Eyelash curling is beneficial for oriental clients who have short lashes that grow downwards. It is now possible to use heated eyelash curlers which accelerate the process.

The lips

Lip cosmetics add colour and draw attention to the lips. As the lips have no protection sebum, the use of lip cosmetics also helps to prevent them from drying and becoming chapped.

It is not uncommon for the lips to be out of proportion in some way. Using lip cosmetics and corrective techniques, symmetrical lips can be created. A careful choice of product and accurate application are required to achieve a professional effect. The main lip cosmetics are lip pencils, lipsticks and lip glosses. Sometimes the lips may be unevenly pigmented. The application of a lip toner or foundation over the lips corrects this.

Lip pencils

A lip pencil is used to define the lips, creating a perfectly symmetrical outline. This is coloured in with another lip cosmetic, either a lipstick or a lip gloss. The lipliner also helps to prevent the lipstick from 'bleeding' into lines around the lips. Lipliner has a wax base, which does not melt and can be applied easily. It contains pigments, which give the pencil its colour. When choosing a lipliner, select one that is the same colour or slightly darker than the lipstick it is going to be used with.

Lipsticks

Lipstick contains a blend of oils and waxes, which give it its firmness, and silicone, essential for easy application. It also contains pigment to add colour; an emollient moisturiser to keep the lips soft and supple; and perfume to improve its appeal. In addition it may include vitamins to condition the lips or sunscreens to protect the lips from ultraviolet rays. Some lipsticks contain a relatively large proportion of water. These moisturise the lips and provide a natural look. The coverage provided by a lipstick depends on its formation.

Lipsticks are available in the following forms: cream, matt, frosted and translucent. Frosted lipstick has good durability, as it is very dry. Some other lipsticks also offer extended durability, and are suitable for clients who are unable to renew their lipstick regularly.

When choosing the colour of lipstick, take into account the natural colour of the client's lips, the skin and hair colours, and the colours selected for the rest of the make-up.

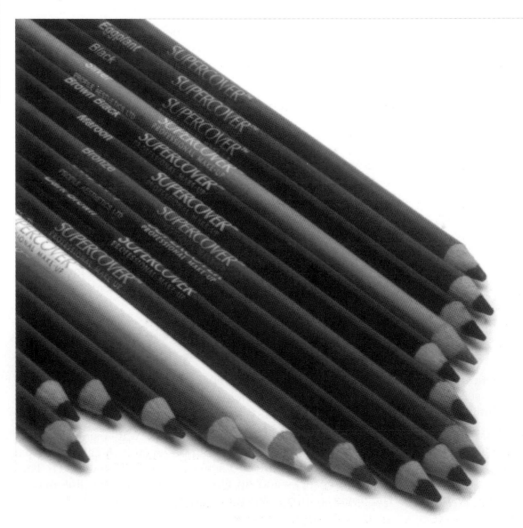

Lip pencils

Lip glosses

Lip gloss provides a moist, shiny look to the lips. It may be worn alone or applied on top of a lipstick. Its effect is short lived. Lip gloss is made of mineral oils, with pigment suspended in the oil. Note that black women often have creases on the lips that extend to the surrounding skin. If lip gloss is used it will bleed into these lines.

Dry lips

Sometimes the lips become dry and chapped. Recommend that the client keeps them moisturised at all times, especially in extremes of heat, cold or wind. Some facial exfolients can be professionally applied over the lips to remove dead skin. If the client does not like to wear make-up during the day, or if the client is male, recommend that the lips be protected with a lip care product.

Corrective lip make-up

Thick lips

- Select natural colours and darker shades, avoiding bright glossy colours.
- Blend foundation over the lips to disguise the natural lip line.
- Apply a darker lipliner inside the natural lip line to create a new line.

Thicker upper or lower lip

- Use the technique described above to make the larger lip appear smaller.
- Apply a slightly darker lipstick to the larger lip.
- If the lips droop at the corners, raise the corners by applying lipliner to the corners of the upper lip, to turn them upwards.

Thin lips

- Select brighter pearlised colours.
- Avoid darker lipsticks which will make the mouth appear smaller.
- Apply a neutral lip liner just outside the natural lip line.

Small mouth

- Extend the line slightly at the corners of the mouth, with both the upper and lower lips.

Uneven lips

- Use a lipliner to draw in a new line.
- Apply lipstick to the area.

Lines around the mouth

- Apply lipliner around the natural lip line.
- Apply a matt cream lipstick to the lips (don't use gloss which might bleed into the lines around the mouth).

Allergies to cosmetics

An allergy to a cosmetic or skin care product will be easy to recognise by the following symptoms:

- Itching.
- Redness or erythema.
- Swelling or oedema.
- Skin rash or urticaria.

These are some of the most well known irritants:

- Lanolin – found in sheep's wool. This is added to many cosmetics and skin care products.
- Eosin – pigment found in lipstick.
- Formaldehyde resin – preservative added to nail enamels.
- Acetone – solvent found in nail enamel removers.

- Cuticle remover – the potassium hydroxide can be caustic.
- Sodium hydroxide – used in soaps. Can cause allergy sensitivity.
- Hydrogen peroxide – used in tinting.
- Ammonia – used in some cleansing products.
- Alcohol – in astringent toners.
- Perfumes/colourants – added to certain cosmetics.
- Titanium dioxide – used in many European skin foundations.
- Alpha hydroxy acids – fruit sugars added to many new skin care products.

Make-up lesson with a client

- Point out to the client their best features.
- Discuss the make-up that they are using at present.
- Write out a colour chart of the colours that you use for the client.
- Commence by applying a day make-up and then adapt it to an evening make-up.
- The client should be seated in front of a mirror so that she can observe the demonstration of techniques and then copy them in front of you.
- Remember to encourage the client during each stage of the make-up.
- Explain aftercare and home care thoroughly to your client.
- Encourage the client to purchase the products you have used on her.
- Keep the client informed of the new products and techniques.

Remedial camouflage

In today's society great emphasis is placed on physical appearance. Whether we like it or not, we are all influenced by media pressure to look the very best that we can, even if this is sometimes an unhealthy attitude to have.

For some this can be made worse by unnatural disfigurement caused either at birth or through illness or accident. While surgery may be an option for some, it is not possible or necessary for others, yet they still feel embarrassment every time they face the outside world. This can have serious repercussions, in some cases making the individual loathe to face anything or anyone new. It can affect career prospects and even the forming of relationships.

The therapist who can provide and instruct on remedial camouflage can greatly enhance an individual's life and gain tremendous job satisfaction.

Role of the cosmetic camouflage therapist
It goes without saying that the therapist working in cosmetic camouflage is entering into a field slightly different from the normal course of work, with the exception, maybe, of electrology. This area of work requires a very discreet approach and a sympathetic attitude so as to prevent the client suffering undue stress or discomfort. The therapist should have a good understanding of the different types of disfigurement possible and be able to identify the client's needs and anticipated outcomes. The experienced therapist should be able to expertly cover any blemishes or disfigurement and most importantly be able to instruct the client on how to do so. This should always be carried out in an atmosphere of peace and tranquillity.

Client consultation
The importance of a correct client consultation cannot be overstated if the treatment is ultimately going to be a success. The first objective is to establish a rapport with the client and instil confidence in the therapist's ability and willingness to help whilst at the same time being realistic in the treatment's outcomes.

It is wise to try to gather information about the scar/disfigurement at the time of booking the consultation so that a general practitioner's note can be provided ahead of time where necessary. This is preferable to referring the client to her/his GP at the time of consultation as it could possibly lead to lost custom through embarrassment or frustration.

It is also most important to allow the client to tell you what is troubling them rather than just presuming. A wrong assessment could cause untold harm to an already sensitive client and this could have serious long-term repercussions on the individual's self-image.

A detailed record card should be completed carefully with the client. On the back of the card the following information should be recorded:
- Products used.
- Shades of creams.
- Number/method of application.
- Results.

Name of client:	Name of doctor:
Address:	Address:
Telephone: Day	Telephone:
Evening:	
Source of referral:	
Type/age of scarring:	
Area(s) of scarring:	
Signature of client:	Signature of therapist:

Example of a remedial camouflage consultation card

A similar card should be given to the client after treatment detailing the products used and the method of application so that it can be used for reference. In some cases it may be necessary to also send a copy of the consultation card to the client's own doctor, especially if consent was required or if there is to be any follow-up medical treatment.

Types of client
Unlike in any other area, the therapist working in remedial camouflage will be dealing with a diverse range of clients: men, women and even children. Some will be new to the clinic, some existing and many will be extremely nervous.

Male approach
Men who come to the clinic for remedial camouflage may often be more inhibited than women. This is partly because they consider salons to be the domain of women, especially if there is feminine-style décor, and because they see cosmetics as a predominantly female medium. When dealing with a male client the main objective is to make the remedial camouflage as undetectable as possible and to ensure appropriate surroundings.

Female approach
The female client will often be more used to cosmetics and therefore less inhibited about using them. She may, however, be more concerned about her appearance than

a male client so may need extra reassurance and even help and guidance with normal cosmetic application.

Child approach

When dealing with children for remedial camouflage it is important not to make them feel that their disfigurement is unacceptable. Often it is a parent who has instigated treatment and this can draw attention in the child's mind to a problem that never really bothered them before. Depending on the age of the child it may be a case of teaching the parent how to apply camouflage techniques. It should be suggested that in this case the child returns at a later date to be given expert advice as well. It is also worth mentioning that some childhood disfigurements disappear with age in some instances.

SELF-CHECKS

1   State the importance of the consultation procedure.

2   Explain how you would handle a child requiring cosmetic camouflage.

Remedial camouflage conditions

Pigmentation disorders

The most common pigmentation disorders are outlined below:

Chloasma

This is a smooth, irregularly shaped patch of brown pigmentation which occurs when there is increased production of the melanocyte stimulating hormone. It occurs most frequently in pregnancy or when taking the contraceptive pill. Exposure to ultraviolet radiation exacerbates the condition.

Vitiligo (leucoderma)

This is an absence of melanin in small patches on the skin caused by the destruction of melanocytes in the basal layer of the epidermis. Sometimes large areas can be affected and the small patches merge into one. The condition is obviously more noticeable on a darker skin. The other key feature of vitiligo is that as there is no protective melanin present, the areas affected are photosensitive and will burn if exposed to UV radiation.

Melanoderma

This is a general term for patchy pigmentation of the skin. There are many reasons for melanoderma but the main cause is allergic reaction to a product being applied to the skin and reacting with UV radiation, e.g. perfume.

Types of naevus

The medical definition of a naevus is a birthmark or circumscribed area of pigmentation due to dilated blood vessels. Many forms of naevus exist including:

- Strawberry naevus. These are normally present at birth or occur shortly afterwards and normally start as a small red spot which enlarges fairly quickly. They are normally raised above the surface of the skin and can become quite large. In most cases they fade with time and will have completely disappeared by the age of about seven when just a red patch remains.
- Angioma (port wine stain). So named because it tends to be dark red or purplish in colour. Angioma can be extremely disfiguring. It is an area of profusely dilated capillaries and often affects the face and neck. The individual is born with this condition.

- Spider naevus (stellate haemangioma). These can appear at any age and are small, red central spots with superficial veins radiating from them. They can occur on any part of the body, but are usually seen on the face and upper cheek area.
- Epidermal benign naevus (moles). Moles can be found all over the body and vary in size and texture. They can be raised or flat, pigmented or normal skin colour, and some contain hairs. Most pigmented moles occur through overgrowth of melanocytes in the basal layer of the epidermis which is an indirect result of exposure to ultraviolet radiation.

Types of scar

A scar is a mark which is left on the skin after it has healed from some form of trauma. There are many different types of scarring, but the main categories are outlined here.

Hypertrophic scar

This is a large unsightly scar which is raised and shiny in appearance.

Ice-pick scar

As the name suggests, this type of scar is rough and pitted. It is a common post-acne blemish.

Keloid scar

This type of scar is fibrous and lumpy as the body continues to produce extra collagen after a wound has healed. Keloid scars are more prevalent on black skin types.

Quiescent scar tissue

This term describes scar tissue which is at rest or has healed. The rate at which a scar heals will vary from one person to another. There are general signs that indicate that a scar is healed:

- There is no evidence of inflammation.
- It is not painful or sensitive to the touch.
- It is not weeping or moist.

Skin disorders

Psoriasis

This is caused by an abnormally fast rate of cell renewal in the epidermis with cells sometimes reaching the stratum corneum in a few days instead of the normal 28–30. This results in clusters of cells forming characteristic oval, dull-red plaques together with silvery scales.

The cause of the condition is not clear but hereditary factors play an important part and it is thought to be exacerbated by stress.

Rosacea

This normally affects the over thirties age group and often women of menopausal age. It begins with a flushed appearance, particularly in response to stress, spicy foods and alcohol. The flushing then becomes permanent as the blood vessels in the area become dilated. This increases the temperature of the skin stimulating sebum production and this in turn leads to papules, pustules and open pores becoming present. It is a chronic disorder of the blood vessels of the face.

Skin conditions

Tattoos

It has long been fashionable for people to have tattoos. A tattoo is where a permanent pigment is put into the skin. Unfortunately many people live to regret having a tattoo and although removal is now possible it is both painful and expensive. Camouflage make-up is an alternative option to successfully hide such marks.

GOOD PRACTICE

Applying the cosmetics with a brush is excellent for thin, 'hairline'-type scars as the cream should not be spread in too large an area.

information point

Camouflage make-up will generally last longer on dry skin types.

Varicose veins

Varicose veins produce a characteristic bulging effect and can be quite disfiguring. They are the result of valves within the veins collapsing through an inherited weakness and/or poor circulation.

SELF-CHECKS

1 List four contraindications to camouflage make-up and explain why each is a contraindication.

2 Describe four types of scar tissue.

3 Name three remedial camouflage conditions which can be successfully camouflaged.

Equipment required for camouflage make-up

A camouflage make-up kit is needed by the therapist and it should be kept in an immaculate and hygienic condition. First, it will be necessary to have a range of skin care products to prepare the skin for treatment. The client may already be wearing some form of make-up but if not it is still necessary to cleanse and remove any traces of sweat, sebum and general dirt. Toner must be used to remove any residue left by the cleansing medium otherwise the camouflage creams may 'slide' on application and also be unstable. Moisturiser should also be applied, but avoid the blemished area for the same reasons.

Secondly, it will be essential to have a good range of cover creams. There are many different types available and it is up to the individual therapist to decide which range is best for them. Great improvements have been made over recent years in the production of camouflage make-up. Many manufacturers produce sample kits of all the colours in their range with replacements available for the colours that are used the most. It will also be important to carry a range of stock for the client to purchase for immediate use.

Within the kit it will be necessary to have a setting or fixing powder. Some manufacturers supply these powders whilst others recommend the use of translucent powder. Retail powder should also be available for the client to purchase. Finally, a range of sponges and good quality sable brushes together with some form of mixing palette will be needed for professional application. Some of the palettes available today are made from clear Perspex with a central magnifier which allows the therapist to blend the creams and hold it up to the skin to check the colour compatibility. (An example of this type of palette is the one produced by Rita Roberts™.)

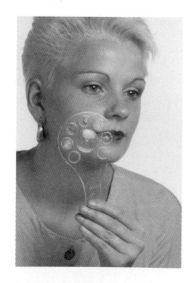

'Blend-in' palette

Lighting

The source and type of lighting is very important when carrying out a camouflage make-up treatment as it will affect the colour of the cosmetics.

The colour of the pigment within the skin will vary depending on the type of light that is illuminating it. Natural daylight is composed of all the colours of the spectrum and will therefore define the face clearly. Artificial (white) light may consist of many hues (colours) some of which may be stronger than others, therefore if the coloured hue falls on a pigment that is able to reflect it, the colour of the lighting is seen. However, if it falls onto pigment and the rays are absorbed then the pigment colour will be distorted.

Example: If white light falls on a red lipstick, the pigment within the product reflects the red light and absorbs the other six colours of the spectrum making the lipstick appear red. However, if pure blue light falls on the lipstick, it will be absorbed and as there is no red light for it to reflect it will appear black.

ACTIVITY

Research the effects of lighting on make-up.

Camouflage make-up creams

When choosing a range of camouflage make-up it is important to consider the following points:

- Colour range. There should be a wide range of colours available to cater for the palest to the darkest skin colouring.
- Even consistency. The products should blend easily on contact with the skin, they should not drag or feel unduly tacky.
- Waterproof. The products should be waterproof to allow the user to participate in normal activities, e.g. swimming.
- UV filters. As scar tissue can be sensitive, cover creams should have in-built UV filters.

Blending techniques

If the therapist is to become skilled in the blending of camouflage make-up, it is essential to have a good understanding of the principles of colour and to practise.

The colour wheel

There are three primary colours: red, blue and yellow. To make a colour you move around the wheel, e.g. red + yellow = orange.

Colourings

The colour of skin can alter through life as it is affected by different factors such as climate, illness and certain products. Skin contains varying amounts of the pigment melanin, which is genetically passed from parent to child. Skin colour can be divided into four basic categories.

- **Caucasian skin**. This is the most fragile of all skin types, prone to sun damage, broken capillaries and pigmentation irregularities. Scarring tends to leave pink pigmentation marks that can be quite noticeable. It has blue and pink tones present from the blood capillaries behind which is a basic tone normally of either yellow or pink. It can vary from being very pale to quite a deep tan depending on UV exposure and hereditary factors.

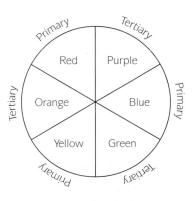

The colour wheel

- **Oriental skin**. This type is more resilient than Caucasian skin and most often is of even tone. However, it can develop pigmentation discoloration if exposed to ultraviolet radiation. This skin type will have more melanin present and be mainly of one colour tone. It has a basic yellow undertone.
- **Asian skin**. This type is normally strong and adaptable. It can have a tendency towards uneven colouring and in particular dark shadows around the eye area. Scarring tends to leave dark pigmentation marks which are slow to fade. It can vary in tone from being quite olive to very dark, but always has a yellow undertone.
- **Black skin**. This skin type has the greatest amount of protective melanin pigment and therefore is the slowest to show signs of ageing. As with Asian skin types scarring tends to leave dark pigmentation marks that are slow to fade. There are many varying colour tones from light brown to deep ebony.

ACTIVITY

Complete a detailed case study on a client with a disfigurement, keeping photographic evidence where possible. Evaluate your findings including client feedback.

Matching skin colour (basic application techniques)

As mentioned previously, when purchasing a camouflage make-up kit it is essential to choose one with a good variety of depths and tones of shades to meet the diverse range of skin colours.

- It will be necessary to establish the depth and tone of the client's skin and to choose the nearest colour to match the client's skin accordingly.
- Neutralise any irregularities present, e.g. green will neutralise red, but it must be remembered that the principle of camouflage make-up is to disguise the abnormality by blending it to the client's skin colour.
- Mix the depths and tones so that when applied to the treatment area it will blend and match the client's skin colour.
- When choosing the correct colour, if the client's skin is midway between two shades, blending equal quantities of both should produce the exact match.
- If a client's skin is closer to one of the shades, blending two parts of the closer to one part of the other should produce a good match.
- Another important point is to write down exactly what has been blended as it is easy to forget.

information point

A dampened cosmetic sponge is used when a light coverage is required. For example, a camouflage treatment for rosacea to give a natural look will allow some of the skin's natural colouring to show through.

Once you have mixed the correct shade it will be necessary to test the cream near the treatment area. If the match is perfect it can be applied to the disfigurement. However, if it is deeply pigmented it may not be sufficient to adequately cover, in which case it will be necessary to apply a thin coat then set it with powder and then apply a second coat and set that.

There are many methods for applying camouflage make-up and whichever method is chosen it will require a lot of practice to become proficient. There are a few basic principles which the therapist should observe:

- Always thoroughly prepare the area before treatment with cleansing, toning and moisturising procedures but avoid putting moisturiser directly over the scar.
- Always study the skin colour and type of disfigurement carefully.

- Always apply camouflage creams sparingly as this will achieve a more natural effect and is less likely to come off on clothing.
- Apply the creams in layers, setting between applications (except where an additional cream is to be added to the basic shade as in the case of toning-in with a surrounding area, in which case the powder is applied at the end).
- Always allow a few minutes for the products to set properly and then brush off the powder in a downward action.
- Blot the area gently with damp cotton wool to remove any detectable traces of powder.
- Use either a brush, dampened cosmetic sponge or even a finger to apply cosmetic camouflage depending on the size and area of the treatment, and always work in a hygienic fashion.
- Use feathering strokes to fade-in the edges around the camouflage area.
- Always explain procedures to the client and give home-care advice on general skin-care, removal, application at home, etc.
- Ask the client to book in for a further consultation so that any queries can be dealt with and you can see how they are progressing with their application techniques.

GOOD PRACTICE

- The finger can be used in several ways: in a rubbing action, a pressing action or in a stippling action. This means that you can control the amount of surface stimulation of the blood capillaries, which is very important in certain conditions.
- Remember to try to contain the cosmetics to the area requiring camouflage for the most natural effect.
- The appearance of stubble will sometimes need to be added to men and this can be achieved by carefully stippling a grey coloured cream.

ACTIVITY

With a colleague, practise camouflaging disfigurements such as freckles, scars, birthmarks, etc. Take the role of the client and therapist and carry out a detailed consultation. Evaluate your findings.

Home-care advice

- Camouflage make-up should be removed thoroughly with an appropriate product.
- Be careful with soap or soap-based products as these can sometimes dislodge the creams.
- When drying with a towel after bathing or swimming always pat dry and do not rub the camouflaged area.
- Climate can have an effect on the durability of the products as heat tends to loosen the creams more readily. For this reason a client will need to take great care whilst in any hot environment.

information point

Artificial freckles sometimes need to be added to restore balance to the face.

Prosthetics

This is the term used to describe any manufactured appendage used to enhance or complete the human body. Obvious examples include artificial limbs, but false nails and eyelashes also fall into the category and an understanding of the filament prostheses available will be of benefit to the camouflage therapist.

ACTIVITY

Research the types of prostheses available.

1. State the main conditions you may encounter in the field of camouflage make-up.

2. Give three important points to consider when selecting camouflage creams.

3. Explain the importance of lighting when carrying out a camouflage make-up treatment.

4. Give four classifications of skin colour and explain two characteristics of each.

Fashion and photographic make-up

It is often a dream of many therapists to become famous make-up artists but many set out with no clear understanding of how hard and unglamorous this job often is. It is not uncommon for make-up artists to be in the middle of a field at 6 a.m. on a cold wet morning trying to recreate a make-up produced the previous afternoon. Its often long hours working with tired, temperamental actors, but if you are determined, hard working, motivated, creative, with lots of people skills, you may well be suited to a career as a make-up artist.

This type of work is a specialist niche market and to ensure this book provides you with the skills and knowledge required we have managed to seek the guidance of a well-established make-up artist who has worked in the USA and UK. Zaf Ansari, who owns Profile Aesthetics Ltd, which provides make-up, training programmes and retails Supercover make-up, has kindly contributed the following information based on his experience.

Photographic make-up

Working and consulting with the photographer and understanding the lighting situation is as important as the make-up techniques. It is important to consider the following questions: Will the shoot be outdoors or indoors? What type of photography will be used? Will it be film, video or a digital camera? Will it be colour or black and white? After answering all of these it is possible to consider the impact and adjust accordingly.

Adjusting make-up for different lighting

Digital cameras, film and photography pick up more colours on skin, clothing and hair and show fairly true to the colours used. While normal video and camera pick up about half of the colour, due to lighting peach colours can appear white and purple may appear black. So it is crucial that a good make-up artist fully understands lighting and photographic mediums.

Today, with new technology, rather than capturing a photograph on film, digital cameras can electronically allow you to download on to your computer or instantly print out on a colour compatible printer. The images created are measured in tiny picture elements known as pixels. The greater the number of pixels, the higher quality and clarity of the picture and the larger the size of the picture can be achieved. This new technology also allows you to sanitise the photos for cosmetic changes and correcting imperfections.

Lighting effects

The amount of light and shadow should relate to the character and appearance of the model. In a portrait, soft smooth skin should be complimented by light and inconspicuous shadows.

---

information point

A good quality digital camera may feature no less than 5 million pixels.

---

information point

For information on Zaf's training courses and products contact Profile Aesthetics Ltd on 0208 781 1311/0845 305 305, via their website, www.supercovermakeup.com or www.profile.eu.com, or at Profile House, 51–53 London Road, West Croydon, Surrey CRO 2RF

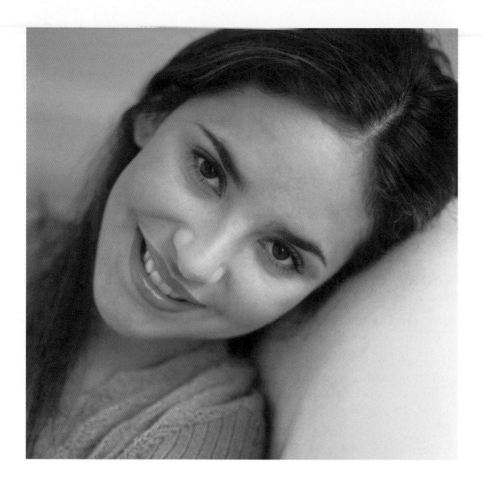

Light, natural day make-up

A camera can see thousands times more than the human eye, therefore all your make-up techniques should be concentrated in blending and smoothing out lines and wrinkles.

Every one is subject to negative lighting. In a film or photographic studio lighting is usually already set up. Generally for evening make-up techniques, especially on more mature clients, you want to use as many highlights as possible on all major depressions in the skin, for the illusion of even skin texture. As with subdued lighting in clubs and restaurants, generally the lines and wrinkles in the skin appear deepened and dark, thereby ageing your clients by maybe 5–10 years.

For catwalk make-up the highlighting and shading for the desired make-up effect can be sharp and anything from 5–7 shades darker or lighter than the colour of the skin.

Colour or black and white photography

Colour photography uses colours as hues, while black and white photography uses grey scale (white, grey and black). For black and white photography, use pale tones of make-up to hide fine lines and wrinkles.

Step-by-step photographic make-up techniques

1 Wash and dry your hands. Sanitise your hands with an instant hand sanitiser. This will instantly remove any germs or bacteria from your hands and fingers.

2 Prepare your model on a make-up chair or couch. Use white capes and a headband to protect the model's hair and clothing.

3 Ask the model if they are allergic to anything, and if they are wearing contact lens. Prepare a fresh skin by cleansing, toning and moisturising using mild

natural products. If they are wearing contact lenses it is best to put them back in before commencing the make-up.

4 Transfer one or two of the nearest colour foundation to the skin from the primary container with a spatula onto the make-up pallet. Transfer the make-up onto a cosmetic make-up sponge and match a base foundation by applying along the jaw line and back behind the ears. The colour should be perfectly matched to the skin and the neck (do not continue with base).

5 Apply a colour correction, blue neutraliser with a small filbert brush no. 6 to dissolve the appearance of any brown to blue discolourations in the skin. Now apply a red neutraliser with a clean filbert no. 6 brush to all areas of the face, neck, etc. to dissolve any major red discolourations.

6 Take your make-up sponge and transfer a liberal amount of make-up base from the pallet to the sponge. Apply make-up to all areas of the face, neck, etc. by patting or stippling the base with a make-up sponge over the colour correction. Blend and smooth out the make-up. The make-up should look as natural as possible.

7 Transfer a small amount of highlighting and shading cream from the primary containers onto another spatula and pallet set.

8 Apply highlight and shadows to all areas of facial anatomy for the desired make-up projection. For example, shading creams on the sides of the bridge of nose, directly under the hollows of the cheeks, hair line, temple areas, puffy eyes, etc. Highlighting creams at cheek bones, nasal lines, cupid bow, etc.

9 Apply cream rouge half an inch behind the apple of the cheeks all the way back to the hair line.

10 Take a professional size powder puff and transfer translucent powder onto the powder puff and set make-up using the powder.

11 Apply colourless powder under the eyes with clean sides of the powder puff to catch any debris of eye shadows. Tissues can also be used.

12 Apply eye shadows, eyeliners, mascara, and colour in brows.

13 Apply a primary blush, apply lipliner and lipstick. (The outside line of the lips are called a collagen line. It is important to cover this with lip liners or shading creams as these lines looks unpleasant in photographs). Blot lips with tissue and apply another coat. Apply lip gloss, as desired.

14 Take a filbert no. 18 brush slightly dampened with water and smooth out any lines or wrinkles which the body heat may have caused.

15 Remove capes and head bands and stand your model on her feet. Look at the type of clothing and style and determine all the skin textures on the chest area, back of neck, arms, legs, etc.

16 Communicate with the photographer the angle of the photos to be taken and look through the camera lens yourself.

17 A thin layer of make-up is now to be applied and set with powder to all exposed areas of skin to be photographed. This is because in a photograph the face can sometimes appear to look light and the chest area dark because the flash reflects light off the face with make-up on, and the raw skin of the chest and neck absorbs light.

18 Your model is now ready to be photographed by a professional photographer. If possible you need to stay during the photo shoot and offer to touch-up any make-up as necessary.

19 The model must not look artificial with heavy powder. You can create a dewy look by use of a hydrator spray in a mist form and spray to any part of face or body and lightly blot with paper towels.

20 Sometimes it is a good idea to keep an inexpensive Polaroid camera so that you can be ahead of the photographer to see how the picture may appear and if you need to make any adjustments to the make-up.

Fashion make-up techniques

Fashion trends are continually changing. They are influenced by seasonal colours along with the lipsticks of the stars or the eye shadows worn by a famous celebrity, which give the product certain glamour and media and household interest. People flock to buy these cosmetics just because someone famous wears them.

Today the main driving force on make-up is fashion. The colours and make-up designs displayed in glossy magazines or used on the catwalk are being imitated. The general public will spend billions of pounds on cosmetics every year and are being 'brain washed' through the media. Professional make-up artists are guided by fashion and an individual's requirement.

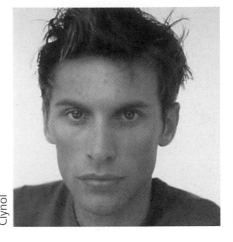

Clynol

Male fashion model

Step-by-step fashion make-up

1 Wash and dry your hands. Sanitise your hands with an instant hand sanitiser. This will instantly remove any germs or bacteria from your hands and fingers.

2 Prepare your model on a make-up chair or couch. Use white capes and a headband to protect the model's hair and clothing.

3 Ask the model if they are allergic to anything, and if they are wearing contact lens. Prepare a fresh skin by cleansing, toning, and moisturising using mild natural products. If they are wearing contact lenses it is best to put them back in before commencing the make-up.

4 Transfer one or two of the nearest colour foundation to the skin from the primary container with a spatula onto the make-up pallet. Transfer the make-up onto a cosmetic make-up sponge and match a base foundation by applying along the jaw line and back behind the ears. The colour should be perfectly matched to the skin and the neck (do not continue with base).

5 Apply a colour correction, blue neutraliser with a small filbert brush no. 6 to dissolve the appearance of any brown to blue discolourations in the skin. Now apply a red neutraliser with a clean filbert no. 6 brush to all areas of the face, neck, etc. to dissolve any major red discolourations.

6 Take your make-up sponge and transfer a liberal amount of make-up base from the pallet to the sponge. Apply make-up to all areas of the face, neck, etc. by patting or stippling the base with a make-up sponge over the colour correction. Blend and smooth out the make-up. The make-up should look as natural as possible.

7 Transfer a small amount of highlighting and shading cream from the primary containers onto another spatula and pallet set.

8 Apply highlight and shadows to all areas of facial anatomy for the desired make-up projection. For example, shading creams on the sides of the bridge of nose, directly under the hollows of the cheeks, hair line, temple areas, puffy eyes, etc. Highlighting creams at cheek bones, nasal lines, cupid bow, etc.

9 Apply cream rouge half an inch behind the apple of the cheeks all the way back to the hair line.

10 Take a professional size powder puff and transfer translucent powder onto the powder puff and set make-up using the powder.

11 Apply a base approximately 3–4 shades deeper than the colour of your model from the jaw bone to the chest area, powder and set the make-up.

12 Apply highlights and shadow creams to collar bones and to cleavage areas. Powder and set.

13 This technique in make-up is known as *facial separation*. What you have achieved is a wonderful highlight lift to the face, where the face is looking much lighter than the rest of the body. This technique is very universal and it is used on many famous faces in film and television make-up techniques and on the catwalk.

14 Apply *wet and dry* method techniques of shimmer or other glittery make-up eye shadows. The wet and dry method is simply using a wet or dampened brush to powder eye shadows and it goes on the skin like a cream or liquid. Using this technique the intensity of colours are much stronger.

15 Create a real drama with your make-up, use blue or green liquid eyeliners or mascaras.

16 Create a smoky or muddy eye effect, which are always in for the fashion make-up concept.

17 Use shimmer blush and glossy lips for that sensual look.

18 Use loose shimmer powder to cheek bones – a nice gold or silver colour. Also brush some of these under the brows, and even to the bottom lips if desired.

19 The final character appearance is the eyebrows: fill in with a soft shimmery eye shadow to keep the flow of the fashion concept going.

20 Dress your model with appropriate dress code. Now apply some loose fine shimmer silver or gold powder to the collar bones and to the cleavage area.

KEY TERMS

You need to know what these words and phrases mean. Go back through the chapter to find out.

Blending techniques

Client consultation

Cosmetic camouflage

Equipment required for camouflage

Fashion make-up

Matching skin colour

Photographic make-up

Prosthetics

Remedial camouflage conditions

Chapter 9 Reception, stock control and health & safety

After working through this chapter you will be able to:

- list different types of infections and infestations
- carry out emergency procedures
- identify hazards and evaluate risks
- reduce health and safety risks
- describe the activities undertaken in the reception area
- deal with telephone messages
- make a number of appointments for clients
- understand the purpose of stock control
- explain the purpose of a consultation
- carry out an effective facial and body consultation.

It is paramount that all the staff working within a salon environment are provided with an induction programme that equips them with the knowledge and skills needed to perform their individual and team role in a safe and effective manner. Health and safety is a legal requirement and it is essential that all staff are active in identifying any potential hazards, are able to evaluate the risks involved and take action to reduce these risks. The salon environment can give rise to a variety of hazards and risks, for example, the use of materials and substances, the use and maintenance of equipment, cross-infection, spillages and breakages, etc.

Hygiene

It is paramount that the therapist ensures the highest standards of hygiene within the salon. Because of the close proximity of therapist and client, good hygiene is essential to prevent infection, cross-infection and infestation.

Protecting against disease

We spend a great deal of our lives surrounded by what are commonly known as 'germs'. Some germs are harmless, some are even beneficial, but others present a danger to us because they cause disease.

The germs which cause disease are usually spread by:

● Unclean hands.
● Contaminated tools.
● Sores and pus.
● Discharges from the nose and mouth.
● Shared use of items such as towels and cups.
● Close contact with infected skin cells.
● Contaminated blood or tissue fluid.

Viruses

Viruses are the tiniest germs, yet they are responsible for an enormous range of human diseases. Viruses can only survive in living cells. The following are examples of viral infections:

● Common cold: the virus is spread by coughing and sneezing and is carried through the air as a droplet infection.
● Herpes simplex (cold sores): the virus remains dormant in the mucous membranes of the skin. It can be activated by sunlight or general debility. Cold sores are most likely to spread when they are weeping.
● Warts: there are several types of wart. Verruca plantaris is a wart which occurs commonly on the soles of the feet and is spread by close contact.

Bacteria

Bacteria are single-celled organisms, which divide in two to reproduce. They grow from spores which are very resistant to attack and multiply very quickly. Bacteria are capable of breeding outside the body and can therefore be caught easily through personal contact or by touching a contaminated article. Bacteria have a cell wall that provides protection and gives rigidity.

Some bacteria cause diseases and infect wounds. The following are examples of bacterial infections:

● Impetigo: bacteria enter the body through broken skin and cause blisters which weep and crust over. The condition is highly infectious and can be spread easily by dirty tools.
● Boils: these can occur when bacteria invade the hair follicle through a surface scratch or by close contact with an infected person.
● Whitlow: this can be caused by the bacteria invading the pad of the finger through a break in the skin which has often been caused by a splinter.

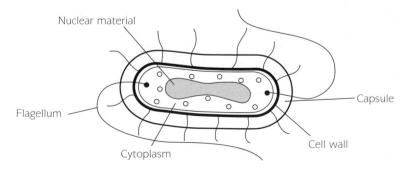

A typical bacteria cell

HEALTH AND BEAUTY THERAPY: A PRACTICAL APPROACH

Fungi

Fungi are yeasts and moulds. Moulds break down all sorts of materials but rarely cause disease. Yeasts are single-celled fungi which can cause disease. Fungal infections are very easily transmitted by personal contact or by touching contaminated articles. The following are examples of fungal infections:

- Tinea pedis (athlete's foot): the fungus thrives in the warm, moist environment between the toes and sometimes on the soles of the feet. The condition is picked up easily by direct contact with recently shed infected skin cells.
- Tinea unguium (ringworm of the nail): may result from contact with the fungus present on other parts of the body, e.g. toenails may become infected during an outbreak of athlete's foot, which if touched could then be spread by contact to the nails.

Animal parasites

Animal parasites are small insects which cause disease by invading the skin and using human blood or protein as a source of nourishment. Diseases caused by animal parasites usually occur as the result of prolonged contact with an infected person. The following are examples of diseases caused by animal parasites:

- Scabies: tiny mites burrow through the outside layer of the epidermis and lay their eggs underneath the skin surface. The condition is very itchy and causes a rash and swelling. Characteristic line formations show where the burrows have been formed.
- Head lice: small parasites which puncture the skin and suck blood. They lay eggs on the hair close to the scalp. The unhatched eggs are called nits and can be seen as shiny, pearl-coloured, oval bodies which cling to the hair shaft.

To protect against the spread of disease you must:

- Provide each client with clean towels and gown.
- Carry out a consultation before each treatment to ensure contraindications are spotted in time.
- Use only tools which have been cleaned and sterilised.
- Use correct treatment techniques to avoid injuring the client.
- Dispose of waste properly after each treatment.
- Wash your own hands before each treatment and as necessary throughout the treatment.
- Maintain high standards of personal hygiene.

GOOD PRACTICE

- Dirt and bacteria accumulate in cracks. You must not use tools with a damaged edge as they cannot be sterilised effectively.
- You have a responsibility to yourself, your clients and your colleagues to always work hygienically and to do everything you can to avoid the spread of infection.
- All work surfaces should be cleaned regularly with hot water and detergent. The treatment couch, trolley, sink and stools should be wiped down at the end of each working day with a solution of disinfectant.
- Waste should not be handled or exposed. Make sure that the waste resulting from your treatments is placed in a lined container, tied up and disposed of in a large sealed refuse sack with other salon waste.

ACTIVITY

Research the different skin conditions caused by bacterial, viral and fungal infections. Note their names and characteristics.

Sterilisation and disinfection

Sterilisation is the destruction of all living organisms. It is very difficult to maintain sterile conditions. Once sterilised items have been exposed to the air they are no longer sterile. Articles which have been sterilised and stored hygienically for a short period are safe to use on the client.

Autoclave

The most effective method of sterilisation is steaming at high pressure in an autoclave. This works on exactly the same principle as a pressure cooker. Steam is produced from a reservoir of water and is contained under pressure at a minimum of 121 °C for 15 minutes. Modern autoclaves use thermochromic indicators which change colour when the required temperature has been reached. Stainless steel and glass items are suitable for sterilisation by this method. A stacking facility is usually provided so that the articles can be placed at different levels in the autoclave. The temperatures used in autoclaves vary from 121 °C to 134 °C and with correct time and heat exposure kill all spores. However, the range of temperature can affect certain materials, e.g. soft plastics. Most hardened plastics are suitable for autoclave exposure but always check first with the manufacturer of the item to be sterilised.

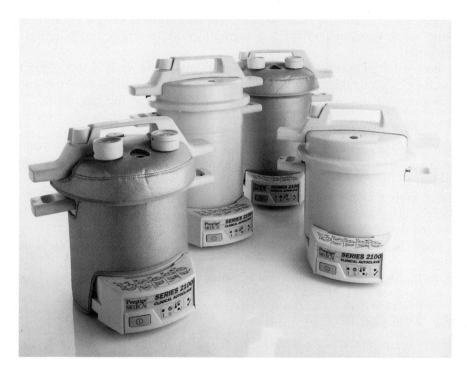

Autoclaves

Sanitisers

Sanitisers operate by irradiating implements with ultraviolet light. This would normally inactivate any bacteria, but as all implements cannot be fully exposed directly to the ultraviolet light, these units are now only recommended for storage of sterilised implements.

Glass bead sterilisers

Glass bead sterilisers reach temperatures between 190 °C and 300 °C (374–572 (°F) depending on the model. This temperature has to be maintained for 30–60 minutes prior to use. If extra items are put into the steriliser during this period, the temperature of the beads drops and the effects are lost. Timing has to begin again.

HEALTH AND BEAUTY THERAPY: A PRACTICAL APPROACH

Glass bead sterilisers can hold only very small items, e.g. tweezers, and the very high temperatures are suitable only for implements made of high-grade stainless steel, otherwise discolouration occurs. They therefore have limited use in the salon.

Chemical methods of sterilisation

Concentrated liquid chemical agents are available which have to be diluted for use. Some chemical agents act as a steriliser, depending on the strength of the solution and the time for which items are kept in contact with them. Some liquid chemical sterilisers are very harmful to the skin and great care is needed when handling them.

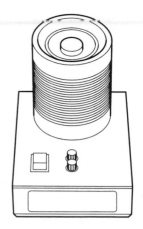

Glass bead steriliser

Disinfection

Disinfectants work against bacteria and fungi, but they just remove contamination; they do not necessarily kill spores. Disinfectants only reduce the number of organisms. Examples of good chemical disinfectants are:

- Gluteraldehyde: a 2% solution is used which remains active for 14–18 days, after which time it must be discarded. Gluteraldehyde is particularly useful for soaking metal instruments and applicators, but must be handled with great care. (See COSHH, Chapter 11.)
- Alcohol: alcohol disinfectants have a very effective bactericidal effect. They must be used once only and then discarded.
- Quartery ammonium compounds: these are bacteriostatic cleansing agents. They prevent bacteria from spreading but are not effective against very resistant organisms.
- Hypochlorites: these products contain sodium or calcium hypochlorite and are often used for general cleaning purposes as they are relatively cheap. Some are corrosive and should not be used for soaking metal instruments.

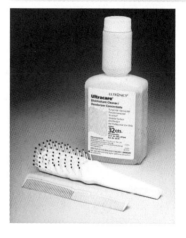

Chemical sterilisation equipment

Antiseptics

Antiseptics are disinfectants used specifically on the skin and for treating wounds. Ready-for-use swabs impregnated with 70% isopropyl alcohol are often used for convenience.

ACTIVITY

Research the different cleaning and sterilising methods used in two salons. Make a note of any special instructions on diluting, using and disposing of the chemical disinfectants and sterilising agents used.

information point

Quartery ammonium compounds are inactivated by soap.

information point

'Aseptic conditions' refers to creating an environment which will avoid infection.

Emergency first aid

You need a basic knowledge of first aid so that you can assist with minor accidental injuries or unexpected situations which happen from time to time in the salon. More serious injuries, for example those involving acute pain or loss of consciousness or serious bleeding, should be dealt with by a qualified first aider, doctor or nurse.

First aid kit

The Health and Safety regulations require the salon to have a first aid kit readily available. The contents are specified and are intended to cover most emergency situations.

The first aid kit must include:

- A first aid guidance card
- Assorted plasters (preferably waterproof)
- Different sizes of sterile dressings
- Bandages
- Sterile eye pads
- Scissors
- Tweezers
- Safety pins.

Useful additions to this list are:

- Surgical adhesive tape
- Antiseptic cleansing products, i.e. liquid and cream
- An eye bath
- Gauze
- Crepe bandages
- Antihistamine cream
- Medical wipes
- Cotton wool.

First aid kit

GOOD PRACTICE

- Contaminated cotton wool and dressings should be disposed of in a plastic bag which has been tied up.
- All accidents which occur in the salon must be recorded in an accident register. This is a requirement of the Health and Safety at Work Act.
- Keep in the first aid box a card which lists names, addresses and phone numbers of the local health centres and hospitals.

information point

Care must be taken to follow COSHH guidelines when storing and handling chemicals.

All staff should know what the first aid box looks like and where it is kept. It is recommended that the box is green with a white cross marked on it and that it is dustproof and free from damp.

If the salon has a fridge with a freezer compartment it is a good idea to keep an ice pack for injuries which produce swelling.

It is advisable to keep a stock of disposable gloves to wear when dealing with open wounds. These give some protection from AIDS and Hepatitis B if an infection is present.

AIDS (Acquired Immune Deficiency Syndrome)

AIDS is caused by the human immuno-deficiency virus (HIV). The virus attacks the body's natural immune system and makes it very vulnerable to other infections, which eventually cause death. Some people are known to be HIV positive, which means that they are carrying the virus without the symptoms of AIDS. HIV carriers

Problem	Priority	Action
Minor cut	To stop the bleeding	Apply pressure over cotton wool taking care to avoid contact with the blood.
Severe cut	To stop the bleeding	Keep applying pressure over a clean towel until qualified help arrives. Put on disposable gloves as soon as possible.
Electric shock	To remove from source of electricity	Do not touch the person until they are disconnected from the electricity supply. If breathing has stopped, artificial respiration will need to be given by a qualified person. Ring for an ambulance.
Dizziness	To restore the flow of blood to the head	Position the person with their head down between their knees and loosen their clothing.
Fainting	To restore the flow of blood to the head	Lie the person down with their feet raised on a cushion.
Nose bleed	To constrict the flow of blood	Sit the client up with the head bent forward. Loosen the clothing around the neck. Pinch the soft part of the nose firmly until bleeding has stopped. Make sure breathing continues through the mouth during this period. If bleeding has not stopped after half an hour, medical attention must be sought.
Burn	To cool the skin and prevent it from breaking	Hold the affected area under cool, running water until the pain is relieved. Serious burns should be covered loosely with a sterile dressing and medical attention sought.
Epilepsy	To prevent self-injury and relieve embarrassment	Do not interfere forcibly with a person during an attack. Gently prevent them from injuring themselves. Ensure the person's airways are clear and wipe away any froth which forms at the mouth. After the attack, cover with a blanket, comfort and give reassurance until recovery is complete.
Objects in the eye	To remove the object without damaging the eye	Expose the invaded area and try stroking the object towards the inside corner of the eye with a dampened twist of cotton wool. If this is not successful, help the person to use an eye bath containing clean warm water.
Fall	To determine if there is spine damage. To treat minor injuries if the fall is not serious	If the person complains of pain in the back or neck, then do not move them: cover with a warm blanket and get medical aid immediately. For less serious falls, treat the bruises, cuts, sprains or grazes as appropriate.
Bruise	To reduce pain and swelling	Apply cold compresses for 30 minutes using a towel wrapped round an ice-pack or very cold tap water. Keep the compress in place with a bandage. Replace it if it dries out.
Graze	To clean wound and prevent infection	Soak a pad of cotton wool with an antiseptic and gently clean the graze, working outwards from the centre. Replace the cotton wool regularly throughout the cleaning. Apply a sterile gauze dressing, preferably a non-adherent type, to protect the wound as it heals. If dirt or foreign matter has become embedded in the graze, the person should be referred to a doctor who may want to give a tetanus injection.
Sprain	To reduce swelling	Apply cold compresses to the area (see treatment for bruises) and support the affected joint with a bandage firmly applied. Refer the person to a doctor.

are able to pass on the virus to someone else through infected blood or tissue fluid, for example through cuts or broken skin. The virus does not live for long outside the body.

Hepatitis B

This is a disease of the liver caused by a virus (HBV) which is transmitted by infected blood and tissue fluids. The virus is very resistant and can survive outside the body. People can be very ill for a long time with a Hepatitis B infection. It is a very weakening disease which can be fatal. Strict hygiene practices are essential to prevent Hepatitis B from spreading in the salon.

ACTIVITY

With a colleague, role play emergency first aid procedures for each of the following:

a nose bleed
b dizziness
c object in the eye
d fainting.

SELF-CHECKS

1 Give an example of each of the following types of infection:

a viral

b bacterial

c fungal

d animal parasite.

2 Define the following:

a sterilisation

b disinfection

c antiseptic.

3 Explain why it is advisable to wear protective gloves when treating an open wound.

4 State the first aid treatment for a client suffering with:

a a burn

b a nose bleed

c an epileptic fit.

Reception

The reception is the central pivot for the staff and clients of the salon. It is an area that everyone has to walk through either as a member of staff entering work and greeting clients or as a client when making and waiting for appointments. Everybody's day revolves around the salon's appointment schedule, and therefore the reception area.

First impressions do count so it is paramount that the reception area is inviting to the client. Therapeutic music rather than a loud, thudding pop record will aid relaxation for the majority of clients, and the use of essential oils either through

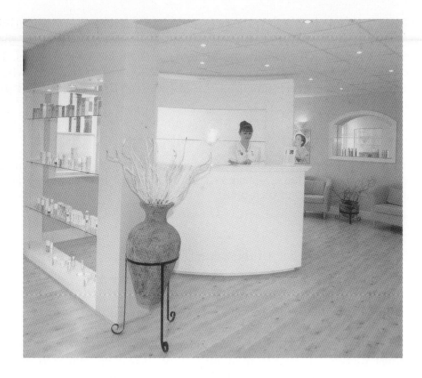

Reception area

burners or fans can saturate the air with a pleasant aroma. The seating should be comfortable in order to allow the client to begin to relax prior to treatment. The décor should reflect the type of premises and clientele the salon is marketing itself to, it should be continually refreshed to keep it in pristine condition and should be kept clean and tidy:

- All surfaces should be dusted and cleaned and waste bins should be emptied on a regular basis.
- Cups and glasses should be removed as soon as possible after use.
- Salon leaflets should be replaced before they become torn or out of date.

GOOD PRACTICE

- The reception is the ideal area to market you and your salon as you have a captive audience. Instead of purchasing magazines which advertise commercial skin care products, produce regular salon leaflets which advertise you, your salon and the professional products you retail.
- Emphasise a healthy lifestyle by displaying information on diet and exercise.
- Serve healthy drinks to your clients, e.g. mineral water and fruit juices rather than only caffeine drinks such as coffee and tea.
- Reference materials should be presented in an attractive but practical manner to withstand regular reading, etc.

The receptionist

Some establishments employ a receptionist, in others the therapists share the responsibility. The receptionist is the first point of contact clients and visitors have with the salon. It is therefore essential that the receptionist has a thorough understanding of the workings of the establishment and is extremely professional in their approach and appearance. It is also beneficial if the receptionist has an understanding of the benefits of the treatments and retail products on offer in the salon.

Many employers are fully aware of the benefits of offering retail products to their staff at cost price together with ensuring that they have experienced all of the salon treatments on offer and having treatments to benefit their individual needs. The image of the salon is reflected by the appearance of the staff. Just think: when was the last time you saw a sales assistant in a top fashion retail outlet dressed in scruffy clothes?

GOOD PRACTICE

It is useful for therapists to have treatments in the salon and role play the treatment as a realistic client, noting the way the reception area looked and how the receptionist and therapist interacted with them and each other.

The reception area is the life-line of the salon. It is here that:

- The appointment book is kept. This is the central control of the salon, everybody plans their activities for the day around this.
- Appointments are made either by telephone or in person.
- Clients are greeted and made welcome by the receptionist.
- Clients and visitors to the salon, e.g. cosmetic company representatives, are taken care of whilst waiting. (It is extremely important, however, that staff do not discuss any business matters in an area where clients may overhear financial purchasing arrangements, etc.)
- Enquiries are dealt with, e.g. information on salon treatments, products, planned salon events, directions to another shop in the area.
- Products are ordered, received, recorded, priced, displayed and sold.
- Salon services are advertised.
- Payment is taken for treatments and retail products.

All of the tasks outlined above are generally undertaken by the receptionist, whose job role mainly involves taking, receiving and recording information either by telephone or in person.

Dealing with clients, visitors and reception enquiries

In order for a receptionist to deal either with clients or visitors to the salon they need to fully understand the workings of the salon including the:

- Roles and responsibilities of each member of staff.
- Recording mechanisms of the salon.
- Treatments offered by the salon and their benefits.
- Retail products sold by the salon.

The receptionist must remain courteous to all clients and visitors and treat them all as equals. Generally clients are polite and friendly. However some people can demand a great deal of attention and at times be aggressive and rude. The receptionist must stay cool, calm and collected; she represents the salon and as the first point of contact will create an impression of the salon to the client or visitor. A friendly smile and voice can often help to calm an aggressive visitor. We all have bad days, but when working in a service industry our moods have to be left at home. Clients and visitors may not always manage to do this so remember that you are probably just an outlet for their emotions, it is likely that it isn't personal and shouldn't be taken as such.

Telephone enquiries

For many clients the telephone is their contact with the business. A good receptionist never forgets that all calls are from individuals and that each one of them is a prospective client.

You should always:

- Answer promptly – on the second or third ring. This gives both sides time to prepare themselves without the caller becoming impatient.
- Be friendly – give the name of the salon and say who you are. Note the client's name so that you can use it in the conversation.
- Smile when you pick up the receiver. Smiles definitely do travel down the telephone!
- Be enthusiastic – ask how you may help the caller. Enthusiasm is infectious and shows you enjoy being helpful.
- Listen attentively – it is very off-putting for a caller if they sense you are being distracted by someone else.
- Leave a good impression. Remember that you are the salon to the caller. Repeat back to them any important points discussed and thank them for calling. Don't forget to use their name!

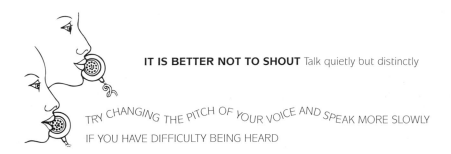

IT IS BETTER NOT TO SHOUT Talk quietly but distinctly

TRY CHANGING THE PITCH OF YOUR VOICE AND SPEAK MORE SLOWLY IF YOU HAVE DIFFICULTY BEING HEARD

Tips for using the telephone

Taking messages

It is essential that all messages are accurately recorded and promptly dealt with. The receptionist or therapist must ensure they record who the message is for, who it is from, the telephone number where the caller can be contacted, the date and time of the message and the actual message, and state whether the caller wants their call returned, will call again or was returning a call. The person taking the message should also record their own name in case there are any queries.

To:	Date:
From:	Time:
Tel. no.:	Taken by:

Message

Please return their call

Will call again

Returning your call

MAKE SURE ALL INFORMATION IS CLEARLY RECORDED AND PASSED ON PROMPTLY.

Message recording sheet

Recording appointments

Recording appointments is an extremely important part of the receptionist's job and it is essential that all staff understand the appointment system that the salon operates. Appointment sheets are always made up in advance, thus enabling clients to book courses of treatments.

The receptionist has to:

- Ensure that the reception desk is supplied with appointment cards, pens, pencils, ruler and rubber.
- Prepare pages in the appointment book at least six weeks in advance, to show the availability of each therapist on a particular day.
- As appointments are arranged, transfer the details to the appointment book in pencil, stating the client's name, their telephone number and the treatment required.
- Make out an appointment card for the client, recording details in pen and stating the date, day, time, therapist's name and treatment booked.
- Check the accuracy of both sets of records before handing over the appointment card to the client.

DATE Monday October 17th   **COMPLEXION**

Time	LOREEN	SAIDA	LIZ	JEAN	PAUL	SUNBED
8.30						
8.45						
9.00			Miss Williams	Mrs Lacey G5		Mrs Turvey C
9.15	Ms. Warner Hydra Plus	Mrs Cogin	AHA	705 7997		646 2216
9.30				Mrs Farmer		Miss Bates
9.45			424 5780	Cellulite treat		777 3434
10.00	221 4477	BODY WRAP	Mrs Rees Ultratone	292 3987	Morning off	Ms. Faulkner
10.15				Mrs Peet		273 2727 DNA
10.30			252 3790	Massage		Miss Laidlaw
10.45	Mrs Perry Dynatone	707 2700	Mrs Christopher Back massage			827 1343
11.00			551 9827	499 2000		Mr Cartwright
11.15	417 9173	Mrs Loy Massage	Mrs Cooke Massage	Mrs Dowding Dynatone		266 0479
11.30	Ms. Harris Massage					
11.45						
12.00		503 2768	448 4790	550 4171		Mr Burke
12.15	335 3939	Mrs Fabes		Miss Lulham		324 1567
12.30		Indian head	LUNCH		Mr Ashford	Mrs Wensley
12.45	LUNCH	923 5625		Hydra Plus	Massage	417 9894
13.00		Ms. Puttick Ultratone				Ms Sullivan
13.15			Mrs Walker	217 9239	842 9111	344 3916
13.30		292 7652	AHA		Mr Lakin Back Massage 978 3493	Mrs Godfrey
13.45	Mrs Turner Massage					237 8999
14.00		LUNCH	506 4455	LUNCH	Mr Ward Massage	Mrs Bona
14.15						462 3911
14.30					320 3493	Ms. C Bailey 121 3790

□	Available Time
⊠	Client has been taken for treatment
◺	Client arrived and is awaiting treatment
DNA	Did Not Attend – Client did not inform: make a note on record card
C	Last minute cancellation

Example of a completed page of an appointment book

- Record the client's arrival at the salon by drawing a diagonal line in pencil across their details in the appointment book.
- When the client has gone through for treatment, draw a diagonal line across the first one to record that they are being attended to.

Clients who arrive unexpectedly may be treated provided that there is a therapist available. The receptionist should always check first and then record the client's details on the day in the appointment book.

In some salons the receptionist prepares a list for each therapist which shows their schedule for the day. This is kept by the therapist and provides a useful quick reference.

GOOD PRACTICE

- It is important that the appointment pages are kept neat and tidy. The correct codes and abbreviations must be used and the start and finish times of treatments made clear.
- Sometimes clients have to cancel or change their appointment. When details are recorded in pencil, they can be rubbed out neatly and the space used for another client.

ACTIVITY

1 Undertake reception duties and keep a log of all the tasks involved.
2 Monitor a colleague undertaking reception duties and identify their strengths along with any areas they need to improve upon. Record the information and present it clearly and logically.
3 With a group of colleagues role play a receptionist, therapist and a client (pleasant and difficult). Video the scenes, analyse and record the receptionist's behaviour highlighting their strengths and weaknesses.

Stock control

Stock is a key term used for all the products which are purchased on a frequent basis and are consumed as part of the treatment. These items are key to running the business.

Good stock management of products/consumables is a key part in running a business effectively. There is a fine balance between holding too much and not enough stock. Both conditions have a detrimental effect on the cash flow of the business.

High level of stock

Holding high levels of stock can have the following effects on the business:

Disadvantages
- Ties up valuable cash which could otherwise be used to invest in new equipment or a wider range of products.
- Increases the risk of the stock being out of date by the time its consumed, wasting money.
- Takes up storage space that could otherwise be used for other equipment or treatment areas.
- Possibly higher insurance premium.

Advantages
- Never run out of the product.
- Easy to manage – there is always plenty of stock.

Low level of stock

Holding low levels of stock has the following effects on the business:

Disadvantages

- Increases the risk of running out of products. Treatments or sales of products will not be available to the client. The immediate effect is loss of sales.
- Client dissatisfaction. The client may consider going elsewhere for their treatments in the future.
- More time and effort is required in managing the stock.

Advantages

- Product ranges can be changed at short notice.
- Better space utilisation.
- Efficient and flexible.

Having the right level of stock is therefore vital to running the business:

- Too much stock – money is tied up unnecessarily.
- Too little stock – shortages and therefore loss of sales.

Managing stock

There are various different ways to approach stock control:

- Fixed re-order stock level.
- Fixed time re-order.
- Economic order quantity (EOQ).
- First in first out (FIFO).

Fixed re-order stock level

This method of stock control is where a re-order level is defined and when the stock reaches this level it is re-ordered. The exact amount and level for re-ordering is determined by how long it will take for the product to arrive from the supplier at the point of ordering it. A simple visual method can be adopted to identify product that needs to be re-ordered – by marking the shelves with fixed re-order lines that show up when the product is lifted off the shelf.

Fixed time re-ordering

This method is exactly as its title suggests. Stock of product is re-ordered at a fixed time each month or week. It can offer a good solution as it represents a routine for the business and ensures that stocks are regularly supplemented. However, it may well mean the level of stocks fluctuating quite a bit depending on the rate they are used up. It is a little inflexible as a system unless used very carefully.

Economic order quantity (EOQ)

There is an optimum level of stock. The precise level will vary from product to product. In order to make the right decision as to how much stock should be held each product needs to be analysed independently. The key is to balance the costs of holding the product in stock (consider space as well as the cost of money being tied up) against the costs of ordering the stock more frequently. Product prices are normally cheaper when they are ordered in bulk.

The stock level that strikes the balance between these two conditions is known as the economic order quantity. If this is taken to be the optimum level of stock for each product it should help to minimise the costs – an important prerequisite to maximising profit.

First in first out

As most products have a shelf life, it is key to ensure that product in stock is rotated properly. This principle is known as FIFO (first in first out), i.e. what gets purchased first gets sold first.

One of the ways in which this principle can be adopted with minimum effort is to store the same product in line on a shelf with purchased product being pushed from the back while sold product is pulled from the front of the line.

Maintaining stock and the retail area

In many salons stock-taking and ordering are undertaken by the receptionist. However, it may be a task given to a therapist or the salon manager. It is extremely important that retail products are accessible and a good stock level is maintained or sales could be lost.

If the receptionist is responsible for the salon's stock they must:

- Keep the retail area clean and tidy: the counter, shelves and stock should be dusted every day and where possible have regular changes of display. Stock which is grubby and dusty will lose its value.
- Inform clients of current promotions: the receptionist should draw special offers to the attention of the clients and make sure the promotional material is displayed where it will catch the client's eye.
- Carry out stock checks: stock checks should be carried out weekly to monitor how well different products are selling and to make sure that popular lines are re-ordered before being sold out.
- Price the retail products: identical products must not be priced differently. Price tickets should be checked as part of regular stock checks. Old price tickets should be removed before putting on new ones so that a lower price is not disguised.
- Store stock correctly so that it does not deteriorate or become damaged. Keep fast-moving lines at the front of the shelves and slower moving ones nearer the back. Do not block aisles or passageways with containers of stock; keep it in a locked cupboard or secure room.
- Display stock attractively: displays should be set up with the minimum disruption to business. If all retail stock is to be displayed, extra space is needed for the fastest selling lines. Shelving should be clean, safe and undamaged and strong enough to take the weight of the products on display. Packaging should be displayed with the product. Take care with flimsy packaging and stack heavier goods lower down than more fragile items.
- Keep accurate stock records. The quality of a product cannot be guaranteed once its expiry date has passed. Stock which has been stored beyond its 'shelf-life' has either to be sold off cheaply or, ideally, disposed of.
- Store stock in a cool, dark place.
- Do not pile boxes too high.
- When an order arrives, bring old stock to the front and store new stock behind. This method of stock control is called FIFO, i.e. first in, first out.

REMEMBER

Storing stock in straight lines makes counting easier.

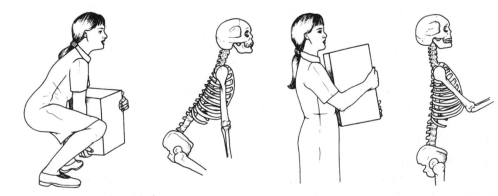

Correct lifting and carrying technique

- Use dummy stock under bright lighting: this way the colour, texture and fragrance of the products will not become spoiled.
- Be careful when unpacking stock. Look out for sharp staple fastenings on boxes and avoid using a knife. Protect your overall when carrying large items. Paper and cardboard packages should be flattened before disposal.
- The salon loses money on old stock which is sold off cheaply or thrown away. Products which are approaching their expiry date should be identified at the stock check and steps taken to sell them before it is too late. This may mean offering a special promotion or reducing the price slightly as an incentive to buy.
- Take care when dismantling a display. Put back equipment where it will not become damaged and keep tools and accessories safe in a box.

The stock sheet lists the number of items in stock per product line. The details of a stock check are recorded on a stock sheet before being transferred to the stock book. The stock book identifies re-order levels, and the receipt and sales of stock.

GOOD PRACTICE

- Ensure a good system of stock control is implemented, highlighting the item, size and minimum and maximum levels of stock required.
- Review the stock control system regularly as requirements may fluctuate due to factors such as the time of year, promotions and changes in current trends. Seek advice from your product supplier who will have experience of these. They may also provide you with a useful stock control system.
- Ensure stock is available or sales will be lost!

Handling stock

The receptionist is the first point of call within the salon where most deliveries will be made. When an order of stock arrives the receptionist/therapist will be expected to sign for the delivery. Most companies will have 'small print' acknowledging all stock is there and that it is in good condition. It is important that if there is insufficient time to count the order or inspect the condition of the stock that the person signing alters the wording to 'not inspected on receipt'. There should be a delivery note with the order which itemises the order in terms of individual product, size and quantity. It is important that the order is processed as soon as possible to check for any discrepancies. The products should be ticked off against the delivery note, then priced and put on the display shelf or in the stock cupboard, ensuring the new stock is behind the existing stock. It is paramount that the delivery note and the original order are compared and any discrepancies between the two noted or any differences in the order delivered and the delivery note or the condition of any of the products delivered are immediately reported to the suppliers. Most suppliers expect salons to notify them of any damage or discrepancies within 48 hours of delivery. There are occasions when the order placed by a salon and the stock delivered are different, such as the suppliers being temporarily out of stock themselves. If this is the case they will usually inform you of this on the delivery note and forward the stock when they have a supply in or may ask you to re-order. Once this is done the details of the new stock can be added to the stock book.

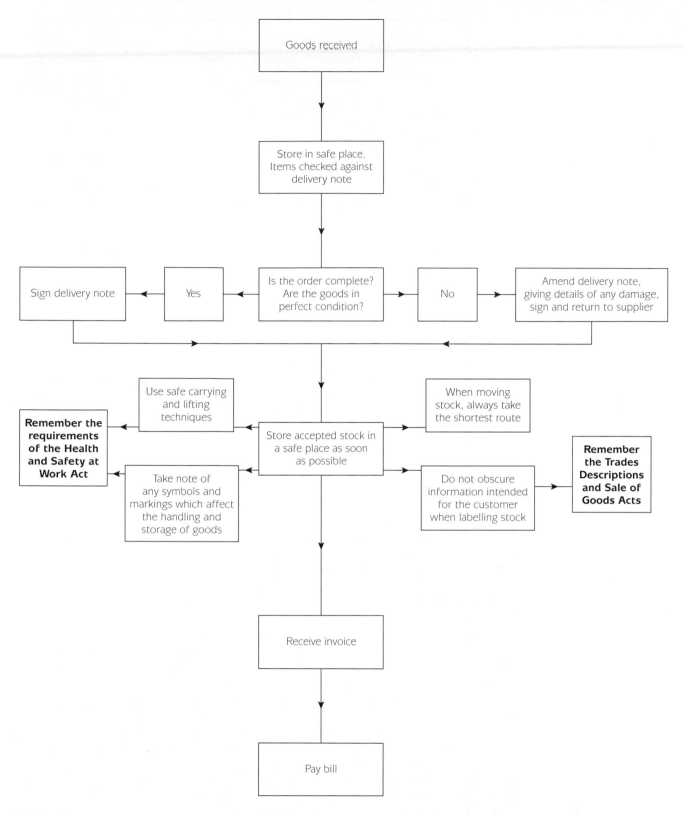

```
                          ┌──────────────────────┐
                          │    Goods received    │
                          └──────────────────────┘
                                      │
                                      ▼
                          ┌──────────────────────┐
                          │  Store in safe place. │
                          │ Items checked against │
                          │     delivery note     │
                          └──────────────────────┘
                                      │
                                      ▼
┌──────────────┐   ┌──────┐   ┌──────────────────┐   ┌──────┐   ┌─────────────────────┐
│Sign delivery │◄──│ Yes  │◄──│Is the order      │──►│  No  │──►│Amend delivery note, │
│    note      │   └──────┘   │complete?         │   └──────┘   │giving details of any│
└──────────────┘             │Are the goods in  │             │damage, sign and     │
                              │perfect condition?│             │return to supplier   │
                              └──────────────────┘             └─────────────────────┘
```

Remember the requirements of the Health and Safety at Work Act

Use safe carrying and lifting techniques

Take note of any symbols and markings which affect the handling and storage of goods

Store accepted stock in a safe place as soon as possible

When moving stock, always take the shortest route

Do not obscure information intended for the customer when labelling stock

Remember the Trades Descriptions and Sale of Goods Acts

Receive invoice

Pay bill

Distribution of stock

	Stock List	
1	Aromatic oil for vapouriser or steam cabinet	30ml
2	Aromatic oil for body massage	30ml
3	Desincrustation gel	250g
4	Ionto gel DS	250g
5	Ionto gel GS	250g
6	Ionto gel SS	250g
7	Ionto gel DC	250g
8		
9		
10		

Example of a stock sheet

No.	PRODUCT CODE	PRODUCT	STOCK LEVEL Min	STOCK LEVEL Max	Date 5/8/04 COUNTER STOCK	STOCK ROOM STOCK	TOTAL STOCK (I)	ORDER	RECEIVED	TOTAL STOCK (II)	SOLD	Date 5/8/04 COUNTER STOCK	STOCK ROOM STOCK	TOTAL STOCK (I)	ORDER	RECEIVED	TOTAL STOCK (II)	SOLD	
1	00070	Aromatic oil for vap/sc 30ml	10	14	6	2	8	2	–	8	–	6	2	8	–	2	10	–	
2	00071	Cellulite cream 150g	6	8	3	3	6	2	–	6	2	3	1	4	2	2	6	1	
3	000072	Stretch mark cream 250g	6	8	4	4	8	–	–	8	1	3	4	7	–	1	8	–	
4	000073																		
5	00074																		
6	00075																		

Example of a stock book

GOOD PRACTICE

- All spillages must be cleaned up straight away to prevent accidents.
- When opening a stock order and products have spilt, notify the supplier straightaway.
- Products deteriorate – always check you store them according to instructions, e.g. below a certain temperature or in air conditioned rooms, and check their life span.

With a colleague, discuss the following and compare your answers with other members of your group:

a What could be the possible reasons for discrepancies at a stock check?

b How do you think that seasonal variations might affect the allocation of space given to stock?

c When are the best times for changing displays and attending to stock?

d Why should the salon aim for a fast turnover of stock?

e What sort of things should be considered when fitting out a stock room?

Computers

Businesses are becoming increasingly aware of the benefits of computerised record keeping. All sorts of information, such as clients' details, appointments, stock records and sales figures can be stored on a disk. The information can be retrieved easily by a trained person. Some manufacturers produce software (programs) specially for use in a salon.

If you use a computer you should copy recorded information on to a second disk to provide back-up in case of loss or damage to the main disk.

Many salons now have their own websites and join those set up by professional bodies.

Risk assessment

In 1999, the Management of Health and Safety at Work Regulations were amended and require all business owners or managers to carry out risk assessments for the health, safety and welfare of both employees and clients. If the salon has more than five employees then formal risk assessment records must be kept. However it is recommended that all employers keep formal records. These regulations also take special notice of employees under the age of 18, requiring employers to carry out risk assessments of their work activities identifying any particular hazard they could be exposed to and then indicating the controls the employer will put in place to ensure the employees' safety. The potential hazards can be considered under three headings: physical, biological and mechanical.

There are five steps involved in carrying out risk assessments:

1 Identify all the potential hazards in all areas of the salon.

2 Determine who could be at risk and how they may be at risk.

3 Evaluate these risks and decide whether the control mechanisms in place are adequate or whether more needs to be done to prevent possible accidents.

4 Formally record all your findings (see pp. 264–68).

5 Monitor and review the risk assessments on a regular basis and ensure all staff are aware of them.

Risk assessment is an essential management tool, which defines what is or could be hazardous and the controls that the employer will put in place to protect its workforce and clients.

GOOD PRACTICE

- Risk assessment will form part of an employee's induction programme but it should not stop there, as it is essential to continually monitor and review risk assessments and update and remind all staff.
- Display your risk assessment records alongside the COSSH regulations within the salon.

REMEMBER

- A hazard is the potential of something to cause harm, e.g. chemicals that may be used in the salon.
- A risk is the likelihood that harm will be caused by exposure to the hazard, e.g. not wearing protective clothing when handling chemicals.

RISK ASSESSMENT

Warwickshire COLLEGE
ROYAL LEAMINGTON SPA & MORETON MORRELL

Programme area/Unit/Department:	Beauty Therapy and Hairdressing			
Logical assessment unit:	Reception			
Completed by:	Dawn Edwards			
Date:	1 May 2001			
Review date:	Oct. 2001			
Authorised by:	Dawn Ward			
Principal:	Ioan Morgan			

PERSONNEL AFFECTED – KEY

Staff	ST	Public	P	Young Persons	YP
Students	S	Contractors	C		

RISK RATING

SEVERITY		LIKELIHOOD	
Fatality	3	Probable	3
Major injury	2	Possible	2
Minor injury	1	Unlikely	1

Activity	Personnel affected	Hazards	Risk (Severity × Likelihood)	Existing control measures	Residual risk (Severity × Likelihood)	Existing control measures
Meeting clients in seated area	P	Large amount of people at any one time	1×2=2	Signing in procedures	1×2=2	
Retail product area	P, ST, S	Chemical	1×2=2	Wearing protective gown	1×2=2	
				Metal cabinet for storage	1×2=2	
				Dummies on display		

Example of a risk assessment record: reception area

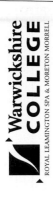

RISK ASSESSMENT

Programme area/Unit/Department: Beauty Therapy and Hairdressing

Logical assessment unit: Hairdressing V406/M408/M407

Completed by: D Edwards

Date: 10 April 200˙

Review date: Sept. 2001

Authorised by: Dawn Ward

Principal: Ioan Morgan

PERSONNEL AFFECTED – KEY

Staff	ST	Public	P	Young Persons	YP
Students	S	Contractors	C		

RISK RATING

SEVERITY		LIKELIHOOD	
Fatality	3	Probable	3
Major injury	2	Possible	2
Minor injury	1	Unlikely	1

Activity	Personnel affected	Hazards	Risk (Severity × Likelihood)	Existing control measures	Residual risk (Severity × Likelihood)	Existing control measures
Use of hairdryer	S ST	Electricity	2×2=4	PAT tested/maintenance Supervision of students Inspection of cables and connections by users	2×1=2	
Use of scissors/ razors	S ST P	Cutting	2×2=4	Supervision of students Safe working practices	1×1=1	
Chemicals: bleach/tint perms	S ST P		2×3=6	Supervision of students Instruction on mixing peroxide Metal cabinet/fridge for storage Skin test for skins prior to all applications	1×1=1	
Hair cutting on floor	S ST P	Slipping up	2×2=4	Supervision/instruction Safe systems of work	1×1=1	
Washing hair	S ST P	Hot/cold water (spillage)	1×2=2	Instruction to students Safe systems of work	1×1=1	
Styling products: gels hairsprays. etc.	S ST P	Flammable products	2×2=4	Metal cabinet for safe storage Safe systems at work	1×1=1	

Example of a risk assessment record: hairdressing department

RISK ASSESSMENT

Warwickshire COLLEGE
ROYAL LEAMINGTON SPA & MORETON MORRELL

Programme area/Unit/Department: Beauty Therapy and Hairdressing

Logical assessment unit: Laundry room

Completed by: Dawn Edwards

Date: 1 May 2001

Review date: Oct. 2001

Authorised by: Dawn Ward

Principal: Ioan Morgan

PERSONNEL AFFECTED – KEY

Staff	ST	Public	P	Young Persons	YP
Students	S	Contractors	C		

RISK RATING

SEVERITY		LIKELIHOOD	
Fatality	3	Probable	3
Major injury	2	Possible	2
Minor injury	1	Unlikely	1

Activity	Personnel affected	Hazards	Risk (Severity × Likelihood)	Existing control measures	Residual risk (Severity × Likelihood)	Existing control measures
Washing towels, etc.	S ST	Electricity	2×2=4	PAT tested, maintenance Service contract Instruction for users	1×2=2	
Tumble dryer	S ST	Electricity	2×2=4	PAT tested. Maintenance Instruction for users	2×1=2	
		Disposal of excess fluff	2×2=4	Extraction for fluff	1×1=1	
Ironing	ST	Electricity	2×1=2	PAT tested Safe practices of work	1×1=1	
Washing towels	ST	Chemical bleach	2×2=4	Safe practices at work Chemical in the metal cabinet Diluted as per instruction	1×1=1	

Example of a risk assessment record: laundry room

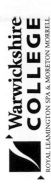

Warwickshire COLLEGE
ROYAL LEAMINGTON SPA & MORETON MORRELL

RISK ASSESSMENT

Programme area/Unit/Department: Beauty Therapy and Hairdressing

Logical assessment unit: Beauty M401/M403/M409/M502

Completed by: Dawn Edwards

Date: 10 April 2001

Review date: Sept. 2001

Authorised by: Dawn Ward

Principal: Ioan Morgan

PERSONNEL AFFECTED – KEY

Staff	ST	Public	P	Young Persons	YP
Students	S	Contractors	C		

RISK RATING

SEVERITY		LIKELIHOOD	
Fatality	3	Probable	3
Major injury	2	Possible	2
Minor injury	1	Unlikely	1

Activity	Personnel affected	Hazards	Risk (Severity × Likelihood)	Existing control measures	Residual risk (Severity × Likelihood)	Existing control measures
Use of hairdryer for mendhi	S ST	Electricity	2×2 = 4	Pat tested/maintenance Supervision of students Inspection of cables and connections by users	1×1 = 1	
Use of autoclave for sterilisation	S ST	Scald with steam Handling hot implements	2×2 = 4	Supervision of students Safe working practices	1×1 = 1	
Electrolysis	S ST P	Needle insertion Needle disposal	2×2 = 4	Supervision of students Safe systems of work Safe disposal in sealed bins collection by council	1×1 = 1	
Electrolysis blend machine	ST P S	Galvanic burn	2×2 = 4	Student supervision Safe systems at work	1×1 = 1	
Galvanic body machine	S ST P	Galvanic burn	2×2 = 4	Safe practices of work Student supervision	1×1 = 1	
Nail extension machine	S ST P	Hygiene/ infection	1×2 = 2	Student supervision induction	1×1 = 1	

Example of a risk assessment record: beauty department

RISK ASSESSMENT

Programme area/Unit/Department: Beauty Therapy and Hairdressing

Logical assessment unit: Stock rooms

Completed by: Dawn Edwards

Date: 1 May 2001

Review date: Oct. 2001

Authorised by: Dawn Ward

Principal: Ioan Morgan

![Warwickshire COLLEGE logo — ROYAL LEAMINGTON SPA & MORETON MORRELL]

PERSONNEL AFFECTED – KEY

Staff	ST	Public	P	Young Persons	YP
Students	S	Contractors	C		

RISK RATING

SEVERITY			LIKELIHOOD	
Fatality	3		Probable	3
Major injury	2		Possible	2
Minor injury	1		Unlikely	1

Activity	Personnel affected	Hazards	Risk (Severity × Likelihood)	Existing control measures	Residual risk (Severity × Likelihood)
Storage of chemicals and aerosols	ST	Flammable	2×2=4	Locked storage room with metal cabinet for flammable chemicals and aerosols	1×1=1
			2×2=4		1×1=1
Storage of equipment	ST		2×1=2	Unused equipment stored on shelves, safety ladder available to reach	1×1=1

Example of a risk assessment record: stock room

ACTION	ACTION BY	TARGET DATE	DATE COMPLETED

Example of a risk assessment action plan

ACTIVITY

1   Make a list of all the hazards in your salon environment and evaluate their potential risk. Draw up a list to reduce the potential risks you have identified.
2   List the safe working practices you observe on a daily basis within the salon and reception area.
3   State what your responsibilities are with regard to health and safety within the salon environment.
4   Name the persons to whom you would report any health and safety issues.
5   Why is it essential to follow manufacturer's and distributor's instructions on the care, maintenance, storage and use of their equipment and products?

Consultation

In order to achieve a beneficial treatment plan for an individual client, it is essential that the therapist carries out a thorough consultation to establish a clear picture of the client's needs and constraints. This can prove to be a lengthy process for the trainee therapist but with time and practice the process will become easier and quicker.

There are many reasons why a client books an appointment for a particular treatment:

- They have heard about its benefits from friends.
- They have read about it or seen advertisements in magazines or local/national papers.
- It has been arranged by a relative or friend as a gift.
- They have, in their eyes, a problem, e.g. excess weight, poor skin condition, cellulite, stretch marks, tension in the muscles.
- They have a problem but don't have the confidence to book the type of treatment needed for this and so they have booked another type of treatment hoping the therapist will boost their confidence and recommend a suitable treatment plan for them.

When carrying out a consultation there are a number of things that the therapist needs to establish: medical details, personal details, body condition, skin analysis.

Medical details

Information regarding the client's past and present medical history should give the therapist clear indicators as to the possible underlying causes of the client's problems such as: the contraceptive pill causing an increase in appetite leading to weight gain; steroid medication for asthma causing weight gain; restricted mobility due to recent scar tissue causing poor muscle tone; previous acne causing skin-pitting-type scarring; childbirth causing poor abdominal muscle tone. Taking medical details also enables the therapist to identify possible contraindications to treatments.

Note: Specific contraindications to individual treatments are dealt with in each chapter.

Personal details

The therapist will take note of personal client details such as name, address and telephone numbers for their client database. A database can be used for a variety of things such as for marketing purposes, e.g. notifying customers of special offers and new product/equipment launches. They are also useful in case of emergencies, such as therapist illness, where an appointment needs to be altered or confirmed.

Taking personal and medical details during the consultation procedure enables the therapist to establish a professional rapport with the client, to put apprehensive clients at ease and to build up a clear picture of the individual client. Information on the client's lifestyle and occupation assist in analysing the client's constraints (time and finances) which have to be taken into consideration when organising a treatment plan for the client. This can also help the therapist in analysing the cause of the client's problem, e.g. a sales representative's job would generally involve a great deal of driving which could led to tension in the trapezius muscle and kyphosis.

A therapist would automatically consider the general health of their client as this can affect many different aspects such as skin condition, posture, etc. It is also useful to consider the client's intake of such things as alcohol, coffee and tea, particularly if the client suffers with cellulite or fluid retention. Tobacco smoking can cause dehydration of the skin as well as generally being an unhealthy habit. Diet plays a large part in our health so this should be taken into consideration as well. A poor diet can affect many of the body functions and systems, e.g. insufficient water could lead to constipation which in turn can bring about poor skin condition.

Female clients may suffer with skin-related problems such as 'breakouts' due to their menstrual cycle, or they may suffer with pre-menstrual syndrome which may affect their general wellbeing and cause many problems such as dehydration of the skin due to stress. The menstrual cycle brings about many changes in the client's body due to the hormonal balance and it is very useful to establish the time of the month prior to treatment, e.g. pre-menstrual, post-menstrual or mid-cycle.

Exposure to ultraviolet radiation is also noted in the consultation process as this can affect the client's skin condition and the sensitivity of the skin.

- A client who suffers with lower backache in the pre-menstrual cycle may benefit from a back massage for relaxation.
- Sunburn in the area of treatment is a contraindication.
- Exposure to ultraviolet radiation can cause dehydration and ageing of the skin.
- A professional therapist will always consider the client as an individual and where needed recommend an alternative therapist for treatments that they are not qualified to offer. For example, if a client has superfluous hair due to hormonal change such as pregnancy, the therapist would recommend electro-epilation, intense pulse light (IPL) or laser treatment.

Body condition

At the initial consultation for body treatments the therapist would establish the client's weight, height, frame size and body type, e.g. ectomorph, endomorph, mesomorph or combination. If the client was extremely sensitive about their

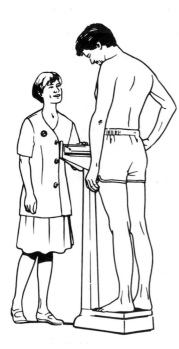

Body condition

Medical details	Personal details
Name of doctor:	Name of client:
Present medication:	Address:
Past medication:	
Number of pregnancies:	Home tel.: Work tel.:
Ages of children:	Date of birth:
Operations: Hysterectomy ( ) Caesarean section ( ) Others	Lifestyle:
	Occupation:
	Smoker (Y/N) Number per week:
Contraindications: Diabetes ( ) Epilepsy ( ) Pacemaker ( ) Heart condition ( ) Asthma ( ) Thrombosis/phlebitis ( ) Metal pins/plates ( ) Skin diseases/disorders ( ) Oedema ( ) Blood pressure (high/low) Recent scars (up to 12 months) ( ) Hepatitis/blood infections (up to 24 months) ( ) Cuts/bruises ( )	

Body condition
Height: Weight: Frame size (small/medium/large)
Body type (ectomorph/endomorph/mesomorph/combination)
Muscle tone (please use the following symbols: +good, =medium, –poor):
Biceps/triceps ( )   Abdominals ( )   Abductors ( )   Adductors ( )   Gluteals ( )   Other
Types of adipose deposit (hard/medium/soft/cellulite)
Areas of adipose deposit:
Areas of cellulite:
Varicose veins/broken capillaries: Circulation (good/poor/fluid retention)
Figure/posture analysis: Scoliosis ( )   Kyphosis ( )   Lordosis ( )   Other
Reason for treatment

Treatment plan	
Recommended retail/home care advice:	Recommended salon treatments:
Eyes	
Face	
Neck	
Décolleté	Recommended salon products:
Bust	Dietary/exercise advice:
Body	

Note. The reverse of this card can be used for recording a client's measurements when undertaking figure improvement programmes.

Indemnity: I confirm that to the best of my knowledge the answers that I have given are correct and that I have not withheld any information.

Signatures of: Client: Date:

                    Therapist: Date:

Example of a trainee's consultation card for body treatments

weight at the initial consultation, the therapist could offer a questionnaire with a number of weight variables to ascertain an approximate guide for organising a treatment plan.

Testing of the client's muscle tone is undertaken to establish any weak areas. The therapist would also note types of adipose tissue, e.g. cellulite, soft tissue and the area of the deposits along with any varicose veins or broken capillaries which may contraindicate treatment and the condition of the client's circulation, e.g. good, poor, fluid retention.

A thorough figure and posture analysis is carried out to highlight any problem areas and the client's reasons for treatment are recorded. All of these points will assist the therapist in establishing a total picture of the client's needs in order to develop a realistic treatment plan for the client.

An example of a trainee's consultation card for body treatments is given on p. 271.

information point

Before stress can be dealt with effectively the therapist must be able to recognise its symptoms.

- Physical symptoms of stress: tension headaches; indigestion; muscle tension; dry mouth and throat; tiredness; menstrual problems; diarrhoea/frequent urination; constipation; clumsiness.
- Emotional symptoms of stress: rapid mood swings; lack of concentration; indecision; feeling tearful.
- Behavioural symptoms of stress: sleep problems; over-eating or loss of appetite; withdrawal from friends and work colleagues; increase in smoking/alcohol intake.

Skin analysis

Analysis of the client's skin condition and turgor (tone) will enable the therapist to evaluate their needs. On a consultation card used for training, a list of the main muscles or areas affecting expression lines could be listed to assist the trainee in recalling the key areas to consider along with possible problems the client might experience, e.g. comedones, areas of flakiness, poor elasticity, acne, rosacea.
An area for the therapist to note additional comments such as if the client has used products like Retinoic A which could contraindicate them to treatments such as waxing, or to note previous treatments and products used. The reason for treatment needs to be established during the consultation procedure to ensure that the therapist can organise an effective treatment plan. Skin analysis can be studied in depth in *A Practical Guide to Beauty Therapy* by Janet Simms published by Nelson Thornes.

An example of a trainee's consultation card for facial treatments is given opposite. After six treatments it is recommended that a new consultation card is completed.

Treatment plan

The therapist is now able to recommend salon treatments, identify a suitable salon range of products and the appropriate retail products for the client and where applicable advise on complementary diet and exercise.

An example of a body treatment record card is given on p. 274.

Medical details	Personal details
Name of doctor:	Name of client:
Present medication:	Address:
Past medication:	
Number of pregnancies:	Home tel.: Work tel.:
Ages of children:	Date of birth:
Operations: Hysterectomy ( ) Caesarean section ( )	Lifestyle:
Others	Occupation:
	Smoker (Y/N) Number per week:
Contraindications: Diabetes ( ) Epilepsy ( ) Pacemaker ( ) Heart condition ( ) Asthma ( ) Thrombosis/phlebitis ( ) Metal pins/plates ( ) Skin diseases/disorders ( ) Oedema ( ) Blood pressure (high/low) Recent scars (up to 12 months) ( ) Hepatitis/blood infections (up to 24 months) ( ) Cuts/bruises ( ) General health (good/poor)	Drink (units per week): Alcohol ( ) Coffee ( ) Tea ( ) Diet: Digestion: General health (good/poor) Exposure to ultraviolet/skin condition:

Skin analysis

Muscle tone (please use the following symbols: +good, =medium, –poor):

Décolleté ( )   Neck ( )   Mandible ( )   Zygomaticus ( )   Orbicularis occuli ( )

Skin turgor (tone):	Areas of pigmentation:
Areas of broken capillaries:	Type of pigmentation/vein:
Skin texture:	
Oedema:	Collagen/elasticity:
Open pores:	Comedones (open/closed/micro):
Papules:	Pustules:
Moles:	Superfluous hair:
Area of flakiness:	Area of shininess:
Seborrhea:	Acne rosacea:
Acne vulgaris:	Dermatitis/eczema:
Psoriasis:	Skin tags:
Dehydration:	Scarring

Skin type:

Comments:

Reason for treatment

Treatment plan

Recommended retail/home care advice:	Recommended salon treatments:
Eyes	
Face	
Neck	
Décolleté	Recommended salon products:
Bust	Dietary/exercise advice:
Body	

Indemnity: I confirm that to the best of my knowledge the answers that I have given are correct and that I have not withheld any information.

Signatures of: Client: Date:

                      Therapist: Date:

Example of a trainee's card for facial treatments

Body treatment record card			
Name of client: _____			
Address: _____		Home tel.: _____	
_____		Work tel.: _____	
	Date	Treatment, products and equipment	Therapist
Client's views on previous treatment			

Example of a body treatment record card

You need to know what these words and phrases mean. Go back through the chapter to find out.

AIDS

Animal parasites

Antiseptics

Autoclave

Bacteria

Chemical methods of sterilisation

Consultation

Dealing with clients, visitors and reception enquiries

Disinfection

Emergency first aid

Fungi

Glass bead steriliser

Hazard

Hepatitis B

Maintaining stock in the retail area

Reception

Receptionist

Risk

Sanitiser

Sterilisation

Viruses

1   Explain why you should consider the following when carrying out a client consultation:
    a personal details
    b medical details
    c body condition
    d skin analysis.

2   What two key areas form a treatment plan?

3   List three examples of:
    a physical symptoms of stress
    b emotional symptoms of stress
    c behavioural symptoms of stress.

4   State the information that should be recorded on a client record card.

Chapter 10 The business environment & related salon administration

After working through this chapter you will:

- have a greater awareness of what is involved in setting up a business
- recognise the roles and responsibilities of the employment structure
- understand the types of resources needed to operate a commercial salon and how to effectively deploy them
- have a greater understanding of the management procedures required to run a successful business.

Beauty therapy is a diverse and exciting career offering many opportunities and working arrangements. There are few professions where so much choice is available. It is essential that the therapist has a good working knowledge of salon administration and related legislation whether they are a junior therapist, manager or self-employed, as the success of the salon ultimately depends on efficient working practices.

Different countries have different legislation governing business practices. This chapter focuses on those business practices in England and Wales and is not intended to be definitive, but more a guide and source of reference.

Forms of business arrangements

Legally all businesses fall into one of the following categories:

- Sole trader.
- Partnership.
- Limited company.
- Franchise.
- Co-operative.

Sole trader

This is the simplest form of business organisation. One person controls finance and decisions. From a legal point of view there is nothing that needs to be done to set up in business as a sole trader.

Advantages

- Easy to set up – no lengthy legal formalities.
- Total control of the business.
- Immediate decision-making.
- Taxed as an individual.
- Should benefit from close relations with suppliers.
- Easy to wind up.

Disadvantages

- Liable for any business losses.
- No legal distinction between the business and personal assets.
- Possible lack of continuity in management if the owner is ill.
- Does not have status.
- Possible lack of finances for expansion.

Partnership

By definition, a partnership is when two or more people go into business together without registering as a limited company or a co-operative.

Again this form of business can be set up without legal formalities, but it is not to be recommended as severe disagreements could jeopardise the business. It is much safer to have a formal partnership agreement drawn up detailing the roles and responsibilities of all partners.

Advantages

- A good way to start up a business that requires more capital than one person alone may have.
- Wider range of complementary skills and knowledge.
- Sharing of workload and general pressures of running a business.
- Sharing of any business losses.

Disadvantages

- All partners are responsible for any business debts even if they are caused by the actions of the other(s).
- Legal costs involved in drawing up a partnership agreement.
- Death or bankruptcy of one partner will automatically dissolve the partnership (unless previous arrangements have been made).
- Possible personality clashes can cause problems.

Limited company

A limited company is formed with a minimum of two shareholders, one of whom must be a director. A company secretary must also be appointed but he/she can be an outsider.

This is a company whereby any business debts are limited to the amount put in. Therefore if the business does go bankrupt, personal possessions cannot be taken to pay the company's debts.

A limited company prior to registration must produce and adhere to two legal documents:

- Memorandum of Association – this sets out the objectives of the company, as well as the company's share capital.

- Articles of Association – sets out additional rules by which the company will be governed.

Advantages
- Limited liability.
- Capital may be increased by selling shares.
- Better definition of management structures.
- Business not affected by death or bankruptcy of any of its shareholders.
- Higher level of status.
- Shareholders are employees of the company and therefore entitled to DWP benefits should the need arise.

Disadvantages
- Costly to set up with time-consuming legal formalities.
- The business will have to make public its accounts.
- As an employee of the company you will be subject to PAYE (see p. 294).

Franchise
A franchise is a business relationship between a franchiser (the owner of a name or method of business) and a franchisee (an operator of that business). The franchisee agrees to pay the franchiser a sum of money for the use of the business name, method of doing business, etc. Often there is an initial fee and an agreed percentage of sales afterwards is paid to the franchiser by the franchisee.

Advantages
- A tried and tested formula.
- A corporate image, instantly recognisable.
- Normally there is a wealth of knowledge available concerning most aspects of the business.
- Back-up services normally provided.
- Sharing of advertising costs.

Disadvantages
- Normally very expensive to set up.
- Business never truly your own.
- Franchiser may lay down certain requirements.
- May not be a flexible enough system to cater for changing needs of a local market.
- Profits normally have to be shared with the franchiser.

Co-operative
A co-operative is a business that is owned and controlled by the people working in it, therefore membership is usually open to all employees. The profits are not shared on the amount of capital put into the business by each individual but are distributed in proportion to the amount of work done by each person.

Choice and type of premises

When setting up in business one of the first things you will need to think about is the premises. The type and location of the premises are extremely important and it will be essential to thoroughly research this. First, you will need to establish that there is going to be a suitable potential market where you are looking. Local competitors will also need to be taken into account as will parking facilities and neighbouring businesses (you hardly want to be situated next door to a betting office!). If the premises you are interested in are not already occupied as a salon you will need to apply to the local council for a change of use.

information point

Never agree to take on premises until you have been granted a change of use.

You then need to decide whether you are going to buy or rent premises. It will probably be the case that finances dictate your ultimate choice, but remember that sometimes large shopping complexes are owned by large companies or councils so the choice may be taken further from you.

Buying

If you decide that you are going to buy your premises you will need to contact a solicitor immediately to deal with the contracts involved and also to organise a land search. This is to check the ownership of the property and any plans in the future for redevelopment, etc. You will also need to establish if the property is freehold, which means that the land and building would be yours if you purchased it, or whether it is leasehold, which would mean that the building would be yours but the land that it is built on belongs to a third party and you would need to pay a ground rent.

Renting

Renting, or leasing as it is correctly known, is when you agree to occupy a building in return for an agreed sum of money. If you decide to rent a property you will again need the services of a solicitor to draw up a lease agreement which should include the following:

- How much rent is to be paid and how often (monthly, quarterly, etc.).
- When the amount of rent paid will be reviewed.
- How long the lease will run for.
- Who will be responsible for repairs, upkeep and decoration of the premises both internally and externally.
- What the rules are regarding subletting.
- Awareness of the Landlord and Tenant Act 1954.

Altering premises

Whether you are the owner of the property or just leasing, if you wish to alter the premises you will need to check the following:

- Planning permission.
- Building and fire regulations.
- Offices, Shops and Railway Premises Act 1963.

information point

Before setting up in business it is essential to prepare a plan, particularly if financial support is needed. Most banks and financial institutions offer guidance and support for small businesses. A business plan should include:

- An Executive Summary – this is a 'taster' which will tempt the reader to continue.
- A Vision/Mission statement, which might be supported by a set of values or codes of conduct.
- Personal details.
- Type of business.
- Business market.
- SWOT analysis (Strengths, Weaknesses, Opportunities and Threats) and the appropriate strategies to address them.
- An appraisal of the market and the environment in which the business will operate.
- A marketing and sales strategy and forecast, which demonstrates how clients will be identified and how the business will be promoted to them. This should also include market research identifying your competitors and clients, your unique selling point (USP), how the products and services will be priced.
- A human resource strategy for the business which demonstrates how suitable skills will be developed or obtained.
- A financial strategy, including profit and loss account and cash flow forecast for the first two years of trading.

BUSINESS DETAILS

Name of business
Address of business

Status of business
Type of business
Telephone
Date business began (if you have already started trading)
Business activities

PERSONAL DETAILS

Name
Address

Telephone (home)	Telephone (work)
Qualifications	
	Date of birth

Relevant work experience

Business experience

Details of personnel (if any)

Name	Name
Position	Position
Address	Address
Date of birth	Date of birth
Qualifications	Qualifications
Relevant work experience	Relevant work experience
Present income	Present income

What skills will you need to buy in during the first two years?

PERSONNEL

Estimate the cost of employing any people or buying any services you may need in the first two years.

Number of people	Job function	Monthly cost	Annual cost

(Remember to include you own salary and those of any you may have in this calculation.)

continued

An example of a business plan

PRODUCT SERVICE

Description of type of products/services to be offered.

Contribution of individual products or services to total turnover

Product   Percentage contribution

                                                                        (The figures in this column should add up to 100.)

Break down the cost of materials (if any)
  PRODUCT 1
  Materials (including packaging, labelling, etc.)   Cost

  *Selling price for Product 1
  PRODUCT 2

  *Selling price for Product 2
  PRODUCT 3

  *Selling price for Product 3
  (*These are assumptions)
Where did you get your estimate from?
Material   Source

MARKET

Describe your market

Where is you market?

Who are your customers?

Is you market growing, static or in decline?

Itemise the competitive products or services
  Name of competitor 1
  Competitor's product/service
  Name   Price
  Strengths   Weakness

  Name of competitor 2
  Competitor's product/service
  Name   Price
  Strengths   Weakness

  Name of competitor 3
  Competitor's product/service
  Name   Price
  Strengths   Weakness

continued

An example of a business plan continued

What is special about your product or service?

Advantages of your product or service over
  Competitor 1

  Competitor 2

  Competitor 3

What is your sales forecast for the
  *1st three months?   Total value
  Treatments/products
  *2nd three months?   Total value
  Treatments/products
  *3rd three months?   Total value
  Treatments/products
  *4th three months   Total value
  Treatments/products
  (*These are assumptions)

Explain how you have calculated these estimates

Give details of any firm orders you have already taken

MARKETING

What sort of marketing do your competitors do?
  Competitor 1

  Competitor 2

  Competitor 3

What sort of marketing or advertising do you intend to do?
Method   Cost

Why do you think that these methods are appropriate for your particular market?

Where did you get your estimates from?
Method   Source

PREMISES/EQUIPMENT/PRODUCT

Where do you intend to locate the business and why?

What sort and size of premises will you need?

What are the details of any lease, licence, rent, rates and when is the next rent review due?

continued

An example of a business plan continued

What equipment and products do you require?

Is equipment bought or leased and how long is the life span?

On what terms will the products be purchased?

RECORDS
Describe records to be kept and how they are to be kept up to date?

OBJECTIVES
What are your personal objectives in running the business?
 Short-term

 Medium-term

 Long-term

How do you intend to achieve them?

What objectives do you have for the business itself?
 Short-term

 Medium-term

 Long-term

How do you intend to achieve them?

FINANCE
Give details of your known orders and sales (if any)

	Date	Orders/sales	Details	Delivery date
1				
2				
3				
4				

Give details of your current business assets (if any)

Item	Value	Life expectancy

continued

An example of a business plan continued

HEALTH AND BEAUTY THERAPY: A PRACTICAL APPROACH

What will you need to buy to start up and then throughout your first year?

Start up

Item	Value

Year I

Item	Value

How will you pay for these?

	Value	Date
Grants		
Own resources		
Loans		
Creditors		

What credit is available from your suppliers?

Supplier	Estimated value of monthly order	Number of days credit

What are your loan or overdraft requirements?

What are you putting in yourself?

What security will you be able to put up?

OTHER

Accountant
Address

Telephone

Solicitor
Address

Telephone

VAT registration
Insurance arrangements

An example of a business plan continued

SELF-CHECKS

1 **a** List four forms of business arrangement.
  b Give two advantages and two disadvantages of each form of business arrangement.

2 State four important points to consider when looking for business premises.

3 Compare and contrast buying and renting as an option when deciding on business premises.

Staff and recruitment

Role of the employer

The employer has overall control of the wellbeing and efficient running of the business whether or not they are directly involved in it.

Role of the manager/manageress

In smaller establishments this role may be performed by the employer. It is not an easy task, requiring a great deal of skill and judgement.

The personal qualities that make a good manager are:

- Enthusiasm about the business and the industry in general.
- Willingness to listen and learn.
- Ability to juggle many tasks at the same time: clients, staff, book-keeping, wages, etc.
- Patience and tact in dealing with both staff and client problems both on a business and a personal level.
- Knowledge of new trends, e.g. attending exhibitions, reading trade journals, etc.
- Excellent personal and interpersonal skills (tact, diplomacy, punctuality, good communicator, working as a member of a team).
- Immaculate appearance.

The role of the therapist

It goes without saying that the therapist should be well trained and qualified. The therapist needs to be enthusiastic about their work and have a willingness to

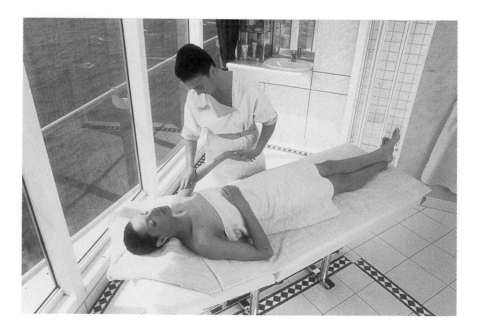

Salon at sea

learn and develop skills. The therapist needs to have a flexible approach and be happy to work as a member of a team, sometimes performing different roles. Again, they should possess excellent personal and interpersonal skills and be of immaculate appearance.

Role of the receptionist

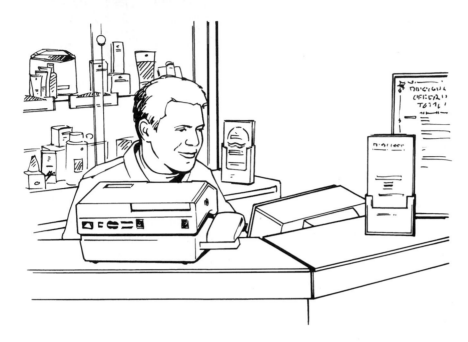

Computerised reception

The receptionist is the first point of contact with the salon and therefore extremely important for the business. The reception area may be staffed by more than one person in larger establishments and by the therapists themselves in smaller concerns. Whoever performs the task needs to be well trained in the workings of the reception area as potential business can be lost through incompetence. (See Chapter 9.)

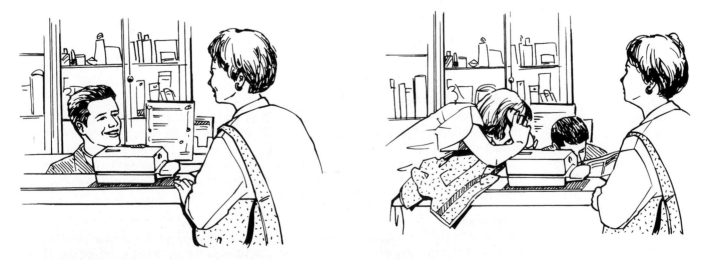

Good and poor reception

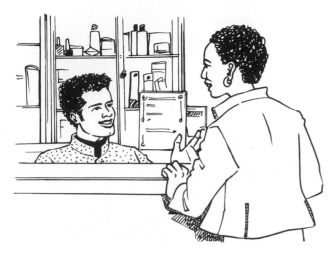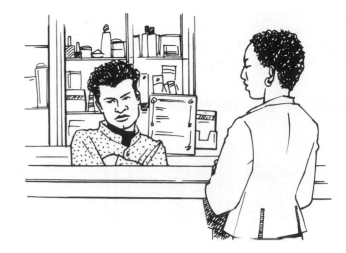

Body language

Support staff

In larger establishments, roles such as cleaning, laundry, handling of stock, preparation of working areas, etc. may be performed by support staff, which will obviously add to the overall efficiency of services provided. However, it is important that everyone in the establishment can deal with these areas if continuity is to be maintained.

Efficient and effective staff practices

Communication

If the salon is ultimately going to be a successful business it will depend upon efficient levels of communication between all employees, thus making the staff more highly motivated and providing a friendly atmosphere for the client. It is also crucial that the communication with clients as well as each other creates a welcoming environment.

- Regular staff meetings should be arranged so all employees know what is happening and are allowed to give comments and express their views.
- Staff should be made to feel that they are an important part of the business.
- Staff should be aware of the range of resources used within the business and how these can be efficiently and effectively utilised to ensure the business is financially sound
- Staff should be rewarded for anything they do well.
- All employees should be treated equally and fairly.
- Gossip should be discouraged either about clients or fellow employees.
- All employees should be treated with respect.

Staff development

The success of the business lies in expansion and not remaining static. New treatments and ideas should be periodically introduced to increase profit margins, attract new clients and to keep abreast of changes. Staff should be regularly sent on training courses whether they be for product knowledge, new skills or further qualifications. This will also help to ensure a highly motivated workforce boosting staff morale.

Appraisal

Appraisal is the term given to a review of an employee's performance over a given period of time, normally annually. The main reason for operating an appraisal system is to help the employee become more effective. It provides the owner/manager with

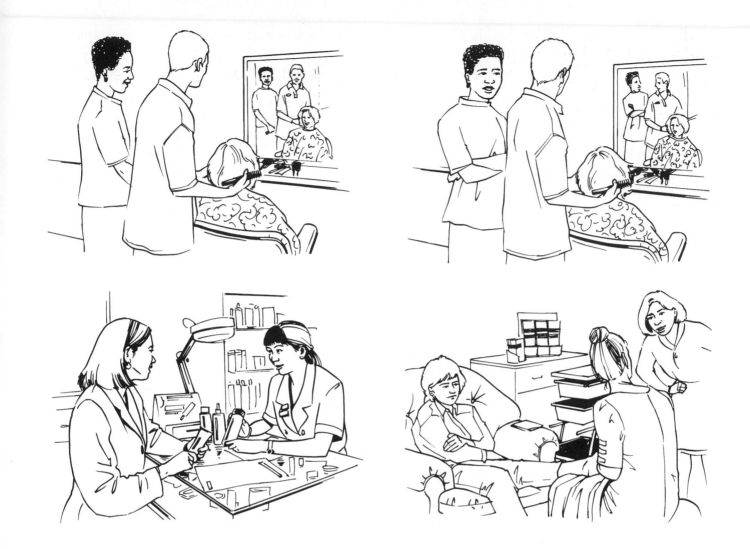

Good and poor practice

the opportunity to review and discuss targets that have been agreed with their employee, such as their productivity (sales/treatment) targets and personal development targets, which contribute to the effectiveness of the business. However, issues should not be left to an annual appraisal, they should be identified and dealt with in the appropriate manner.

The appraisal is normally categorised into the following areas:

- Review. Looking back over the period concerned, what is the appraisee's job? Has it altered in any way? Is it being performed effectively? Are there any problems?
- Action. What needs to be done? Should there be any training and development? Does the employee need more support/guidance?
- Monitoring. Are the actions being carried out? Are targets being achieved?

Costing of treatments

Many salons do not properly cost out their services so therefore they do not make an adequate profit and wonder why the business is not doing very well even though the appointment book is always full. Costing is very important and should encompass materials, overheads, wages and a profit margin.

The following shows an example of a back massage treatment with an explanation underneath:

Back massage treatment (30 minutes) £15.00

Material	£1.00
Electricity	£0.80
Laundry	£1.00
Overhead	£1.20
Labour	£6.00
Profit @ 50%	£5.00

- The figures for the materials used are obtained by dividing how much the product would cost at retail by the number of times you can use that product.
- The electricity and overheads costs are calculated by taking the quarterly bills, dividing to find the hourly rate and then dividing again by the number of therapists.
- Laundry is calculated in the same way.
- Labour in this incidence is calculated on the therapist working for £12.00 per hour.
- Profit is calculated on 50% of the total other costs.

SELF-CHECKS

1. Identify the important legislative requirements necessary to conduct a successful business.

2. What is the main purpose of a contract of employment? Outline the important points such a contract should cover.

3. State the roles and responsibilities of:
   a the employer
   b the manager
   c the therapist
   d the receptionist.

4. What do you understand by the term 'appraisal'?

ACTIVITY

Cost out a range of salon services based on the example given.

Marketing and promotion

Many salon owners may wonder why business is not better when they feel they are offering an excellent service, using top quality products and employing well-qualified and highly competent staff. The answer probably lies in the fact that they are not marketing themselves sufficiently.

Marketing is not just about placing an advertisement in the local paper, it is the whole product, the image that the salon wishes to create. In the business of aesthetics this is never more important, attention to detail counts. Marketing your services and appropriate skin-care products to the right audience requires foresight, empathy, knowledge, enthusiasm and above all, understanding.

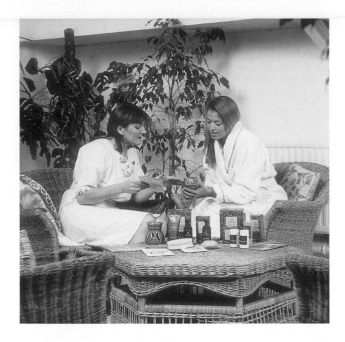
Consultation area

Retailing in the salon

Selling is a very important aspect of salon operations. Profits made on the sales of products and services make the business successful, which will ultimately increase the earning potential of all the employees.

The majority of sales in a salon are lost by therapists who think it is not their job to 'sell'. However, a professional therapist realises that a client is not only paying for a service but for the experience and knowledge the therapist has to offer. Many clients are reluctant to ask the therapist which products and treatments are right for them but they desperately want to know. It is an essential part of a therapist's job to provide their clients with advice on how to take care of themselves and this includes advice on treatments and products. A therapist must look at each client individually and ensure they link suitable treatments and products not only to the service the client has booked but perhaps also to the client's lifestyle. For example, if a client booked for a back massage informs the therapist she is getting married in nine months, the therapist could link a range of treatments such as facials, waxing, manicures, slimming and toning treatments and make-up to help her prepare for her big day. Remember, therapists train for a long time and every year of industrial experience with additional training expands the breadth of knowledge that can be offered to a client.

Cerebral profile of a client

It is paramount that a therapist can identify an individual client's cerebral profile in order to meet their retailing needs. Asking questions and listening to the client's responses can assess this. The therapist must then choose products to match the client's needs and select the appropriate vocabulary (to suit her cerebral profile) to gain a 'yes' response to retailing. A client may actually have several profiles to match her lifestyle, for example one for work and one for her private home life. A therapist must also assess their own profile in order to learn how to identify and strengthen their own weaknesses.

Research has identified four different client profiles:

1   **The rational (intellectual, technical) client**: will analyse every piece of information available, will not want to know about packaging or product texture, but will want pure factual information on ingredients and their effects. The sale

of goods to this client will be made more quickly if you give precise information and the correct products and ingredients to gain the appropriate results. This type of client will spend a lot of money if the quality is right.

2   **The insecure client**: needs security, so the therapist must reassure them, be extremely patient and proceed step by step. This client will need a lot of written documentation to peruse (finding security in written rather than spoken information), will want to know how long the product brand has been around, the number of countries where it is available and whether it has been tested, for example in hospitals, etc. This client will have a mental budget before entering the salon and will know what they have available to spend.

Always reassure this type of client; slowly tell them step by step that they have made a good choice, the right choice and that they will be very pleased with their purchase. This client will need to be given trial sizes with leaflets and brochures. However unwittingly, do not mislead the client. The sale will take time but once you have established trust and confidence this client will maintain their trust in you.

3   **The 'original' (artist) client**: wants the latest product and wants to be the only one with it! It is important to stimulate this client's imagination; they will not want technical information as they are after the designer 'tag' and like to take risks. As long as you do not mislead you could use phrases like: 'this product is revolutionary', 'extraordinary', 'outstanding' or better still 'it's unique', 'just for you'. The sale to this client does not take so long and they will not have a fixed budget.

4   **The sentimental client**: is extremely talkative, wants to be your friend and to do exactly the same as you. This client is generally very emotional and will talk about their spouse, children, grandparents, animals and so on. It is important to be very attentive, paying close attention to details such as noting their birthday, likes and dislikes, etc. If the client talks about their next family holiday, for example, you could direct them to the skin-care products they could purchase for use in the sun, discussing the texture, colour and aroma of the product which they will enjoy talking about. The sale with this client may take a long time but they have no mental budget and they will trust your advice.

Objections to sales

In learning to retail, the therapist needs to understand why the various objections to sales are made and whether an objection has occurred because of a misunderstanding. The therapist must put in place a 'discovery step' to establish what is behind the objection and whether it is authentic. To do this the therapist and client need to be face to face, for eye contact, so that the therapist can ascertain the real reason for the objection from the client. That it is a 'real' objection may be evident from the client's non-verbal communication – their body language may be relaxed while they answer questions. A client making a 'fake' objection may be less relaxed and may seek reassurance by frequently touching their face. The therapist should take a positive approach to the challenge of an objection by trying to discover whether there is a misunderstanding, by staying calm and not becoming aggressive, and by respecting the client's wishes and needs.

There are several common objections to making a purchase.

● **Costs**. You could establish why the client thinks the product is expensive by asking them with what they are comparing the product. Perhaps the product seems expensive compared to the brand the client currently uses, so you could compare active ingredients of that brand to the one being recommended or discuss which will give the greater results in a shorter space of time. Never belittle a competitor but state the obvious, for example if the client is using a product with which you are familiar, you may be able to tell her the product is less suitable for her at the moment as her skin is currently dehydrated. Ask the client about her skin and whether she is seeing an improvement in her skin, as generally in retail outlets there is no follow-up to check on any improvement once a client has purchased a product. You, however, can provide a professional service and can evaluate and review home-care on a monthly basis and recommend the use of high quality professional products with active ingredients prescribed by a professional therapist. Remember, if cost is a problem to a client do not recommend several products to them, prioritise just one.

- **Time**. Establish why the client believes they have no time for skin care by asking what they mean by a long time. Respond that it takes only 5–10 minutes a day for basic skin care to maintain the youthful appearance of the skin.
- **Efficiency**. Generally, a client who uses this as an objection will have either a 'rational' or an 'insecure' profile so the therapist needs to respond with the appropriate vocabulary to reassure them. Establish what they mean by 'not efficient' and respond with the appropriate information such as quoting past case studies or data on efficiency tests carried out by the manufacturer.
- **Texture/Aroma**. If the client raises an objection over these points then the therapist is at fault, as they have not listened adequately to the client's preferences, noting the textures and aromas they like, before recommending products.
- **Sensitivity**. If a client states that they are sensitive to products, the therapists must determine what they mean by sensitive. Discuss what ingredients they are sensitive to and respond with information supplied by the manufacturer on dermatological tests they have carried out. Always offer this client a trial size product (it is not a gift to complement a sale but a trial for allergy testing to reassure them) and record this on their record card ensuring a follow-up on its performance at the next visit.

The therapist's body language, volume and speed of voice, appearance and perfume and the salon environment (the temperature, lighting, aroma, etc.) will all play an important part in establishing a professional relationship with clients, therefore ultimately affecting the total revenue into the salon from treatments and retail.

To gain information from the client, a therapist must use open questions which allow the client to respond and closed questions to confirm information and gain a 'yes' response to a question. For example, if a client indicates they want to purchase an efficient slimming cream, the therapist should respond by asking what the client means by 'efficient'. The client's response will provide the therapist with a guide to either a further open question or a closed one to take the sale forward. After gaining several 'yes' responses, the therapist must close the sale by asking whether the client would like to buy the product(s) today.

GOOD PRACTICE

- Ensure you offer each client retail and salon treatment advice.
- Listen to each client to identify their profile and select the appropriate vocabulary to gain a 'yes' response.
- Keep up-to-date with all the commercial and professional products on the market.
- Record all sales and trial sizes on each client's records and evaluate and review the client's progress at their next visit.

It is important to have a thorough understanding of all the products and treatments available in the salon. Many skin-care companies offer product knowledge workshops to familiarise the therapist with the products and methods they offer. If this is not available then it will be essential to read all the information available about the products you intend to sell.

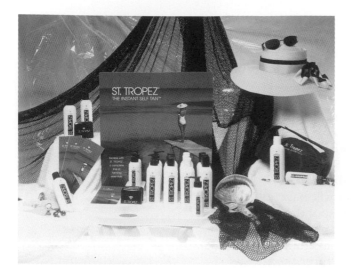
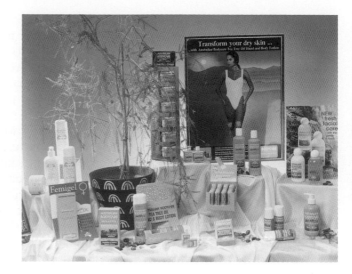

Promotional displays

Advice for successful selling

1   Find out exactly what the client needs. This means asking questions and listening carefully to the answers. Use closed questions to get short, straightforward answers (usually yes or no); these help to confirm or eliminate information and ideas. Use open questions to invite fuller and more detailed answers. Open questions help to develop the conversation and provide more personal information.

2   Give the client advice. Always relate the benefits of the product specifically to the client.

3   Always smile and talk confidently and positively about the product which you have chosen. Where possible tell the client about your personal experiences with the product.

4   Explain how the product should be used. If possible let the client feel, smell or hold the product. Remember that if the client touches the product and asks the price, then the item is practically sold.

5   Close the sale. Look for signals that tell you the client has decided to take your advice and buy the product; head nodding in agreement, smiles and friendly eye contact are positive buying signals.

6   Where appropriate, explain the benefits of the different sizes available in the product. These will usually be linked to the price. Hesitation or reluctance to mention the price will give the client the impression that you consider the product too expensive.

7   Gain agreement with the client. This is achieved either immediately or after a short period of 'thinking' time. Do not be afraid of silences at this stage. Just keep quiet and wait patiently for the patient to make a decision. Do not talk yourself out of a sale.

8   Use link selling to encourage your client to buy complementary products from the same range, e.g. cleansers and toners, body exfoliants and lotions, etc.

9   Once you have sold the product, wrap it up and process the payment. As you hand over the purchase, check once more that the client understands how to use the product.

10 Enter the details of the purchase on the client's record card and be sure to ask next time how the client is finding the product.

Sales and selling pointers

- Offer trial sizes to unsure clients to help gain a sale.
- Offer trial sizes when clients purchase a product to introduce them to an additional or complementary product within that range.
- Introduce a client referral scheme into the salon – if a regular client introduces a friend then some kind of incentive such as a discount could be given.
- Introduce a referral scheme with other practitioners – offer incentives to possible sources of client referrals such as hairdressing salons or health clinics.
- If a therapist goes on maternity leave, send a card informing her regular clients and perhaps offer them a discount for treatments with another therapist until she returns.
- Acknowledge all clients' birthdays – in the month of their birthday send each client an incentive to visit the salon.
- Organise new treatment promotions.
- Have new treatment information printed and hand it out to every client.
- Offer special treatment packages – holidays, Christmas, etc.
- Change display areas very regularly.
- Change salon price lists yearly and date them.
- Change salon décor regularly.
- Set out to promote a product every week knowing all its benefits, effects and ingredients (you will soon know your whole range very thoroughly).
- Organise a salon anniversary promotion yearly inviting local press along.
- Make a feature out of a 'slow' day of the week – give it a name and offer extra incentives when people have an appointment on that day.
- Change your own image regularly.

GOOD PRACTICE

- Use the seasons to your advantage when promoting treatments and highlight the treatments' seasonal benefits to your clients, such as detoxifying treatments for summer exposure.
- Regular newsletters are a way of keeping your clients up-to-date on your services and staff, as well as a way of reminding them of the benefits of existing treatments.
- Enter professional competitions and use these for promoting your business.
- Remember that pre- and post-natal clients need a lot of care and attention. Do not assume them to be contraindicated to all treatments as there are a great many treatments that will benefit them, ranging from pre-birth relaxing and skin- and nail-care treatments to post-birth slimming, toning and relaxing treatments.

Taxation

Tax can be defined as a compulsory financial contribution imposed by the government in order to raise revenue to support the public services that are used and shared by everyone. There are many forms of taxation – on individual earnings, on the profits of a business, Value Added Tax (VAT) and National Insurance (NI). VAT and NI are explained briefly below.

Value Added Tax (VAT)

This is a tax that is levied by the Government on most business transactions known as 'taxable supplies'. If a business has a taxable turnover greater than a certain

information point

- The Government has the right to decide which products/ services are liable to VAT charges. Those which are not, are referred to as *zero rated*. Products which are zero rated include books, brochures, children's clothing. Services that are exempt from VAT include education, medical services, banking and insurance.
- Full current details can be viewed on the Customs and Excise website, www.hmce.gov.uk

amount (enquire at your local tax office for the current level) it must register for VAT, filling out the appropriate form from the VAT office. A registration number will then be issued and detailed records will need to be kept of all business transactions. The salon owner will need to charge VAT on services provided and products sold, currently standing at 17.5%, and will be liable to pay VAT on equipment and products purchased from VAT registered companies. These are referred to as outputs and inputs respectively. Every three months (VAT tax period) it will be necessary to fill in a form known as a VAT return. Where output tax exceeds input tax the difference will need to be paid to Customs and Excise, and the reverse where input tax is greater than the output – then it may be reclaimed from Customs and Excise.

Example of VAT input/output tax costings

Input tax		Output tax	
Purchases		Sales	
Products for treatment	£8.00	Chakra Journey sales cost	£60.00
Net cost	£8.00		
Plus VAT @ 17.5%	£2.80	Plus VAT @ 17.5%	£10.50
Gross business cost	£10.80	Cost to client	£70.50

PAYE (Pay As You Earn)

It is a legal requirement to register all employed staff with your local tax office. On registering staff the tax office forward the employer a reference number and an employers' pack which includes a CD and tax deduction tables and details on National Insurance contributions.

National Insurance contributions

This is a tax paid by every working person to the Inland Revenue to support public services, the unemployed and to help towards the payment of a pension in old age. The contributions should be collected by the employer in the case of employees.

Payroll system

All business need a payroll system to record and pay staff and the Inland Revenue accordingly. In today's technology-driven world this tends to be carried out electronically although some people still prefer to maintain manual records. In setting up this system the employer needs to prepare the following:

- A P11 working sheet for each employee. This records their name, National Insurance number, tax paid to date and salary paid to date. It is important that this is accurately updated each time the employee is paid.
- A payslip which shows an employee's gross salary; how this is calculated, i.e. made up of basic pay, overtime, commission, etc.; deductions made, i.e. tax, National Insurance, pension, etc.; and their net salary.
- A P32 employer's payment record form which logs the total payments made by the employer to the Inland Revenue.

- A P14 end of year summary form which itemises each of the business's employees and all payments made to them alongside any deductions from their salary.
- A P35 employers' annual return form which lists all the employees' PAYE deductions for the year.

Basic business terminology

Banking

Bank statement

A bank statement is a document issued by a bank to all account holders normally on a monthly basis showing all the transactions that have occurred for that period. It will detail how much money is in the account, how much has been put in and taken out.

Cash flow

This can be defined as the flow of money in and out of a business. A cash flow statement is compulsory for all large companies.

Cheque guarantee card

This card will be requested every time you write a cheque as it is a guarantee to the retailer that the bank will honour the cheque to the value shown on the card. If the card limit is for £50.00 then the bank will only honour a cheque drawn to that amount or less.

Credit card

Credit cards offer a method of paying for goods and services without cash. It can be used as a form of credit (in which case interest will be paid) or the amount can be paid off monthly. A statement of account will be sent out detailing exactly how much you have spent each month.

Credit card statements

These are monthly reports detailing purchases made, payments received, any interest payable, monies owed, minimum repayment and balance available.

Current account

This is a bank account that traditionally does not pay interest on any money deposited within it but does give the recipient a cheque book and cheque guarantee card to draw from the account.

Deposit account

This is a bank account that pays interest on any monies deposited in it. There may be clauses attached as to how much notice needs to be given for withdrawals without forfeiting interest.

Standing order

A method of paying for regular expenditure such as bills. The bank will ask you to fill in a form detailing the person to whom payment is to be made, their bank details

DATE _____			PAID IN BY _____	bank giro credit		

Main Street Bank
Babystreet Branch

A Hair and Beauty Salon Ltd

	Notes £50		
	£20		
	£10		
	£5		
	Coins £1		
	Other Coins		

CASHIER'S STAMP

CASHIER'S STAMP

A/C _____

CASH _____

CHEQUES _____

£

FEE BOX

CHEQUES

20-40-40	24680099	23
Branch Sort Code	*Account Number*	*Transaction Code*

Total Cash £

Cheques, etc £

£

Main Street Bank plc.   Please do not fold this counterfoil or write or mark below this line

C000120C 20D4040A 24680099C 23

Paying-in slip

and the amount payable. This amount will then be deducted on a regular basis until the bank is notified otherwise.

Direct debit

This is similar to a standing order only this time it is the person requesting the money who instructs the bank to deduct from your account. You will need to fill out a mandate sanctioning the request. Direct debit is very useful where the sum involved may change monthly.

Overdraft

The account holder and the bank agree a limit to which the account may be overdrawn giving a flexible form of finance. Interest will be paid on the amount overdrawn.

Loans

A loan is a formal arrangement with a bank or financial institution allowing an agreed sum of money to be lent to the account holder for an agreed period of time. This is normally for a longer period than an overdraft.

ACTIVITY

Collect information from banks and other financial institutions on the services they offer.

Orders

Advice note

This is a document sent by the supplier to advise when goods will be delivered.

Credit note

This is given by a supplier in exchange for faulty goods and is normally offset against the next invoice.

Delivery note

This document (which is often produced in triplicate) is issued when goods have been ordered and are packed ready for delivery, itemising every product. When the driver delivers the goods you are asked to sign the document to confirm that you have received them. One copy is normally given to you, one retained by the supplier and one by the driver.

Pro-forma invoice

This document is issued in particular for a new customer when their credit worthiness is not yet known. It requests payment for goods before they are dispatched.

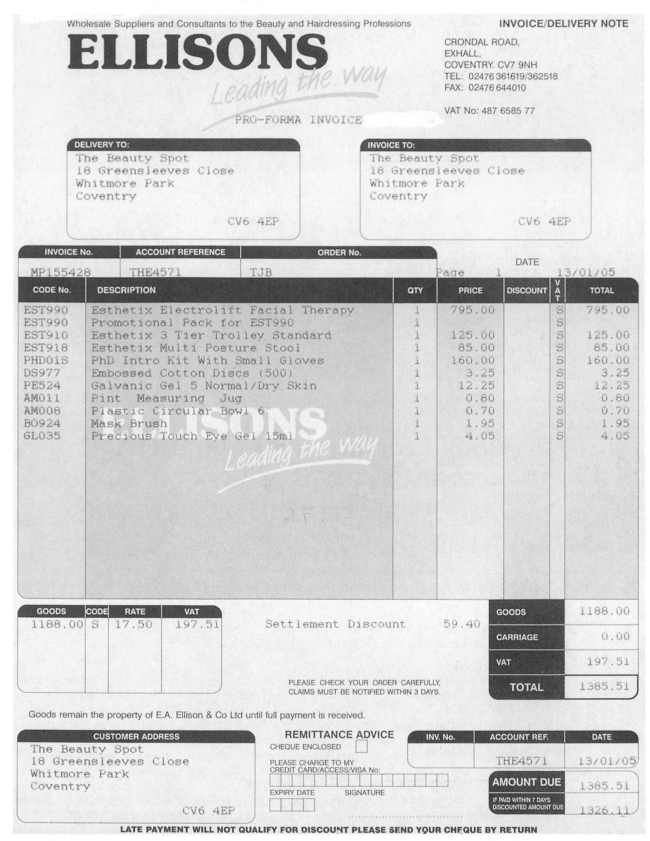

Pro-forma invoice

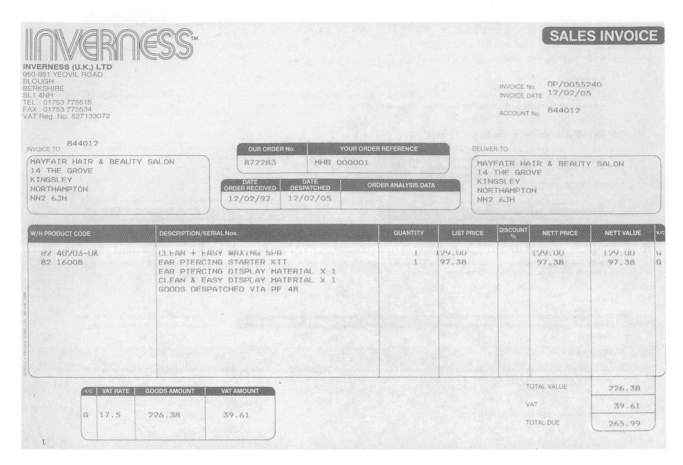

Invoice

Book-keeping and computerised account systems

When setting up in business it will be necessary to keep records of every transaction in a detailed and formal way. The reasons for this are first to have documentation of the business's financial position and secondly to allow for an interpretation of the results. It is important to be able to ascertain why things may not be going too well and respond to them. Whilst it is possible to buy 'off the shelf' book-keeping systems, many people who are not expert in the field contract the work out to specialists.

If you are going to undertake the role of book-keeper yourself then certain business documents and information will need to be entered into what are known as *ledgers*.

There are three ledger accounts:

- Sales ledger – this gives the accounts of debtors (credit customers).
- Purchase ledger – this gives the accounts of creditors (credit suppliers).
- General ledger – this gives the accounts for sales, purchases, returns, income and expense accounts and asset and liability accounts. The cashbook, which consists of cash and bank accounts, is sometimes referred to in a separate section.

Drawing up the sales ledger

All businesses will be required to keep an account for each customer, or *debtor* as they are called. In the hair and beauty industry money is normally paid at the end of a treatment so the business should not have a situation where many customers owe money.

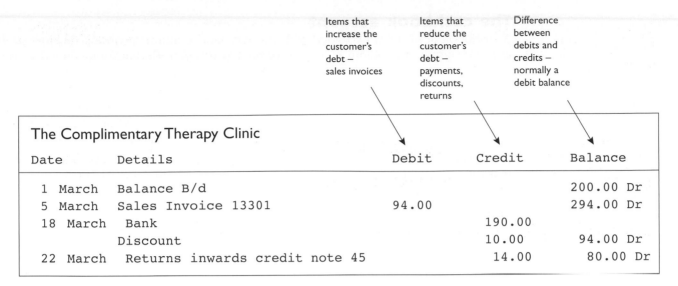

The Complimentary Therapy Clinic		Debit	Credit	Balance
Date	Details			
1 March	Balance B/d			200.00 Dr
5 March	Sales Invoice 13301	94.00		294.00 Dr
18 March	Bank		190.00	
	Discount		10.00	94.00 Dr
22 March	Returns inwards credit note 45		14.00	80.00 Dr

Sales ledger

Drawing up the purchase ledger

The manager will need to be aware of what the business owes to suppliers (*creditors*). Although monthly statements may be received it is important to keep the business's own record up-to-date. The entries would be the opposite way round to those in the sales ledger.

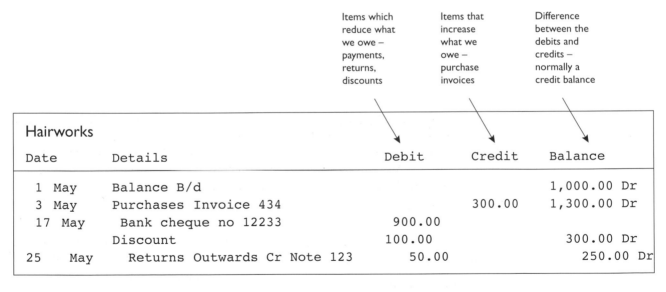

Hairworks		Debit	Credit	Balance
Date	Details			
1 May	Balance B/d			1,000.00 Dr
3 May	Purchases Invoice 434		300.00	1,300.00 Dr
17 May	Bank cheque no 12233	900.00		
	Discount	100.00		300.00 Dr
25 May	Returns Outwards Cr Note 123	50.00		250.00 Dr

Purchase ledger

Drawing up the general ledger

The manager will need to know the business's total sales, purchases and returns for any one year of trading. This information can be obtained from invoices and credit notes. First, the details from the invoices, credit notes, cheques, petty cash vouchers, paying-in slips, receipts, wage slips, etc. will need to be entered into a *day book*. Each month the total from the day book should be entered or posted into the relevant accounts in the general ledger.

The cashbook account

A cashbook account is two-sided with the left-hand column recording receipts (*debit*) and the right-hand column recording payments (*credit*). Certain points need to be considered when filling out the cashbook:

- The date that the transaction took place.
- Where the money came from or where the money went to (if possible name the account). Cheque numbers, accounts references, etc. should also be noted.
- Was the money paid out of the business or received into it?

The cashbook will need to be balanced on a regular basis, e.g. monthly, and this means that the balances of the creditors' and debtors' accounts are worked out. The cashbook should show the difference between the amount paid and the amount withdrawn.

The single-entry system of book-keeping

The single-entry system uses the standard practice of one entry column and, providing there are analysis columns in the cashbook and the petty cashbook, it is easy to total the income and expenditure to see where the money is coming from and going to. A profit and loss account can easily be calculated from this information.

The double-entry system of book-keeping

Double-entry systems take place between the ledger accounts and must clearly show that wherever there is a debit in one account there must be a corresponding credit in another account. The double-entry system expresses both sides of every transaction and two entries are made each time.

The trial balance

The trial balance is the name given to the list of balances that is calculated by checking the debits and credits within the ledger. If there is a debit entry for every credit entry, as in the double-entry system, then the total value of the debit and credit entries should be the same. This is then known as the trial balance and if the total debit and credit entries are not the same then there has been an error in the book-keeping process.

The final balance

The figures from the trial balance are used to draw up the final accounts for the end of the trading year. The final accounts will consist of a profit and loss account and a balance sheet. The profit and loss account will show the profits over losses for the trading period and this is done by calculating the total value of sales minus the total value of expenses incurred. The balance sheet will show the value of the business at the end of the trading period and this is calculated from its assets, liabilities and capital held.

The final accounts ultimately provide information about the financial performance of the business and will be of use for securing or maintaining finance in the future, for those people with a vested interest in the business and for monitoring business performance.

Balance sheet

This is a statement detailing all the assets and liabilities of a business.

Cash book

This book is used to record all payments and receipts carried out on a daily basis together with what has been paid into and taken out of the bank account. It should be periodically checked against bank statements.

Gross profit

This is the term used to describe all profit made before necessary deductions have been taken off.

Net profit

This is a term used to describe the final profit made after all necessary deductions have been made.

Where the money has gone to – we debit an account that receives

Where the money has come from – we credit an account that gives

Debit   Credit

EXPENSES	INCOMES

Used for profit and loss account

ASSETS	LIABILITIES CAPITAL

Used for balance sheet

Balance as at 31st December 2004

	£	£
Cash	294.00	
Bank	2 883.70	
Petty Cash	40.00	
Debtors	1 061.50	
Creditors		178.60
Travel	8.40	
Stationery	5.96	
Light & Heat	157.00	
Wages	280.00	
General Expenses	17.64	
Purchases	460.00	
Sales		2 100.00
Returns Inwards	98.00	
Returns Outwards		114.00
Discount Allowed	25.00	
Discount Received		9.70
VAT		28.90
Capital		34 000.00
Drawings	250.00	
Premises	30 000.00	
Office Equipment	850.00	
Total	36 431.20	36 431.20

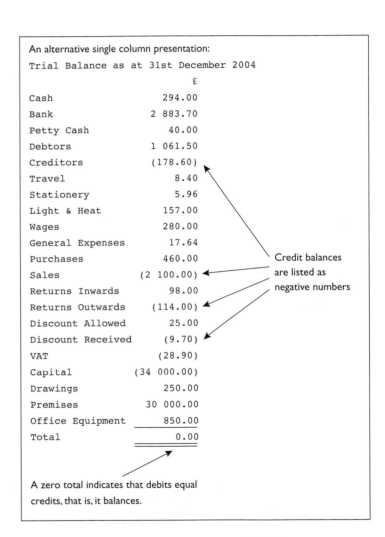

An alternative single column presentation:

Trial Balance as at 31st December 2004

	£
Cash	294.00
Bank	2 883.70
Petty Cash	40.00
Debtors	1 061.50
Creditors	(178.60)
Travel	8.40
Stationery	5.96
Light & Heat	157.00
Wages	280.00
General Expenses	17.64
Purchases	460.00
Sales	(2 100.00)
Returns Inwards	98.00
Returns Outwards	(114.00)
Discount Allowed	25.00
Discount Received	(9.70)
VAT	(28.90)
Capital	(34 000.00)
Drawings	250.00
Premises	30 000.00
Office Equipment	850.00
Total	0.00

Credit balances are listed as negative numbers

A zero total indicates that debits equal credits, that is, it balances.

Trial balance

Petty cash book

All minor cash transactions including the date, the amount of cash used and the purpose of the transaction are recorded in this book.

Profit and loss account

This document summarises all business transactions for a given period (normally one year).

Purchase day book

This allows you to keep a record of any monies that you owe concerning purchases. It should also detail when goods were supplied and the date by which they must be paid for.

Wages book

This is a record of wage/salary details of every employee and will often include personnel information such as NI number, PAYE number, pension and other deductions.

ACTIVITY

Examine a successful business in your area and try to define the reasons why they have become successful.

SELF-CHECKS

1　Explain the importance of marketing and promotion in the salon.

2　What do you understand by the term 'value added tax'?

3　List the key principles involved in setting up a business.

Insolvency

This is a term used to describe either a business or a person who is unable to pay their debts (bankrupt).

Liquidation

This refers to the winding up of a business to pay off its debts.

KEY TERMS

You will need to know what these words and phrases mean. Go back through the chapter to find out.

Basic business legislation

Basic business terminology

Business plan

Choice and type of premises

Competition

Development targets

Forms of business arrangement

Marketing and promotion

Personal learning

Productivity targets

Resources

Staff and recruitment

Taxation

Professional standards (ethics)

Every profession has a code of conduct and beauty therapy is no exception. The code stipulates how the therapist should conduct him/herself in order to obtain a high professional standard.

Medical problems

- Do not carry out any medical treatments.
- Do not give injections.
- Do not cut or sever the skin in any way.
- Do not prescribe oral medication.
- Never treat a client under a doctor's care without obtaining written permission.
- Do not criticise any treatment being given by a doctor.
- Always refer to a doctor if you think a client has a medical problem.
- Try to foster good relations with your local medical practitioners.

Salon manners

- Do not enter into discussions on sex, religion, politics or any other potentially controversial subjects with your clients.
- Never discuss one client with another.
- Do not repeat information you have been told in confidence.
- Avoid repeating bad publicity about other therapists or salons.
- Do not act in a manner that may bring the profession into disrepute.

Advertising

- Never make false claims.
- Do not practise undercutting of prices.
- Do not compare yourself in advertisements with other salons.

Chapter 11

Related business legislation

After working through this chapter you will be able to:

- understand the diversity of legislation that impacts on the successful operation of a business
- be able to identify the important legislative requirements necessary to conduct a successful business
- understand the importance of getting up-to-date advice on the law and regulation.

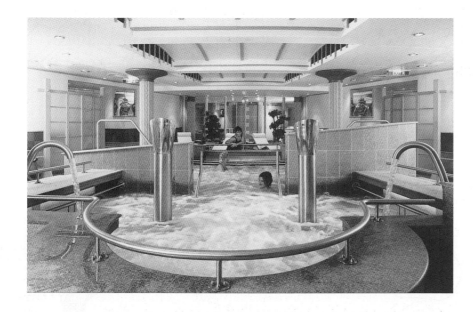

Spa at sea

Basic business legislation

Trade Descriptions Act 1968 and 1972

This Act makes it a criminal offence to describe goods falsely, and to sell or offer for sale goods which have been so described. It covers many things including advertisements, display cards and oral descriptions and applies to quality, quantity, fitness for purpose and price. The part of the Act passed in 1972 deals with labelling of the country of origin; a product must be clearly labelled so that the consumer can see where it was made.

The Landlord and Tenant Act 1954

This piece of legislation gives the tenant security of tenure, which means that you cannot be removed from the premises you are leasing unless the landlord can show a justified reason (not paying the rent, etc.). If the landlord wishes to remove you to sell the premises you will be entitled to compensation.

Related health and safety legislation

Offices, Shops and Railway Premises Act 1963

This piece of legislation relates in particular to hygiene, health and safety of the premises and covers such things as:

- Washing facilities.
- Toilets for both sexes and for client use.
- Sanitation.
- Safety on stairways.

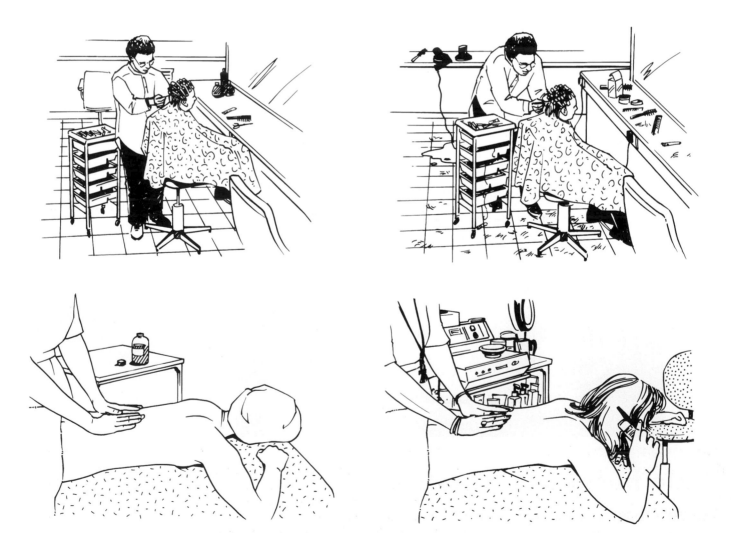

Examples of good and poor standards

- Eating and drinking facilities for staff required to stay on the premises at break-times.
- Adequate space for each employee (at least 400 cubic feet if the ceiling is 10 ft high).
- Fire exits and adequate fire-fighting equipment.

The Management of Health and Safety at Work Regulations Act 1999

In 1999, the Management of Health and Safety at Work Regulations were amended and require all business owners or managers to carry out risk assessments for the health, safety and welfare of both employees and clients. If the salon has more than five employees then formal risk assessment records must be kept, however it is recommended that all employers keep formal records. These regulations also take special notice of employees under the age of 18 requiring employers to carry out risk assessments of their work activities identifying any particular hazard they could be exposed to and then indicating the controls the employer will put in place to ensure the employees' safety.

Further details and examples of risk assessment records are covered in Chapter 9 in this book.

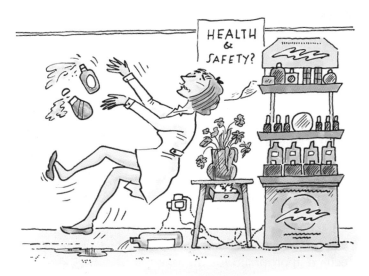

Accidents can happen at any time!

REMEMBER

- A hazard is the potential of something to cause harm, e.g. chemicals that may be used in the salon.
- A risk is the likelihood that harm will be caused by exposure to the hazard, e.g. not wearing protective clothing when handling chemicals.

The Health and Safety (Young Persons) Regulations 1997

These regulations amend the Management of Health and Safety at Work Regulations 1992. They place new responsibilities on employers employing people aged under 18. Under these regulations employers are expected to carry out risk assessments to ascertain the risk to any young person before they start work. The aim is to ensure that no young person can be employed to undertake duties that are beyond their physical or psychological capability.

The Fire Precautions (Workplace) Regulations 1997

These regulations set minimum safety standards in the workplace and ensure that risk of fire in the workplace is assessed and action taken. Where there are five or more employees the risk assessment must be formally recorded.

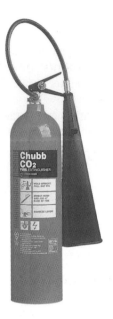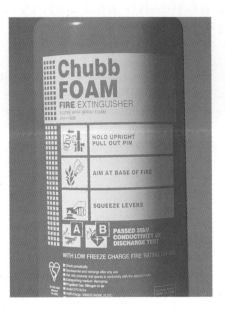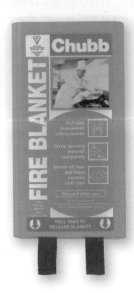

Fire-fighting equipment

The Safety Representatives and Safety Committees Regulations 1997

This is to allow the appointment of a safety representative, from a trade union that is recognised by the employer, to consult with their employees on matters relating to health and safety. The number of representatives will be reflective of the variety of occupations, the total number of the employees and the different types of activities undertaken. The appointed representative has the right to time off for attending training that is deemed appropriate for the job.

The Health and Safety (Consultation with Employees) Regulations 1996

Under these regulations the employer must consult on health and safety issues with any employees who are not members of any group covered by a trade union.

The Reporting of Injuries, Diseases and Dangerous Occurrences Regulations 1995

These regulations are commonly referred to as RIDDOR. They cover all employees and members of the public who as a result of work-based activity suffer a condition or an injury. The HSE operates as the enforcing body and any accident resulting in more than three consecutive days absence due to a work-related injury must be reported within ten days. In April 2001 the HSE established a new incident contact centre (ICC) for all incidents reportable under RIDDOR.

Health and safety legislation – the 'six pack' 1992

The new health and safety at work legislation is commonly referred to as the 'six pack' and was introduced to fulfil European Union directives. It is composed of the following six regulations.

HEALTH AND BEAUTY THERAPY: A PRACTICAL APPROACH

1 The Management of Health and Safety at Work Regulations 1992

This is to ensure that the correct systems are in place to co-ordinate, control and monitor health and safety management. This regulation requires the employer to:

- assess the health and safety risks to employees, clients and other visitors to the business premises
- plan, implement, monitor and review preventative measures
- maintain accurate health and safety records, e.g. servicing and repair of equipment
- select and appoint appropriate people to implement fire evacuation procedures and first aid
- ensure that all employees are provided with detailed information on the company's health and safety procedures and are adequately trained and updated in these.

2 Provision and Use of Work Equipment Regulations 1992

The aim of this legislation is to clarify and join together the many regulations relating to equipment. This legislation ensures that all equipment, whether new or second-hand, must be properly maintained and all employees must be correctly trained in how to use and maintain it. It also ensures that written records regarding its maintenance are accurately kept.

3 Manual Handling Operations Regulations 1992

This is to ensure that proper procedures are laid down by the employer for the manual handling of goods, etc. within the workplace to prevent injuries such as repetitive strain, back injuries, sprains, and strains, e.g. lifting heavy loads which often results in industrial injury.

4 Workplace (Health, Safety and Welfare) Regulations 1992

These are to clarify and link together previous legislation relating to the working environment, safety facilities and 'housekeeping'.

5 Personal Protective Equipment at Work (PPE) Regulations 1992

These are to clarify and join together previous legislation including the use, type and storage of personal protective equipment. It is the employer's responsibility to ensure that all employees who may be at risk of being exposed to health risks or injury are provided, free of charge, with appropriate protective equipment. They must also ensure that such equipment is maintained in good working order and that all employees are trained in its use.

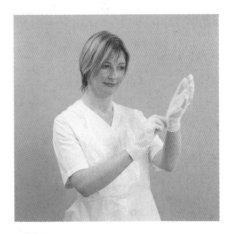

Wearing disposable gloves

6 Health and Safety (Display Screen Equipment) Regulations 1992

These are to clearly identify rules and regulations to protect the health and safety of employees who use display screen equipment. As the use of computers in businesses has rapidly expanded, these regulations were needed to ensure employees are protected from eye strain, muscular pain, etc. These regulations apply to both new and second-hand equipment and require employers to assess the work area and equipment to prevent risk of strain or injury to employees and to provide suitable desks, chairs and, if needed, spectacles, along with the appropriate training.

Electricity at Work Regulations Act 1990

This piece of legislation states that all pieces of electrical equipment in the workplace should be checked annually by a qualified electrician. In particular, businesses should discontinue use of any equipment that is broken or damaged, displays exposed wires or worn flexes or has a cracked or broken plug.

Also, you should take care never to overload sockets. Within a health and beauty and hairdressing business there is likely to be a great deal of portable equipment, e.g. hairdriers, epilation units, etc., which it is essential to have tested annually.

GOOD PRACTICE

Many establishments take out a contract with either the equipment providers or a local company to undertake maintenance and testing of electrical equipment. If in doubt, contact your local trade wholesaler for recommendations of suitable people.

The Control of Substances Hazardous to Health Regulations (COSHH) 1988

These regulations lay down the ways in which substances which can be deemed hazardous to health should be used and stored. Employers are responsible for assessing risks from hazardous substances and deciding upon action to reduce them. The majority of manufacturers issue clear instructions on the handling of products that fall within these regulations. It is essential that all employees should be made aware of the risks of such substances and where necessary be given training in such areas. Employees should always follow safety guidelines and take the precautions identified by their employer.

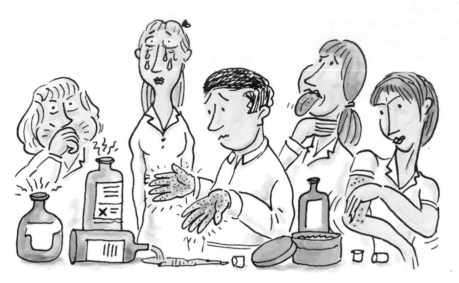

Know how to protect yourself from potentially hazardous substances

Some examples of hazardous substances that may be found within a health, beauty or hairdressing environment are listed below under the following categories: highly flammable, explosive, harmful/irritant products.

Highly flammable

Highly flammable substances, e.g. acetone and solvents, are deemed hazardous to health because if their vapours are exposed to naked flames or other means of extreme heat they can ignite.

Recommended storage

These products much be kept sealed and stored in a cool place. It is important not to store large quantities together as in the event of a fire they would cause a large explosion.

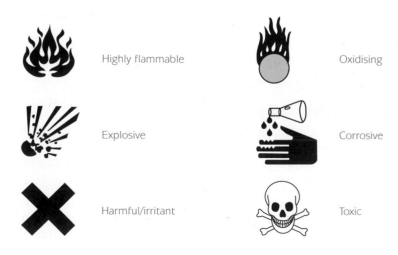

Common symbols used for substances hazardous to health

You should also be aware that some products are more flammable than others, e.g. ethanol-based products such as witch-hazel are far less flammable than acetone-based products such as nail enamel remover.

Recommended handling and usage

It is important to use flammable products in an area that is well ventilated and not to dispense them in an area where there is a risk of fire, e.g. whilst someone is smoking, near a naked flame or near an area of extreme heat. Extreme care must be taken when transferring products into dispensing containers to ensure that the labels are clear and correct. Care must be taken when using the product to avoid excessive inhalation, or contact with eyes and skin.

In the event that the product comes into contact with the eyes or skin, emergency first aid of rinsing with water should be given immediately.

If the casualty continues to have any sign of irritation they must be referred for medical advice. Medical advice must be sought if the product has been in contact with the eye or ingested. In the case of inhalation the person must be moved into fresh air.

Recommended disposal

These types of products must not be disposed of via sanitary systems as this leads to pollution. Advice on disposal should be sought from the practitioner's local environment health and trading standards department.

Recommended action

In the event of a fire evacuate the premises and notify the fire brigade of the location of stored flammables.

information point

- Acetone is used as a solvent in nail enamel removers. It can cause splitting and peeling of the nails and skin rashes on the fingers and hands. Inhalation of acetone can irritate the lungs.
- Alkyl sodium sulphates are used in shampoos for their cleaning ability and ease of rinsing from the hair. They may cause irritation to the skin.
- Ethanol is a colourless, clear and very flammable cosmetic ingredient. It is used as an antibacterial agent in mouth washes, liquid lip rouge, nail enamel, astringents, etc. It is also used medicinally as a topical antiseptic, blood vessel dilator and sedative.
- Ethanolamide of lauric acid is used in soapless shampoos and is a mild skin irritant.
- Ether is used as a solvent in nail enamel. It is a mild skin irritant.
- Ethoxyethanol is used as a solvent and plasticiser for nail enamels. It is toxic when applied direct to the skin.
- Hydrogen peroxide is an ingredient used in lash and brow tinting, skin bleaches, hair bleaches, permanent colours and cold permanent waves for its oxidising and bleaching ability. If used undiluted it can cause burns to the skin.
- Salicylic acid is obtained from sweet birch, wintergreen leaves and other plants. It is used in small percentages as an anti-microbial and preservative in cosmetics such as face masks, hair tonics, hair dye removers, deodorants, suntan lotions, etc. In medicines it is used in higher quantities in ointments, plasters, powders and lotions. Absorption via the skin may cause irritation such as skin rashes, vomiting, increased respiration and abdominal pain.

ACTIVITY

1   Select ten cosmetics from a bathroom, list their ingredients and research the effect of each.
2   List the products that due to their ingredients should be stored out of direct sunlight.

Explosive

Aerosols, e.g. hairspray, nail dry sprays, deodorants and air fresheners, are deemed hazardous to health as they are flammable and are explosive under certain heat-induced conditions.

Recommended storage

These products must be stored in a dry, cool place and away from direct sunlight.

Recommended handling and usage

Any product considered to be flammable should only be used within an area that is well ventilated. Care must be taken when handling such products to avoid contact with the eyes.

It is important when using aerosol/spray containers not to heat the canister or to tamper with the actuator. Care must be taken when using the product to avoid excessive inhalation and not to dispense it on to or near a naked flame or a very hot surface, which might cause combustion and fire.

Recommended disposal

In the event of a spillage, ventilate the area then, wearing disposable gloves and using a cloth or tissue, wipe up the spillage immediately.

Unless stated by the manufacturer dispose of small quantities in the normal manner ensuring that the canister cannot be pierced or placed in extreme heat.

Recommended action

In the event of a fire evacuate the premises and notify the fire brigade of the location of stored aerosols.

Harmful/irritant products

Products such as hydrogen peroxide are deemed hazardous to health as they may cause irritation whether through direct contact, inhalation or absorption.

Recommended storage

These products should be stored carefully in a cool place within the business premises to avoid unnecessary exposure and possible irritation. The products must retain their lids and labels.

Recommended handling and usage

Care must be taken when handling harmful products including the wearing of gloves to protect the hands. Spillages must be removed immediately.

Recommended disposal

The majority of these products used within the health, beauty and hairdressing environment can be disposed of in the normal manner. It is important to observe manufacturers' instructions and if necessary seek the advice of the environmental health and trading standards department within the local authority.

Recommended action

Observe standard first aid procedures if ingredients come into contact with the eyes or skin or if inhaled or ingested.

The Health and Safety (First Aid) Regulations 1981

These regulations lay down the minimum requirements for the provision of first aid in the workplace. The requirements will obviously vary according to the number of employees and the type of work performed within the business. There should be at least one employee who has received training in first aid and continues to keep their skills current, e.g. a St John's Ambulance First Aid certificate has to be renewed every three years.

The contents of a standard first aid box are listed in Chapter 9. It is important to note that from time to time regulations may change or be updated. The container must be clearly labelled in accordance with current regulations.

Health and Safety at Work Act (HASAWA) 1977

This piece of legislation gives rights to both employers and employees. Employers must provide:

- a safe and healthy workplace including maintenance of a reasonable working temperature of not less than 16 °C after the first opening hour, effective ventilation, suitable lighting and humidity levels and adequate toilets and washing facilities
- proper safety procedures – fire exits, notices, drills, handling and recording of accidents, etc.
- safe equipment which is regularly serviced
- adequate training for all staff in safety procedures
- access to a written local health and safety policy.

Employees must:

- follow health and safety procedures
- act to protect themselves and others
- treat all equipment properly and report any faults.

Fire Precautions Act 1971

This piece of legislation states that all employees should be trained and aware of emergency fire evacuation procedures. This should include such things as:

- the nearest fire exit (this should remain unlocked with clear access during working hours)
- the appropriate assembly point that everyone should meet at once the building has been evacuated
- in the event of a fire lifts must not be used
- where possible all windows and doors should be closed on leaving the premises
- all personal belongings should be left behind when evacuating the premises
- an awareness of the location and type of fire fighting equipment available on the premises.

GOOD PRACTICE

Each business should hold regular fire drills to ensure that their employees are fully prepared for their own safety and that of the clients in the event of a fire.

Diversity and equality related legislation

The Employment Equality Regulations 2003

There are two sets of regulations: the Employment Equality (Sexual Orientation) Regulations 2003 and the Employment Equality (Religion or Belief) Regulations 2003, which outlaw any form of discrimination in employment or vocational training which is based on the grounds of sexual orientation, religion or belief. These regulations deal with direct discrimination, whereby a person is treated less favourably than another on the grounds of sexual orientation, religion or belief, as well as dealing with the indirect form of discrimination, whereby a provision, criterion or practice disadvantages people of a particular sexual orientation, religion of belief. They also deal with any harassment or victimisation of an individual or groups.

The first aid requirements of a workplace will vary according to:

- the number of employees
- the nature of the work undertaken within the business
- the size and layout of the business premises
- the employer's first aid policy.

Unfortunately, despite legislation and employers' efforts to prevent accidents within the workplace, they do happen whether through human error or environmental causes. It is therefore important for procedures in the case of accidents to be included as part of staff induction. This should include information on risk assessment, handling possible accidents, names of first aiders, location of first aid box and procedure for recording such occurrences in the business accident book.

Maternity and Parental Leave Regulations
Maternity rights

In England and Wales women employees who satisfy the relevant qualifying conditions are entitled to the following statutory rights:

- Paid time off to receive antenatal care. A woman who is advised by a properly qualified person to attend an antenatal clinic has the right not to be unreasonably refused time off during her working hours to enable her to keep an appointment.
- Maternity pay, which is currently payable for 26 weeks, to a woman absent from work because of her pregnancy (there are certain qualifying requirements).
- The right to return to work after confinement. A woman can currently return to work at any time before the end of the leave period.

New fathers have a right to two weeks' leave and statutory paternity pay.

Parents who are adopting have the right to time off and statutory adoption pay.

Since 15 December 1999, employees who have completed one year of service with their employer have been entitled to 13 weeks' parental leave for each child born or adopted after this date. They will be able to take this leave up until the child's fifth birthday or until five years have elapsed following placement in the case of adoption. Parents of disabled children will be able to use their leave over a longer period until the child's eighteenth birthday.

The Disability Discrimination Act 1995

This Act covers people who have any disability. The disability of a person is defined in the Act as either a physical or mental impairment which has a substantial long-term effect on an individual's ability to carry out what are considered to be normal day-to-day activities. This Act has four parts related to access, employment, goods and services and education making it unlawful for employers who have two or more staff to discriminate against any current or prospective employee or client because of a reason relating to their disability. It also gives rights to clients for ease of access to the goods and services offered. Responsibilities of employers include such things as making reasonable changes to the working environment and general employment arrangements so that the disabled employee/client is not disadvantaged compared to anyone else.

The Sex Discrimination Acts 1975 and the Race Relations Act 1976

The aims or these acts are to prevent direct or indirect discrimination against candidates when applying for work on the grounds of race, sex, or martial status. The Equal Opportunities Commission will investigate complaints made on any of the above grounds and it monitors job advertisements as well.

Equal Pay Act 1970

The aim of this Act was to ensure that people who undertake the same work must be employed on the same terms and pay.

---

information point

- A woman is automatically held to be unfairly dismissed if the sole reason or principal reason for the dismissal is either that she is pregnant or any other reason connected with the pregnancy.
- An employer should carry out a risk assessment on a pregnant employee.

---

information point

- By 2006 it will be illegal to discriminate on the grounds of a person's age.
- The rights of gay and lesbian persons are now covered in the Human Rights Acts. From December 2003 it became unlawful to discriminate on the grounds of a person's preferred sexuality. In the same month it became unlawful to discriminate on the grounds of a person's religion or belief.
- The Race Relations Amendment Act and the Disability Discrimination Act are both vicarious. This means that an employer is responsible for the actions of their employees unless the employee has received training.

---

information point

An employee can seek unfair dismissal on grounds of sex discrimination through an industrial tribunal irrespective of length of service.

Legal rights of an employee and related legislation

Contract of Employment Act 1972

This is a legally binding document drawn up by the employer when a new member of staff is appointed. The reason for such a document is to give both the employer and the employee a certain degree of protection and security and to formalise specific points. By law any person working 16 hours or more a week must be given a contract of employment within eight weeks of the starting date.

The contract should cover the following points:

- Name of the company and the employee.
- Date when employment began.
- Job description.
- Hours of work.
- Pay scale, how payment will be made and at what intervals (weekly, monthly, etc.).
- Holiday entitlement.
- Pension arrangements.
- Sickness and sick pay conditions.
- Length of notice which an employee is entitled to give and receive.
- Disciplinary procedures.

There are other conditions which may be added, such as working at different locations, confidentiality, medical examination, etc. and these are sometimes presented in a separate staff handbook.

The National Minimum Wage Act 1998

This Act took effect from 1 April 1999 and it enforces the following pay rates (at time of print):

- a minimum level of £4.85 an hour for workers aged 22 and over
- a development rate of £4.10 an hour for 18–21-year-olds and for those aged 22 or over who receive accredited training for six months.

Exemptions from the national minimum wage include:

- self-employed
- anyone under 18
- unpaid voluntary workers
- au pairs
- share fishermen
- some apprentices and trainees
- university or college students on placement with an employer as part of their course.

information point

An employer must by law take out employee liability insurance

Working Time Regulations (1998)

On 1 October 1998 regulations to implement the European Working Time Directive came into force. The regulations provide the following new rights.

- A limit on the hours which a worker can be required to work from an average of 48 hours per week though some may choose to work longer.
- A right to four weeks paid leave per year.
- A right to 11 consecutive hours rest in any 24-hour period.
- A right to an in-work rest break if their working day is longer than 6 hours.
- A right to one day off each week.
- A limit on normal working hours of night workers to an average of 8 hours in any 24-hour period and entitlement for night workers to receive regular health checks.

CONTRACT OF EMPLOYMENT

THIS AGREEMENT dated _____
is made **BETWEEN**

(1) *Salon's name* _____ "The Business"

(2) *Employee's name* _____ "The Employee"

1 Definitions

"Business" the business carried on from time to time by The Business name

"Confidential Information" any trade secrets or any other confidential Information relating to the Business (including information relating to any of the Business customers or anyone else the Business deals with)

"Employment" The Employee's permanent employment under this Agreement

"Incapacity" any illness or similar reason preventing the employee from properly carrying out the employment

"Proprietor" the Proprietor of the Business or from time to time the person having control over the Business. The proprietor at the date of this contract is

_____

2 Job title and length of employment

2.1 The Employee agrees to waive any rights to a redundancy payment and any claim in respect of unfair dismissal under the Employment Protection (Consolidation) Act 1978

2.2 The Business agrees to employ the Employee as a Beauty Therapist from: date _____

2.3 The employment may be brought to an end;

2.3.1 by either party giving the other weeks written notice; or

2.3.2 by the business under Clause 15

2.4 No employment with a previous employer counts as part of the Employee's continuous employment with the Business.

3 Duties

The Employee must:–

3.1 do all in her power to promote, develop and extend the Business

3.2 comply with the directions of the Proprietor

3.3 work in any place which the Proprietor may (reasonably) require.

4 To devote full time

4.1 The Employee must (unless prevented by incapacity) devote his/her whole time and attention to the Business

4.2 The Employee must not without the prior consent of the Proprietor take part in or have an interest in any other business which is simiar or competes with the Business.

5 Pay

The Business agrees to pay the Employee a fixed salary accruing from day to day at the basic rate of £____ per year payable in arrears by equal monthly (weekly, quarterly) instalments on the _____day of each month (week, quarter).

6 Commission

6.1 On the sale of individual courses of treatment to clients commission will be paid to the Employee. The total value of treatments will be calculated on sales within the specified period and commission will be paid at the following rates:–
(a)   Rates of commission to be inserted here

6.2 The Employee will be paid commission on sales of any product sold directly by the employee that is supplied by the Business

6.3 Commission will be based on the sale price of the product less VAT and paid at the following rates:–
(a)   Rate of commission to be inserted here

6.4 Commission will be calculated on sales directly attributable to the Employee in a specified monthly (weekly, quarter) period and the commission will be paid on the day basic salary is paid.

Continued

Example of a contract of employment

7 Training courses

Employees will be given regular training courses to update skills and product knowledge.

7.1 If any employee terminates her employment with the Business within a period of One month of completion of a training course, the Employee will be required to refund to the Business 100% (one hundred per cent) of training costs and expenses incurred by the Business.

7.2 If an Employee terminates his/her employment within three months of completing a training course, the Employee will be required to repay the Business 50% (fifty per cent) of training costs/expenses incurred by the Business.

7.3 If an Employee terminates his/her employment within Six months of completion of a training course, the Employee will be required to contribute 25% (twenty-five per cent) of the training costs and expenses incurred by the Business.

7.4 If the Proprietor terminates the Employee's employment, the Employee will not be required to refund any training costs and expenses.

8 Expenses

8.1 The Business agrees to pay the Employee all reasonable expenses wholly and exclusively incurred by him/her in the performance of the employment

8.2 The Employee must give receipts or other evidence of these expenses.

9 Holidays

9.1 The Business holiday year runs from
_____ to _____

9.2 The Employee is entitled to_____working days holiday in each holiday year (in addition to the usual public holidays) to be taken when convenient to the Business

9.3 The Employee must not without consent of the Proprietor carry forward any unused part of his/her holiday to a subsequent holiday year

9.4 The Employee may be required to work on some Bank Holidays and the Employee will be given seven days notice of the requirement to work on a Public/Bank holiday and will be given a proportionate amount of time off in lieu.

10 Hours of employment

Details of hours to worked each week to be stated clearly at this point in the contract

The Employee will be required to work for absenteeism of colleagues at the request of the Proprietor and the Employee covering for absent colleagues will be given a proportionate amount of leave to that extra work undertaken by the Employee to cover for absent colleagues. Alternately, the Employee working additional hours to cover for absent colleagues at the request of the Proprietor may be paid for such additional hours at a rate agreed prior to undertaking the said work agreed with the Proprietor.

11 Pension

The Business has no Pension Scheme which supplies to the Employee or include details of Company Pension Scheme if applicable.

12 Confidentiality during the employment

12.1 The Employee is aware that in the course of the employment he/she may be given or come across confidential information

12.2 The Employee must not disclose or use any confidential information (Except in the proper course of his/her duties)

12.3 The Employee must use his/her best endeavours to prevent any disclosure of any confidential information

12.4 All notes of any confidential information which the Employee acquires or makes during the employment are the property of the Business. When the employment ends (or at any time during the employment, should the Proprietor so request) the employee must hand over these notes to someone duly authorised by the Proprietor to receive them.

13 Confidentiality after the employment ends

After the employment ends the Employee must not disclose or use any Business trade secrets or any other information which is of a sufficiently high degree of confidentially as amounts to a trade secret.

continued overleaf

Example of a contract of employment continued

14 Unfair competition after the employment ends

14.1 The Business is entitled to protect its confidential information, its goodwill and its trade connection from any unfair competition by the Employee. Therefore:

14.1.1 For six months after the employment ends the Employee agrees not to:

(a) seek business from any person, firm or company who at any time during the six months immediately preceding the ending of the employment has been a customer of the Business and with whom the Employee has had personal contact or:

(b) attempt to persuade away from the Business any person who has at any time during the twelve months immediately preceding the ending of the employment been employed by the Business.

Insert salon address

_____

_____

(c) work within three miles of any other premises of the Business where the Employee was employed for at least Six months in the last eighteen months of Employment.

15 Incapacity

15.1 If the Employee cannot work because of incapacity he/she must immediately tell the Proprietor. The Employee must provide a medical certificate specifying the nature of the incapacity and its likely duration after four days of the start of his/her absence and then at weekly intervals.

15.2 The Employee will be paid during absence due to incapacity Statutory Sick Pay.

16 Grievance procedure

If the Employee has any questions or grievance relating to the employment:

16.1 In the first instance he/she should discuss the matter informally with his/her immediate superior

16.2 If the matter is still unresolved or if the Employee still thinks that he/she has not been fairly treated, he/she may appeal in writing within seven days of the informal discussion.

17 Disciplinary procedure

A copy of the current edition of the Disciplinary Procedure affecting the Employee is available for inspection from the Proprietor at any time.

18 Ending the employment

The Business may end the employment without notice or pay in lieu of the notice on the following circumstances:

18.1 If the Employee has committed a serious or repeated breach of any of his/her obligations under this Agreement (or the Business has reasonable grounds for believing he/she has done so) or:

18.2 If the Employee:–

18.2.1 becomes bankrupt: or:

18.2.2 enters into a voluntary arrangement under the Insolvency Act 1986; or

18.2.3 becomes of unsound mind or becomes a patient under the Mental Health Act 1983: or:

18.2.4 If the Employee has been absent for a period of twenty six weeks (whether consecutive or in aggregated) in any period of two years as a result of incapacity.

19 Effect of ending the employment

19.1 The Employee must still comply with his/her obligations under clauses 12, 13 and 14 of the Agreement even if the Business has committed a breach of this Agreement, however serious

19.2 The ending of the Employment will not affect any rights the Business has against the Employee (or the Employee has against the Business) arising from any breach of this Agreement which occurred before the employment ended.

Signed _____

Dated _____ day of _____

Example of a contract of employment continued

The Employment Rights Act 1996

This Act supersedes some of the points in the Trade Union and Employment Rights Act 1993 which was designed to improve the employment rights of part-time workers. It entitled all female employees to take up to 14 weeks' maternity leave irrespective of their length of service with the organisation. It also gave all employees, after a period of time, the right to be given written terms and conditions of employment and it enabled all employees to appeal against unfair dismissal.

Ms Simone Horton began employment as a hairstylist with Mrs Delvis Bona proprietor of Hairworks, 23 High Street, Sheffield on 1st June 1997.

Duties

As a hairstylist you will be expected to perform all services (cutting, colouring, perming, relaxing, setting and blow drying) on all female and male clients of all ages and assist in maintaining the tidiness of the salon.

Place of work

Your main place of work will be at the Sheffield salon. However, from time to time you may be asked to undertake demonstrations to the public at various venues around Sheffield to promote the business.

Salary

Your basic pay will be £145.00 per week plus 5% commission of all retail sales and 10% commission after £145 per week on all services. Your pay will be transferred directly to your bank on the 1st day of the month (commencing 1st July 1997). Travel expenses at a rate of 33p per mile will be paid whenever you incur expenditure on behalf of the salon, i.e. demonstrations at venues other than the salon.

Hours/Holiday/Sick leave/Pay/Pension

Your working hours will be:

Tuesday–Thursday	9.00 – 5.30
Friday	11.00 – 8.30
Saturday	9.00 – 4.00

You are entitled to 14 days holiday per year plus the statutory public holidays. Sick leave and pay is subject to statutory sick pay. There is no company pension scheme.

Notice

The amount of notice of termination of your employment you are entitled to receive is one month and you are also required to give us one month's notice. Your employment is permanent subject to your general rights of termination under the law.

Disciplinary/Grievance procedure

You are asked to note the company's disciplinary procedure enclosed with this statement.

DISCIPLINARY PROCEDURE

1.   A breach of the following rules may result in instant dismissal without warning upon the decision of any two of the salon Directors:-

   1.1 Improper acquisition, use of or disclosure of information concerning the business or its clients which may come into your knowledge by reason of employment.

   1.2 Any conduct which in the opinion of the salon Directors may have the effect of bringing the integrity and reputation of the salon into disrepute.

2.   In the event of the salon Manager being dissatisfied with your work, conduct, time keeping or any other aspect of your employment you may be given a verbal warning as to the matter causing dissatisfaction by a Director of the salon or his/her representative. If after a reasonable period the salon Manager remains dissatisfied with the matter complained of, the matter may be referred to the salon Directors and you may be given a written warning. If the salon Manager continues to be dissatisfied with the matter complained of, the matter will again be referred to the salon Directors and you may be given the statutory minimum notice of dismissal to which you are entiled by virtue of the length of your employment with the salon.

3.   If during the course of your employment you receive more than one verbal warning under Clause 2 for any one or number of matters, then you may be given a final written warning that if any matter subsequently warrants further verbal warning you may be dismissed.

4.   No disciplinary action will be taken until your case has been investigated by the salon Director. If there is any disciplinary decision relating to you, or you have any grievance relating to your employment, you may apply in writing within fourteen days of such decision or the occasion of such grievance to the salon Directors and you may be accompanied by any one employee of your choice from the salon.

Example of a written statement of employment

The Employment Rights Act of 1996 states that an employee is entitled to ask for a written statement of their terms and conditions of employment after one month's employment, and have the right to receive this after the expiry of two months from the date of commencement of employment. This Act does not refer to a contract of employment but does give an employer a legal obligation to supply a written statement which should contain details of the salary or wages, hours of work, notice entitlements and obligations, holiday entitlement, date of commencement of employment, job description and workplace location. This Act does not require the employer to title the document as a contract, although in employment law the employee is deemed to have a contract of employment when the offer by the employer of the job and the acceptance by the employee indicates an intention to enter into a legally binding relationship.

If the employer does not provide the written statement then the employee has the right to make an application to an industrial tribunal who can order the employer to produce the written statement.

Unfair dismissal – the Employment Protection (Consolidation) Act 1978

Under the Employment Protection Act 1978 an employee may claim unfair dismissal if they can prove that the employer has acted in an unlawful manner. The employee must have worked for the organisation for at least one year.

Unfair dismissal can also be sought, irrespective of the employee's length of service, on the grounds of:

- pregnancy
- discrimination due to the sex, race, religion or belief, sexual orientation or marital status of an individual.

All of these rights are not affected by the signing of a contract of employment, which usually states 'this contract does not affect your statutory rights'.

Misrepresentation Act 1967

This legislation protects a person who enters into a contract and allows them the opportunity to make a claim based on misrepresentation of terms which causes them to suffer damage.

Statutory rights

An employee's statutory rights generally include the following:

- a detailed pay statement indicating what they have earned and what deductions the employer has made
- for them not to be discriminated against
- equal pay for equal work
- at least one week's notice of dismissal if they have been employed for two months
- statutory sick pay
- statutory maternity pay
- a healthy and safe working environment
- after two years of employment with the same company they have the right to redundancy payment
- the right to complain to an industrial tribunal if they feel that they have been unfairly dismissed
- the right to retain their employment under the same conditions should the business be taken over by another company
- the right to be a member of a trade union.

These rights are not affected by the signing of a contract of employment, which usually states 'this contract does not affect your statutory rights'.

Statutory sick pay (SSP)

All employees over the age of 16 years of age are entitled to the payment of statutory sick pay (SSP) from their employer after they have been off work through illness for four consecutive days. The employer by law must pay this minimum amount to the employee and they must maintain records of SSP and the employee sickness for inspection by the Department of Social Security (DWP). These records must include details of the dates of absenteeism due to sickness and the days that the employee would normally be at work, i.e. the qualifying days, which are generally Monday–Friday but in the health, beauty and hairdressing industries are highly likely to be different.

REMEMBER

An employee is not entitled to SSP if they are off work for less than four consecutive days.

Disciplinary procedures

All employees should receive a copy of the company's disciplinary procedure with their contract of employment. This will detail the company's policy for dealing with what it considers to be misconduct. The employee should be given a breakdown of the areas of misconduct. There should also be a description of the disciplinary action taken, i.e. verbal warning, written warning, etc., the level of management to be involved in such a scenario together with an appeals procedure.

The majority of employers will stipulate that an employee will be given one verbal warning of misconduct followed by a formal (verbal and written) warning and a final written (verbal and written) warning followed by dismissal. Immediate suspension may take place if gross misconduct occurs, e.g. theft.

GOOD PRACTICE

A written disciplinary procedure should:

- indicate who it applies to
- ensure it allows for swift action
- state clearly the stages of disciplinary action
- state clearly which managerial staff have responsibility for disciplinary procedures
- allow for employees to be notified of any complaints against them
- allow for employees to put forward their case
- allow the employees to be accompanied by a representative, e.g. from a trade union, or another employee
- allow for full investigation before the disciplinary action is taken
- allow the employee the right to appeal.

information point

- Large companies tend to have their own clearly defined grievance and disciplinary procedures.
- The Department of Trade and Industry (DTI) publishes a booklet entitled *Individual Rights of Employees* available at Job Centres.

Termination of employment and redundancy

The manager at some time during their career may have to consider action or even possible termination of an employee's employment. It is paramount that they must consider carefully the legal implications such as unfair dismissal and ensure that they observe fully the employer's and employee's rights. It is wise to contact the local Advisory, Conciliation and Arbitration Service (ACAS) office for current legislation and advice.

GOOD PRACTICE

- A contract of employment can be used to the employer's advantage if probationary periods and performance targets have been included, agreed upon and are not fulfilled.
- It is essential for the manager to keep abreast of any changes in the employment law. It may be in the case of a small business due to restricted legal knowledge that they decide to take advice from a legal business adviser.

GOOD PRACTICE

The employer should:

- always investigate alleged misconduct
- involve all parties concerned
- allow time for improved conduct before taking further steps
- ensure that apart from an extremely serious offence no employee should be dismissed on the first occasion
- ensure that dismissal is fair before taking action.

ACTIVITY

Design a grievance/disciplinary procedure suitable for a large hair and beauty chain ensuring that the following points are taken into consideration:

- protection of and respect for the physical and human resources of the company
- accurate, truthful completion of records, e.g. bookings, time-keeping, stock-taking, etc.
- employee's attendance, e.g. time-keeping, illness, etc.
- confidentiality
- rules and regulations relating to food, drink, etc.

Treatment and consumer legislation

This legislation relates to services offered within the business and its environment.

Local bye-laws concerning body massage treatments

In England and Wales licensing is controlled by the local authorities. Anyone wishing to set up a clinic offering body massage treatments may need a licence to practise, depending upon the area of the country in which their business is located. This license is obtained from the local authority through the Environmental Health and Trading Standards Department (EHTS). To qualify for such a licence the applicant normally submits information concerning their premises, staff and qualifications. Inspection of the premises is then carried out and once approved by the authority an annual fee, which varies from authority to authority, is paid.

Local Government (Miscellaneous Provisions) Act 1982

This Act is monitored through the local Environmental Health and Trading Standards Department. Any practitioner using needles for treatments, such as acupuncture, epilation, sclerotherapy, collagen injections, semi-permanent make-up or ear piercing, must apply for a licence to practise under the above Act. This is to ensure that correct hygienic practices are used for storage, use and disposable of 'sharp' implements.

The Sale and Supply of Goods Act 1994

This Act replaces the Supply of Goods and Services Act 1982 and the Sale of Goods Act 1979. It relates to all goods including food regardless of where they are purchased. Terms under the Act state that the seller has to ensure that the goods are:

- of satisfactory quality: this is defined as the standard that would be regarded by a reasonable person as satisfactory having taken into account the description of the goods, the price and any other relevant circumstances
- reasonably fit: the goods must be able to meet whatever the seller claims they do, e.g. a car must reach 0–60 miles per hour in the number of minutes stated.

Once the contract has been made between the seller and the buyer this Act can be enforced. Verbal and written contracts are both classed as valid contracts and a buyer is entitled to have either their money back or goods replaced if the contract is broken.

Office of Fair Trading (OFT)

The Office of Fair Trading (OFT) is responsible for the administration of policy competition in the UK. It controls monopolies, mergers and consumer protection, e.g. it investigates consumers' complaints about inaccurate trade descriptions.

Trade Descriptions Act 1968, 1972

This Act makes it a criminal offence to describe goods falsely, and to sell or offer for sale goods which have been so described. It covers many things including advertisements, display cards, oral descriptions and applies to quality, quantity, fitness for purpose and price. The part of the Act passed in 1972 deals with labelling of the country of origin; a product must be clearly labelled so that the consumer can see where it was made.

The Consumer Credit Act 1974

This Act ensures that the actual rate of interest charged for credit facilities must be highlighted to a borrower.

The Prices Act 1974

This ensures that prices should be displayed so as not to give a false impression to potential buyers.

The Resale Prices Act 1964, 1976

This Act prevents manufacturers from enforcing retailers of their products to charge a certain price. However, it does not prevent them from supplying a recommended retail price.

The Consumer Safety Act 1978

This Act identifies the standards for legal safety to reduce the possible risk to consumers from products that may be potentially dangerous or harmful.

The Consumer Protection Act 1987

This Act deals with three main subjects: product liability, general safety requirements and misleading prices. It follows European directives to safeguard the consumer from unsafe products.

Environmental Health and Trading Standards Departments (EHTS)

Trading standards officers are employed by local authorities and their remit is to investigate complaints from consumers against businesses. Having investigated the complaint they have the authority to take the business to court to prevent reccurrence of the complaint.

The British Standards Institution (kite marks and safety standards)

The British Standard Institution (BSI) is an independent body which sets voluntary standards of reliability and quality. Its objectives are to:

- establish quality standards
- promote health and safety
- protect the environment.

Manufacturers submit their products voluntarily for them to be tested on such things as their safety, quality, strength, etc. The kite marks of the Institution are displayed by

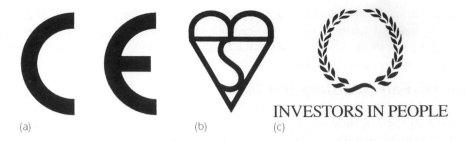

Quality marks (a) European quality specification; (b) BSI kite mark and (c) Investors in People Award

many businesses to provide the consumer with a guarantee that they have recognition from the board, indicating that the product has been tested and approved. Examples of such quality marks include the BSI kite mark, the British Gas Seal of Service and the Investors in People Award.

Data Protection Act 1984

Practitioners using computers to store personal data on their clients must comply with the Data Protection Act of 1984 which requires them to register with the Data Protection Registrar, or they are liable to face prosecution. The Act only applies to computer information stored relating to living persons. It does not cover manually stored records unless these are made under the Consumer Credit Act.

Information and forms are available from Post Offices and there is a fee for a 3-year licence. However small businesses can complete a simplified registration form. The application requires information on what is stored on the computer, its uses, sources and to whom the data may be disclosed.

Anyone who feels that they are affected by lost or incorrect information or disclosure of personally held computer data without their consent may make a claim to the Registrar. They can be told who holds data on them and for a nominal fee are entitled to see these records within 40 days of payment. NB when completing client records careful consideration should be given to the terminology used.

In-salon entertainment

Many hairdressing and beauty salons play background music within their establishments to create the appropriate type of ambience. In beauty and health clinics it is often intended to create a relaxing environment whereas the environment of the hair salon is much more lively. If the owner decides to play recorded music they will need to pay a fee, whereas if they use a television or radio broadcast they will need to buy a licence.

Insurance

Insurance is a way of protecting people and property against unforeseen circumstances. It is possible to insure against almost any risk for a sum of money called a premium. In return for this payment, should the risk which you are insuring against occur, you will receive compensation to indemnify you for the loss (to be put back in the position you were in before the loss).

When operating in a business certain forms of insurance are compulsory by law. They are as follows.

Public liability insurance

This insurance covers claims relating to injury, disease or damage to the property of a third party (the client). It can be extended to cover liability arising out of goods sold or supplied or if the business involves work away from the premises.

GOOD PRACTICE

Contact the public enquiry sector of the Health and Safety Executive for published material relating to health and safety.

information point

For information on current fees contact:
Performing Rights Society Ltd
Phonographic Performance Ltd

information point

The EU directive to list product ingredients became effective on 1 January 1997.

Many professional beauty therapy organisations can arrange group cover which is normally included in some form of membership fee which will generally encompass other benefits. It is sensible to look at having a £1 million cover against any injury arising out of the treatments offered.

Employer's liability insurance

Any business employing staff is legally obliged to have this form of insurance. If an employee is injured at work it is normally the employer who is held responsible whether personally at fault or not. The insurance certificate must be prominently displayed. Any injuries that do occur must be recorded in an accident book.

Although not compulsory by law it is sensible to have insurance to cover:

- Theft.
- Damage to premises, stock and equipment by fire, flood, etc.
- Loss of profits through damage to premises.
- Fidelity bonding (insurance cover to protect against the dishonesty of employees).
- Personal accident insurance.
- Life assurance.

ACTIVITY

Draft a plan of a salon layout and decide on the type of establishment and the number of staff to be employed. Pay particular attention to health, safety, hygiene and legislation.

KEY TERMS

You will need to know what these words and phrases mean. Go back through the chapter to find out.

COSHH

Disability discrimination

Disciplinary procedures

Employment legislation

Fire precautions

Sex discrimination

Termination of employment

The 'six pack'

Treatment and consumer legislation

Unfair dismissal

Chapter 12 Anatomy and physiology

After working through this chapter you will be able to:

- have a greater awareness of the structure and functions of the human body
- be able to give a brief outline of the structure and functions of the various systems of the body
- be able to relate this knowledge to the practical treatment situation where appropriate
- name and describe the location and the function of the bone structure of the:
    - cranium and face
    - arm and hand
    - lower leg and foot
- name and describe the location and the function of the superficial muscles of the face and neck
- name and describe the location and the function of the following nerves:
    - 5th cranial nerve
    - 7th cranial nerve
    - 11th cranial nerve
- locate the motor points of the face and neck
- understand the circulatory system and composition of the blood
- name and describe the location of the arteries and veins of the head and neck
- understand the composition and functions of the lymphatic system
- name and describe the location of the lymph nodes of the face and neck.

In order for the therapist to plan and perform effective treatment programmes for individual client's needs, it is essential to have an understanding of the structure and functions of the body. This chapter is designed to give an overview for therapists who have previous knowledge of anatomy and physiology and it is recommended that further study is undertaken from specialist sources.

Cells and tissues

The human body develops from a single cell called the *zygote*, which results from the fusion of an *ovum* and *sperm*. Cell multiplication follows and as the foetus grows, cells with different structural and functional characteristics develop. However, all cells carry the same genetic 'blue-print' as the initial zygote.

Structure of the cell

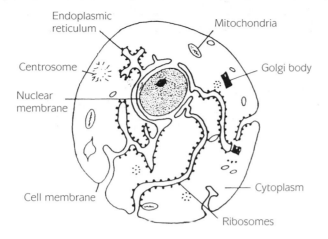

Endoplasmic reticulum
Mitochondria
Centrosome
Golgi body
Nuclear membrane
Cell membrane
Cytoplasm
Ribosomes

An animal cell

All animal cells are composed of the following basic structures.

Cell membrane

This is really the cell wall and it keeps the cell contents intact. Substances can pass into and out of the cell across the membrane. It is a flexible structure and can change shape.

Cell fluid

Known as *cytoplasm*, cell fluid is a jelly-like substance that suspends all the cell's contents. Found within the cell fluid are folded membranes forming tubes known as *endoplasmic reticulum*, structures which function as transportation channels.

In addition to the internal system of membranes there are other structures within the cytoplasm:

Mitochondria

Food substances such as sugar are broken down chemically in the mitochondria to release energy that is needed to drive the reactions in the cell.

Ribosomes

Ribosomes play a part in building up proteins from which all cells and tissues are constructed.

Golgi bodies

Golgi bodies are specialised structures found near the nucleus. Their main function is to add carbohydrate to cell protein.

Nucleus

The nucleus is the most important part of the cell. It is a large spherical body enclosed in a special cell fluid called protoplasm, but separated from it by a nuclear membrane. In the nucleus there are a number of thread-like bodies called *chromosomes*. There are 46 chromosomes in every human cell which are arranged in pairs, one from each pair being inherited from the male parent and the other from the female. The chromosomes contain the basic hereditary information which determines the individual's characteristics and traits, such as hair and eye colour, the structure of bones and teeth, etc.

Mitosis

Mitosis is the process of cell multiplication that occurs throughout life whereby cells are formed to replace those that have died. Mitosis is divided into four phases.

1 Prophase

A structure called a *centrosome* divides into two *centrioles* which migrate to opposite sides of the cell remaining attached by thread-like *spindles*.

2 Metaphase

The nuclear membrane disappears and the chromosomes arrange themselves at the centre of the cell. They are attached to the spindles of the centrioles.

3 Anaphase

The *centromere*, a structure that connects pairs of chromosomes, divides and the identical chromosomes move apart, breaking the spindle structure.

4 Telophase

The spindles disappear completely while the nuclear membrane reappears around each of the two groups of chromosomes. A constriction occurs around the middle of the cell body until eventually the cell divides into two. The two cells are known as *daughter* cells.

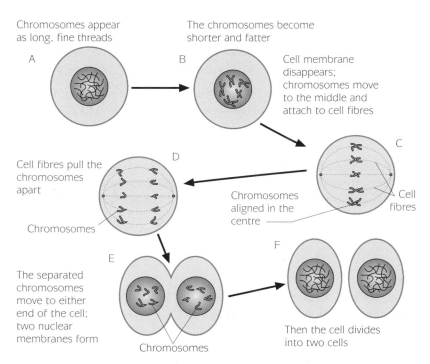

Cell division by mitosis

Types of tissues

Cells unite to form tissues within the body. There are four main types:

- Epithelial.
- Connective.
- Muscular.
- Nerve.

Epithelial tissue

This is the simplest form of tissue and consists of one layer of cells in the case of simple epithelium and two or more layers in the case of stratified epithelium.
This type of tissue forms the skin and is found within the linings of certain organs.

Connective tissue

There are many forms of connective tissue in the body. Adipose, bone and fibrous tissues are a few examples. Connective tissues can generally be thought of as tissue that unites other tissues together or gives support.

HEALTH AND BEAUTY THERAPY: A PRACTICAL APPROACH

Muscular and nerve tissue

See pp. 336–41 for muscular tissue and pp. 347–50 for nerve tissue.

See pp. 336–41 for muscular tissue and pp. 347–50 for nerve tissue.

ACTIVITY

Research the different types of epithelial, connective, muscular and nerve tissue.

SELF-CHECKS

1 Describe epithelial tissue.

2 Explain briefly the process of cell division by mitosis.

The skin

The human skin is the largest organ of the body covering an area of approximately 1.2–2 square metres. Its main purpose is one of protection. It keeps the internal structures of the body covered and intact and it has to be able to withstand daily wear and tear. It also protects the body against invasion by bacteria, chemicals and other foreign substances.

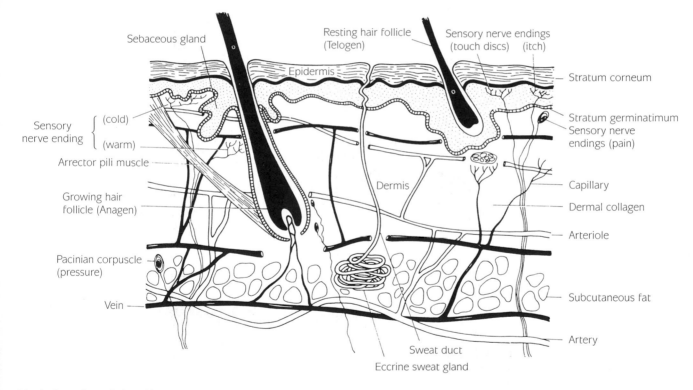

Vertical section of the skin

The structure of the skin

Skin is composed of three main layers:

- Epidermis.
- Dermis.
- Subcutis.

Epidermis

This is the outer, visible layer of the skin and is itself composed of five distinctive layers. It takes approximately 30 days for this layer to renew itself and will vary in thickness on different parts of the body.

The five distinct layers of the epidermis are:

1 **Stratum germinativum** (sometimes referred to as the basal layer). This is the deepest layer of the epidermis and consists of columnar cells which are mitotically active. The new cells produced by mitosis in the stratum germinativum are continually pushed up into the subsequent layers of the skin. *Melanocytes* are present within this layer and are responsible for producing the pigment melanin.

2 **Stratum spinosum** (sometimes referred to as the prickle cell layer). This layer is immediately above the basal layer and consists of cells with prickle-like projections which are connected to each other. They are living cells, each containing a nucleus.

3 **Stratum granulosum**. This layer is formed from rows of flattened cells which contain a granular protoplasm. The dark granules present are *keratohyaline* which is involved in the first stage of keratinisation.

4 **Stratum lucidum**. This layer consists of light-permeable, transparent cells which contain droplets of a substance called *eleidin*. Eleidin is formed from keratohyaline and transforms into *keratin*.

5 **Stratum corneum**. This is the visible layer of the epidermis. Its cells are completely flattened, keratinised structures with no nucleus. Cells are shed from the stratum corneum and replaced on a continuous basis. The stratum corneum usually consists of many flattened cells.

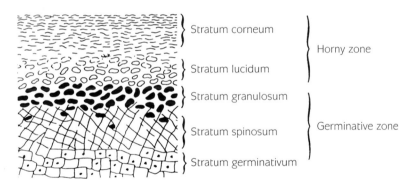

The layers of the epidermis

information point

- The moisture content of the stratum germinativum is on average 83%.
- The moisture content of the stratum corneum varies on average between 9–16%.
- The average thickness of the stratum corneum can be compared to the thickness of a tissue.
- Ultraviolet radiation causes the skin to protect itself by causing thickening of the stratum corneum. This may give the skin an uneven surface.
- On average the body loses 5 billion dead skin cells per day.

Dermis

The dermis lies directly below the epidermis and is the thickest layer of the skin. It consists of two main layers known as the *superficial papillary layer* and the *reticular layer*. Found within the dermis are the following structures:

- **Collagen and elastin fibres**. Collagen is a protein constituent and is responsible for giving the skin its firm contours. Elastin is formed from connective tissue. The yellow elastin fibres give the skin its suppleness. Collagen and elastin both deteriorate with the natural ageing process.
- **Hair and hair follicles**. The hair follicle is a natural indentation within the dermis consisting of a downward extension of epidermal cells. The hair follicle is composed of an inner and outer root sheath which is surrounded by a connective tissue sheath. This sheath has a loosely knit mesh of papillary cells overlying it, interspersed with nerves and blood capillaries. At the base of the follicle is a cluster of cells called the *dermal papilla* which provides the sole source of nourishment for the hair.
- **Sudoriferous glands**. These are found in abundance within the dermis and are composed of epithelial cells. They produce a watery substance known as sweat, which travels via a duct to the surface of the skin through a pore, or otherwise open into hair follicles. There are two main types of sudoriferous gland; *eccrine glands* and *apocrine glands*. The latter do not become active until puberty. Both play a part in the heat regulation of the body.
- **Sebaceous glands**. These are also found in abundance within the dermis and are composed of secretory epithelial cells. They produce a fatty substance called *sebum* and normally open into a hair follicle. Sebum keeps the hair lubricated and gives some protection to the surface of the skin.
- **Arrector pilorum muscles**. These are tiny, involuntary muscles attached to the hair follicle. The muscles respond to cold and fear causing them to contract and forcing the hairs within the follicles to stand on end, giving the skin the appearance of goose flesh.
- **Sensory nerve endings**. Within the dermis are nerve endings which respond to pain, pressure, heat, cold and touch. The nerves carry impulses to the brain. Without the responses made to impulses from the sensory nerve endings serious mechanical damage could occur to the skin and the body as a whole.
- **Lymph vessels**. These are found in abundance throughout the dermis. Lymph vessels help to drain excess fluid.

Subcutis

The subcutis is the third layer of the skin and is a type of connective tissue which divides the dermis from the muscular layer. It has a rich blood supply and contains some sensory nerve endings. The majority of the cells in this layer are fat cells which act as a buffer to prevent damage to the underlying structures and also insulate the body against heat loss. The thickness of the subcutis varies on different parts of the body, for example it is thicker on the gluteal area than the forehead. It is generally thicker on women than on men.

Natural moisturising factor

The skin has a natural moisturising factor which is created within the cell regeneration and the production of the skin's acid mantle. It helps to prevent moisture loss from the epidermis. As the cells move upwards towards the surface of the skin, moisture is pushed from the inside of the cells outwards thus coating each cell with a sticky intercellular glue. This has the effect of holding the stratum corneum together.

The functions of the skin

The skin serves many important functions. The main ones are:

- **S**ecretion.
- **H**eat regulation.
- **A**bsorption.
- **P**rotection.
- **E**limination.
- **S**ensation.

Secretion

The two main substances the skin secretes are *sebum* and *sweat*.

Sebum is produced by the sebaceous glands which are situated in the dermis between the angle of the follicle and the arrector pilorum muscle. Sebum is a fatty substance which lubricates the skin's surface and the hair. Sebum is also bactericidal and so prevents bacterial infection.

Sweat is produced by the sudoriferous glands which are coiled tubules situated in the dermis. Sudoriferous glands open onto the skin's surface via a small duct (the sweat duct) and pore.

There are two types of sweat gland:

- Eccrine glands are found in abundance all over the body. They secrete a clear, watery fluid.
- Apocrine glands are found under the arms (axillae) and in the groin area (inguinal). They produce a milky fluid. Apocrine glands start working from puberty onwards.

Heat regulation

Body temperature in good health is 36.9 °C. For this temperature to remain constant a heat loss/production balance must be maintained. This is sometimes referred to as *homeostasis*.

Heat loss is affected by two main factors: the amount of blood circulating in the capillaries and the amount of sweat formed and its rate of evaporation.

Any increase in body temperature will have the following effects:

- *Vasodilation* occurs. The capillaries near the skin's surface dilate, allowing more blood to circulate nearer to the surface where heat will be lost by radiation and convection thus giving the skin a flushed look.
- Increased amounts of sweat are produced. This has a cooling effect as it evaporates from the surface of the skin.

A decrease in body temperature will have the opposite effects:

- *Vasoconstriction* occurs. Capillaries near the skin's surface constrict. Less blood flows near the surface and therefore less heat is lost.
- Sweat production diminishes.

Absorption

As one of the skin's main functions is to protect against the intrusion of foreign substances, the skin absorbs very little. Only tiny quantities of water and oil-soluble substances are absorbed.

However, the skin can be said to absorb radiation, in particular ultraviolet radiation. Ultraviolet rays penetrate the skin and act on a substance called *ergosterol* which is present in the subcutis of the skin, producing vitamin D.

Protection
The skin has several protection mechanisms:

- The stratum corneum (horny layer) of the epidermis contains keratinised cells which act as a buffer and are impervious to most substances.
- Sweat is acidic and has the effect of inhibiting organism growth.
- Sebum, as well as being bactericidal, acts as a lubricant preventing the surface of the skin from cracking. This also helps to prevent invasion by bacteria.
- Adipose tissue in the subcutis insulates the body and protects the underlying structures from bumps and knocks.
- Sensory nerve endings in the skin respond to painful stimuli to protect the body from mechanical and environmental damage.
- Melanin is produced in the skin in response to ultraviolet radiation. Certain types of ultraviolet radiation can cause damage to the skin, such as premature ageing and skin cancers. Melanin is produced to limit this damage.

Elimination
As has been previously mentioned the skin secretes sweat and sebum. These contain waste products that the body needs to eliminate.

Sensation
The sensory nerve endings found within the dermis protect the body from serious environmental and mechanical damage by reacting to pain, pressure, heat, cold and touch.

pH of the skin
pH is the measurement of acidity or alkalinity. The pH scale ranges from 0–14 with 7 being neutral. The lower the number the more acidic and the higher the number the more alkaline. The skin has a pH between 4.5 and 6 making it acidic.

ACTIVITY
Describe the physiological effects of massage on the skin.

SELF-CHECKS
1 Name the layers of the epidermis and give a brief description of each.
2 List the main functions of the skin.

information point
- Sweat contains: 99.4% water, 0.4% water-soluble substances such as urea and salt, 0.2% trace minerals and has a pH of 7.3.
- Sebum contains: lipids (oils and fats – typically squalene, glycerol and cholesterol), carbohydrates and water and has a pH of 4.5.

information point
The skin is pH buffered, meaning that the pH of the skin does not change very easily (a buffer is acid and salt, the skin is lactic acid and lactate).

The skeletal system

There are two types of skeleton:

- Exoskeleton – this is where hard material is formed mainly on the outside of the body. Crustaceans normally have an exoskeleton.
- Endoskeleton – this is where the skeleton is formed inside the soft tissue. The skeleton is made of bone and cartilage such as in human beings.

Functions of the skeleton
The skeleton has four main functions:

- Support.
- Protection.
- Muscle attachment.
- Movement (locomotion).

Support

The skeleton supports and raises the body from the ground and allows movement. Vital organs are suspended from the skeleton thus preventing them from crushing each other.

Protection

The skeleton is uniquely designed to protect the internal organs. In particular it protects:

- the brain, which is encased in the cranium
- the spinal cord, which is encased in the vertebral column
- the heart and lungs, which are surrounded by the rib cage.

The organs are protected by the skeleton from distortion resulting from pressure, and from injury resulting from impact.

Muscle attachment

The skeleton acts as a framework for the voluntary muscular system. For movement to take place a muscle must be held in place firmly at one end (this is known as the origin of the muscle) and be free to move at the other end (this is known as the insertion of the muscle). The origins and insertions of most of the body's muscles are located on the bones of the skeleton.

Movement (locomotion)

Many bones of the skeleton act as levers. When muscles pull on these levers they produce movement, such as the chewing action of the jaw, the flexing of the biceps and the inhalation/exhalation movements of the ribs. All these movements require a system of joints and muscle attachments.

Composition of the skeleton

The skeleton consists of some 204 bones in adult life.

- 22 form the cranium.
- 25 form the thorax.
- 33 form the spine.
- 120 form the upper and lower limbs.
- 4 form the pelvis.

Types of bone tissue

There are two types of bone tissue: *compact* and *cancellous*.

Compact bone

Compact bone contains large numbers of structures called *Haversian systems*. A Haversian system consists of a central longitudinal canal, called the *Haversian canal*, rich in blood, lymph and nerves, surrounded by plates of bone arranged concentrically, called *lamellae*. Spaces between lamellae contain osteocytes or bone cells called *lacunae*. The Haversian systems are covered with a tough, fibrous sheeting called *periosteum*. This tubular formation makes this type of bone strong and rigid.

Cancellous bone

Cancellous bone appears more 'spongy' than compact bone. It has larger Haversian canals with less lamellae, giving a latticework appearance. Cancellous bone contains red bone marrow.

Periosteum

Periosteum is the fibrous sheeting which covers the bone surface. It is composed of two layers. The inner layer produces new cells for bone growth. The outer, fibrous layer has a rich vascular supply.

HEALTH AND BEAUTY THERAPY: A PRACTICAL APPROACH

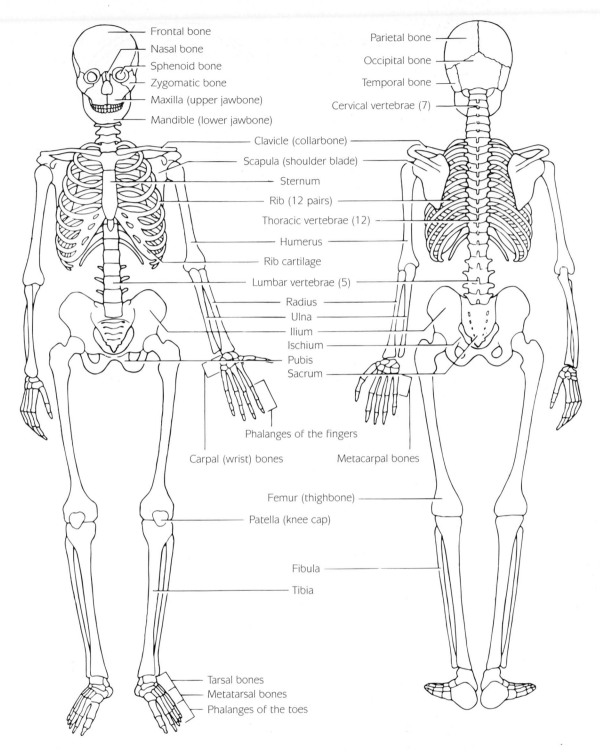

The skeleton

Labels (front view, left to right):
- Frontal bone
- Nasal bone
- Sphenoid bone
- Zygomatic bone
- Maxilla (upper jawbone)
- Mandible (lower jawbone)

- Clavicle (collarbone)
- Scapula (shoulder blade)
- Sternum
- Rib (12 pairs)
- Thoracic vertebrae (12)
- Humerus
- Rib cartilage
- Lumbar vertebrae (5)
- Radius
- Ulna
- Ilium
- Ischium
- Pubis
- Sacrum

- Phalanges of the fingers
- Carpal (wrist) bones
- Metacarpal bones

- Femur (thighbone)
- Patella (knee cap)

- Fibula
- Tibia

- Tarsal bones
- Metatarsal bones
- Phalanges of the toes

Labels (back view):
- Parietal bone
- Occipital bone
- Temporal bone
- Cervical vertebrae (7)

Classification of bones

Long bones

The strongest bones of the skeleton, long bones are composed of a shaft (diaphysis) and two ends (epiphyses). The diaphysis is formed from compact bone while the epiphyses have an outer covering of compact bone with cancellous bone found within. An example of a long bone is the femur.

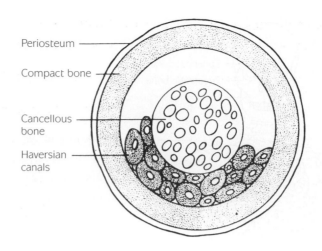

Cross-section through a long bone

Periosteum
Compact bone
Cancellous bone
Haversian canals

Short bones

Short bones are the small bones found in the wrists and ankles. They consist of a relatively thin outer layer of compact bone with cancellous bone inside. Examples of short bones are the metatarsals.

Flat bones

Flat bones consist of two thin layers of compact bone joined by a layer of cancellous bone and covered by periosteum. Two sets of blood vessels pass into the bone to supply the spongy and compact tissues. Examples of flat bones include the frontal and parietal bones of the cranium.

Irregular bones

Irregular bones consist of a mass of cancellous bone covered by a thin layer of compact bone overlaid with periosteum. Examples of irregular bones are the vertebrae.

Sesamoid bones

Sesamoid bones are rounded masses of bone tissue found in certain tendons. The best example of a sesamoid bone is the patella.

Joints

Where two or more bones come together a joint is formed. There are three main classifications of joint: *cartilaginous*, *fibrous* and *synovial*.

Cartilaginous joints are slightly moveable joints. They are held together by strong ligaments. The bones are separated by pads of white fibro-cartilage which allow only slight movement when the fibro-cartilage pad is compressed. Examples of this type of joint include the sacro-iliac joint and the symphysis pubis.

Fibrous joints are fixed joints. They do not allow any form of movement. Fibrous tissue is found between the bones in these joints. Examples of fibrous joints are the sutures between the bones of the skull.

Synovial joints are freely moveable joints. They allow a considerable amount of movement. The joint is enclosed in a fibrous capsule supported by ligaments. The capsule is lined by a synovial membrane which secretes synovial fluid into the capsule. Synovial fluid prevents friction between articulating surfaces of the joint which are both covered in hyaline cartilage for smooth operation.

The types of synovial joint are:

- Ball and socket joints.
- Hinge joints.
- Pivot articulations.
- Gliding joints.

information point

Three times as many women as men are affected by rheumatoid arthritis, which leads to joint inflammation and pain.

HEALTH AND BEAUTY THERAPY: A PRACTICAL APPROACH

Synovial joints are capable of the following types of movement:

- Extension – when a limb is extended, two parts of the limb are pulled away from each other.
- Flexion – when a limb is flexed, two parts of the limb are pulled towards each other.
- Abduction – when a limb is pulled away from the midline (median line) of the body.
- Adduction – when a limb is pulled towards the midline of the body.

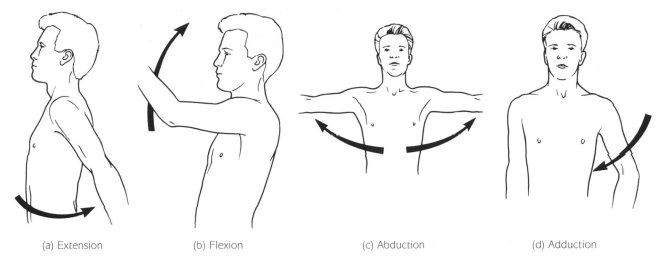

| (a) Extension | (b) Flexion | (c) Abduction | (d) Adduction |

Movements of the upper limb

- Circumduction – combination of flexion, extension, abduction and adduction.
- Rotation – movement round the long axis of bone.
- Pronation – when a limb is turned to face downwards.
- Supination – when a limb is turned to face upwards.
- Inversion – when a limb is turned to face inwards.
- Eversion – when a limb is turned to face outwards.

Ball and socket joints
These joints are capable of flexion, extension, abduction, adduction, rotation and circumduction. Examples of ball and socket joints include the hip and shoulder.

Hinge joints
These joints allow for flexion and extension. Examples of hinge joints include the knee, elbow, ankle and the joint between the atlas and occipital bone in the head.

Pivot articulations
These joints allow for rotation only. Examples include the joint between the radius and ulna and the axis joint of the head.

Gliding joints
In these joints the articular surfaces glide over each other. Examples of gliding joints are the tarsal joint of the ankle and the carpal joint of the wrist.

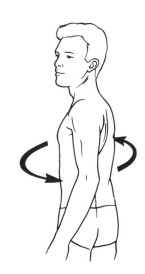

Rotation

ACTIVITY

With a colleague, undertake the following activities, noting which bones and types of joints are being used:

a walking up stairs

b catching a ball

c rotating the head.

information point

Flat feet are caused by weaknesses in the lower leg muscles, not in the feet.

SELF-CHECKS

1 Give the functions of the skeleton.

2 Name two classifications of joints.

The muscular system

Roughly one-fifth of body weight is made up of muscle. It is muscle which forms the flesh of the body and moves the body with the aid of the skeleton. Whilst most muscles are attached to bones, there are exceptions, such as the epicranial aponeurosis. Both ends of the epicranial aponeurosis are attached to the skin. The muscle causes movements such as frowning, raising of the eyebrows, etc.

The naming of muscles is complicated. They can be named according to:

- Function, e.g. flexor or extensor, adductor or abductor, supinator or pronator.
- Attachments, e.g. sternocleidomastoid.
- Shape, e.g. trapezius.
- Formation, e.g. biceps (2 heads), triceps (3 heads), quadriceps (4 heads).
- Position, e.g. intercostal muscles (between the ribs).

Types of muscular tissue

information point

The composition of muscular tissue is:

- 75% water
- 25% solids, of which the most important is a protein called myosin.

There are three types of muscular tissue: *voluntary*, *involuntary* and *cardiac*.

Voluntary muscular tissue

Voluntary muscle is also called striated muscle and forms the flesh of the limbs and trunk. It consists of long fibres, made of multi-nucleate cells, which vary considerably in length according to the individual muscle. Each fibre contains numerous thread-like structures called *myofibrils*. Myofibrils are alternately striped in regular light and dark bands which is why voluntary muscle is sometimes called striated muscle. Muscle fibres are surrounded by a membrane called the *endomysium*. The fibres are bound together in bundles called *fasciculi* and surrounded by a sheath called the *perimysium*. The fasciculi in turn form a bigger bundle enclosed by a sheath called the *epimysium* which ultimately forms an individual muscle.

As the name suggests, voluntary muscle is under conscious control. It contracts quickly when stimulated by nerve impulses but tires rather quickly as well.

Involuntary muscular tissue

This type of muscle is found in the walls of the internal organs, e.g. stomach, bowel, uterus, etc. It consists of spindle-shaped cells, each of which contain a nucleus. These cells are unstriped and have no sheath but are bound together by connective tissue. They are not under control of will and are designed for slow contraction over a long period. Involuntary muscle, therefore, does not fatigue easily.

Cardiac muscle

This type of muscle is found only in the heart wall and is both involuntary and irregularly striped. It consists of short, cylindrical, branched fibres with a centrally placed nucleus. Cardiac muscle has no sheath but is bound together by connective tissue. It is not under control of will and contracts automatically throughout life in a rhythmical pattern. The rate of these contractions is controlled by nerves which quicken or slow down the action. This is the strongest type of muscular tissue within the human body.

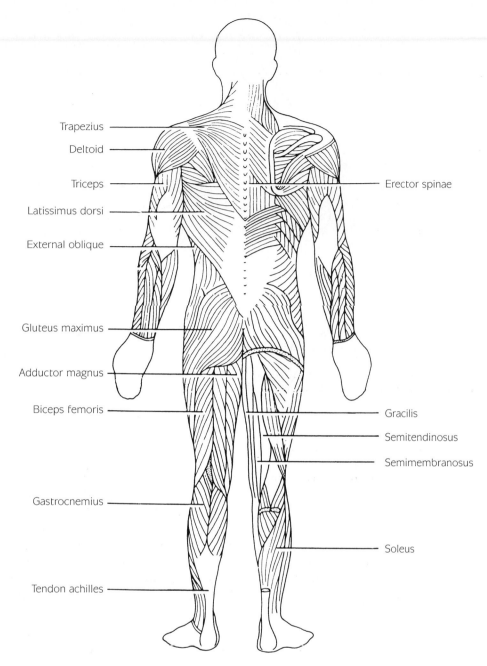

Trapezius

Deltoid

Triceps

Latissimus dorsi

External oblique

Gluteus maximus

Adductor magnus

Biceps femoris

Gastrocnemius

Tendon achilles

Erector spinae

Gracilis

Semitendinosus

Semimembranosus

Soleus

Muscles of the body – posterior view

The properties of muscular tissue

Muscle has four main properties:

- The power of contraction.
- Elasticity.
- Fatigue.
- Muscle tone.

The power of contraction

Voluntary muscle contracts as a result of stimuli reaching it from the nervous system and many nerves have their endings in muscles. Messages passing down a nerve from the brain cause the muscle to contract when they reach it. Other stimuli such as electrical currents applied directly to the muscle or its nerve will also cause contraction.

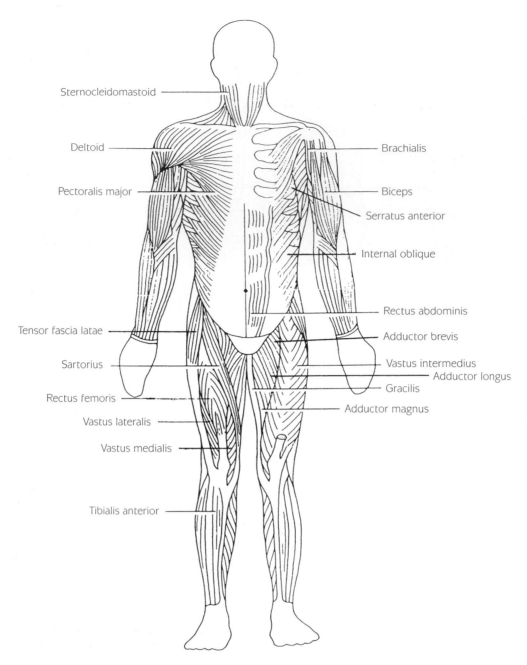

Muscles of the body – anterior view

The labels on the diagram, reading top to bottom, left side:
- Sternocleidomastoid
- Deltoid
- Pectoralis major
- Tensor fascia latae
- Sartorius
- Rectus femoris
- Vastus lateralis
- Vastus medialis
- Tibialis anterior

Right side:
- Brachialis
- Biceps
- Serratus anterior
- Internal oblique
- Rectus abdominis
- Adductor brevis
- Vastus intermedius
- Adductor longus
- Gracilis
- Adductor magnus

Elasticity and fatigue

When a muscle contracts, it uses energy which is derived mainly from the respiration of glucose. Glucose is supplied to the muscle via the blood. The blood also carries oxygen which the muscle uses to 'burn up' the glucose. During normal activity, the glucose is respired aerobically, that is the glucose is broken down to form water and carbon dioxide. The water and carbon dioxide are removed from the muscle and it does not tire.

During heavy exercise glucose is required anaerobically. Anaerobic respiration produces lactic acid which is ultimately broken down to form carbon dioxide and water. However, lactic acid is not broken down very fast. After a certain number of contractions lactic acid begins to accumulate in the muscle. The muscle then becomes tired and is unable to contract with the same degree of efficiency. This affects the elasticity of the muscle and ultimately results in fatigue.

	Position	Origin	Insertion	Action
Muscles of the neck and back				
Sternocleidomastoid	Front of the neck	Sternum and clavicle	Mastoid process	Used separately, turns the head to opposite side; used together, flexes the neck
Trapezius	Back of the neck and chest	Occiput and spines of the thoracic vertebrae	Spine of the scapula and clavicle	Draws scapula back, bracing the shoulders; pulls the occiput, extending the neck
Latissimus dorsi	Crosses the back from the lumbar region to the shoulder	Lumbar vertebrae, sacrum and back of iliac crest	Humerus	Adduction of the shoulder, drawing the arm back and downwards
Erector spinae	Between the transverse and spinal processes of the vertebrae	Sacrum	Occipital bone	Keeps the body in an upright position and produces extension of the vertebral column
Serratus anterior	Lateral chest wall	Upper nine ribs	Vertebral border of scapula	Draws shoulder forwards and rotates scapula
Muscles of the chest				
Pectoralis major	Front of the chest	Sternum and clavicle	Humerus, outer edge of the bicipital groove	Adduction of the shoulder, drawing the arm across the thorax
Muscles of the arm				
Biceps	Front of arm	By two heads from the scapula (coracoid process and above the glenoid cavity)	Radial tuberosity	Flexion of the elbow and shoulder; supinates hand
Triceps	Back of arm	By one head from the scapula and by two heads from the shaft of the humerus	Olecranon process of ulna	Extension of the elbow and shoulder
Deltoid	Over the shoulder	Spine of scapula and clavicle	Deltoid tubercle of humerus	Abducts the shoulder to a right angle
Brachiali	Crosses front of elbow	Humerus	Ulna	Flexion of the elbow
Muscles of the abdomen				
Rectus abdominis	Front of the abdominal wall	Upper border of pubic bone	5th, 6th and 7th costal cartilages and xiphoid process	Flexes the spine and aids respiration
External oblique	Forms the outer coat of the side abdominal wall	Lower ribs	Iliac crest	Flexes trunk together with internal oblique
Internal oblique	Forms the second coat of the side wall of the abdomen	Iliac crest	Lower ribs and fascia of the rectus abdominis	Flexes trunk together with external oblique. Produces rotation when used with the external oblique of the opposite side

continued

	Position	Origin	Insertion	Action
Muscles of the buttocks				
Gluteus maximus	Large quadrilateral mass forming the prominence of the buttocks	Outer surface of ilium, also sacrum and coccyx	Upper end of femur	Extends the hip joint and rotates it laterally
Gluteus medius	Lies below the gluteus maximus	Gluteal surface of ilium	Greater trochanter of femur	Abduction of the hip joint
Muscles of the hip and upper leg				
Quadriceps	This extensive muscle mass forms the bulk of the anterior region of the thigh and is divided here into four separate muscles: the rectus femoris, vastus lateralis, vastus medialis and vastus intermedius			
Rectus femoris	Front of thigh	Ilium	Upper border of patella	Flexes the hip joint
Vastus lateralis	Lateral side of femur	Greater trochanter and linea aspera of femur	Tibial tubercle	Extends the knee joint
Vastus medialis	Medial side of femur	Lesser trochanter of femur	Tibial tubercle	Extends the knee joint
Vastus intermedius	Covers front of femur	Upper end of femur	Tibial tubercle	Extends the knee joint
Abductors of hip	Outer side of thigh	Anterior aspect of ilium	Between the two layers of a fascia lata	Abducts the hip
Adductors of hip (pectineus, adductor brevis, adductor longus, adductor magnus, gracilis)	The group lies on the medial side of the thigh	Pubic bone	Linea aspera of femur	Adducts the femur
Hamstrings (biceps femoris, semimembranosus, semitendinosus)	Back of thigh	Ischial tuberosity and femur	Tibia and fibula of knee	Extension of hip and flexion
Sartorius	Crosses over the front of the thigh	Anterior superior iliac spine	Upper part of the tibia	Weak flexor of both hip and knee joints
Tensor fascia latae	Lateral aspect of upper thigh	Outer part of iliac crest	Fascia latae	Abducts and rotates the femur and extends the knee
Muscles of the lower leg				
Tibialis anterior	Front of leg	Lateral surface of upper end of tibia	Medial cuneiform bone	Flexion and inversion of the foot
Gastrocnemius	Posterior calf area	Condyles of femur	Calcaneum	Flexes foot
Soleus	Posterior of calf area	Head and upper part of fibula and tibia	Calcaneum	Flexes foot

Muscular tone

Even when a muscle appears to be at rest it is always partially contracted and therefore ready for immediate action. This state of partial contraction is called muscular tone.

Tendons

Tendons are tough, fibrous and inelastic. They are found at the ends of muscles and their main purpose is to provide attachment to bones.

Ligaments

Like the tendons above, ligaments are strong, fibrous and do not stretch. Their function is to connect bones together.

SELF-CHECKS

1   Draw and label diagrams of the main muscles of the body.
2   State the four properties of muscular tissue.

The circulatory system

The circulatory system consists of:

- Heart
- Blood
- Blood vessels
- Lymph
- Lymph vessels.

The heart

The heart is a hollow organ with walls made of cardiac muscle. It is approximately 10 cm long and weighs about 225 g in women and 240 g in men. The heart is situated in the thoracic cavity protected by the rib cage and it lies obliquely to the left-hand side.

The heart is composed of three distinct layers:

1   **Pericardium**. This is a smooth, membranous covering which is formed of an outer fibrous layer and an inner, serous coat. Between these layers a serous fluid is secreted which allows for ease of movement between the two layers.

2   **Myocardium**. This is the muscular layer of the heart and is formed of a specialised, involuntary muscular tissue. This cardiac muscle is exceptionally strong. The fibres are bonded together in branches and it has to be able to contract rhythmically throughout life.

3   **Endocardium**. This is the inner, lining membrane of the myocardium layer. It is very thin and consists of flattened epithelial cells.

Internal structure of the heart

The heart is divided into a right and left side with a layer of myocardium called the *septum* separating them. Each side is divided into two chambers. There are four

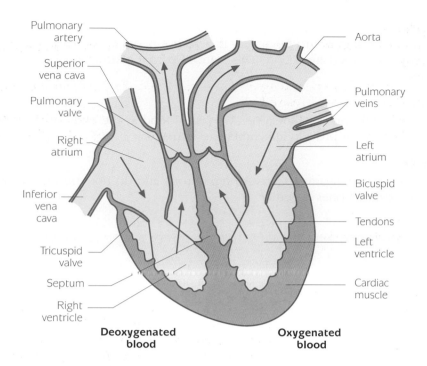

Pulmonary artery

Superior vena cava

Pulmonary valve

Right atrium

Inferior vena cava

Tricuspid valve

Septum

Right ventricle

Aorta

Pulmonary veins

Left atrium

Bicuspid valve

Tendons

Left ventricle

Cardiac muscle

Deoxygenated blood

Oxygenated blood

The heart

chambers in total; the right and left *atria* and the right and left *ventricles*. Valves separate the chambers on each side of the heart from each other. The valve separating the right atrium and ventricle is called the *tricuspid valve*. The valve separating the left atrium and ventricle is called the *bicuspid* or *mitral valve*. These valves open and close when the pressure changes within the chambers.

When cardiac muscle contracts it squeezes blood out of the heart and into the arteries which carry it to all parts of the body. When cardiac muscle relaxes the heart fills with blood from the veins. This mechanism of contraction and relaxation is known as the heart beat.

Flow of blood through the heart

Deoxygenated blood returns from the body to the right atrium of the heart via the largest veins of the body, the superior and inferior vena cavae. This blood is then squeezed through the tricuspid valve into the right ventricle from where it is then forced through the pulmonary artery which carries the deoxygenated blood to the lungs. Gaseous exchange takes place between the blood and the air in the lungs; carbon dioxide is excreted and oxygen is absorbed. The now oxygenated blood returns to the heart via the pulmonary veins which empty the blood into the left atrium. It passes through the bicuspid valve and into the left ventricle, then is forced into the largest artery of the body, the aorta, which carries the oxygenated blood to the rest of the body.

Cardiac cycle

The contraction and relaxation of the heart is called the cardiac cycle and is divided into two phases:

- **Diastole** – when blood is passing from the veins into the atria and then into the ventricles. Heart muscle is relaxed.
- **Systole** – when the ventricles contract during systole the valves in the heart are pushed closed causing the pressure in the arteries to increase. This gives the pulse.

Blood

Blood consists of:

- Erythrocytes (red blood cells).
- Leucocytes (white blood cells).
- Platelets.
- Plasma.

Erythrocytes (red blood cells)

Erythrocytes are minute, biconcave discs made from spongy cytoplasm surrounded by an elastic membrane. Their red colour comes from *haemoglobin* combined with oxygen. Haemoglobin is a protein which contains iron and has a natural affinity with oxygen. Haemoglobin combines with oxygen to form *oxyhaemoglobin*. Red blood cells are the mechanism by which oxygen is transported around the body. Red blood cells are made in red bone marrow. Cell formation takes approximately seven days, during which time the nucleus disappears and they cease to be true cells. The life span of a red blood cell is roughly four months, after which time the cell is destroyed in the liver or the spleen.

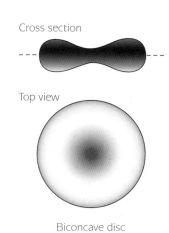

Cross section

Top view

Biconcave disc

Erythrocyte (red blood cell)

Leucocytes (white blood cells)

Leucocytes are colourless cells each containing a nucleus. There are far fewer white cells than red cells; approximately one to every six hundred red cells. The main function of white cells is to fight infection and protect the body against viruses, toxins and bacteria. There are different types of leucocytes and they have different functions within the body.

Granulocytes form approximately 75% of the total number of white cells. They ingest bacteria by encapsulating them and digesting them slowly – a process called phagocytosis. Granulocytes have a life span of about one week and are made in bone marrow.

Lymphocytes form roughly 23% of the total number of white cells. They are formed in lymph nodes and produce antibodies which kill foreign proteins. They can live for up to one hundred days.

Monocytes form approximately 2% of white cells. They can ingest foreign proteins in the blood.

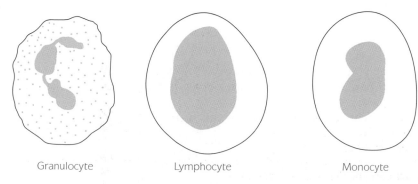

Granulocyte   Lymphocyte   Monocyte

Leucocytes (white blood cells)

Platelets

Platelets are formed in the red bone marrow and are fragments of red blood cells. They play an important part in the clotting process of blood.

Plasma

Plasma is a slightly alkaline, yellowish fluid in which the blood cells float. It consists of 96% water together with other important compounds such as:

- Proteins, e.g. albumem, fibrogen, globulin.
- Antibodies.
- Soluble salts, e.g. sodium chloride, potassium chloride, calcium phosphate.
- Food substances, e.g. amino acids, glucose, fatty acids, glycerol.
- Waste products, e.g. urea, carbon dioxide.
- Hormones.

Functions of blood

- Transport of oxygen from the lungs to the body tissues.
- Transport of carbon dioxide from the body tissues to the lungs.
- Transport of excretory products.
- Transport of digested food.
- Distribution of hormones.
- Distribution of heat.
- Clotting process of blood (this occurs to prevent loss of blood from a wound).

The blood clotting process in damaged tissue

Platelets produce a substance called *thrombokinase* which acts on *prothrombin* (which is already circulating in the blood) to change it to *thrombin*. Thrombin reacts with calcium ions in the blood producing *fibrinogen* – fibres of protein which radiate across the wound tangling red and white cells together with platelets – thus preventing blood loss.

Arteries and veins

Arteries and veins are hollow elastic tubes that transport blood which has been pumped by the heart around the body. They differ slightly in structure.

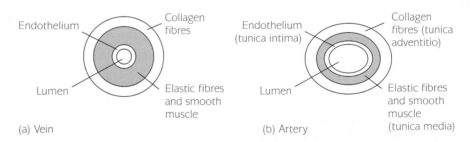

Cross-sections of an artery and a vein

Veins:

- have thinner walls than arteries
- contain valves to prevent the back-flow of blood
- carry deoxygenated blood (with the exception of the pulmonary vein mentioned earlier)
- have walls consisting of three layers – the tunica adventia, tunica media and tunica intima.

Arteries:

- have thicker walls than veins
- do not contain valves

- carry oxygenated blood (with the exception of the pulmonary artery mentioned earlier)
- have walls consisting of the same three layers as veins, but they are thicker than in veins.

Blood pressure

Blood pressure is the amount of pressure exerted on the arteries by blood as it flows through them. It is measured in millimetres of mercury (mmHg) using a *sphygmomanometer*.

The lymphatic system

The lymphatic system is a subsidiary or second circulatory system which drains the tissue fluid. It consists of a series of fluid-filled tubes beginning as fine, blind-ended capillaries which spread throughout most of the tissues of the body. These pass into larger lymphatic vessels which eventually drain into the great veins of the neck. The principal function of the lymphatic system is to fight infection within the body.

Lymphatic fluid

Lymph is a clear, straw-coloured liquid with a similar composition to blood plasma. Its main composition is water with some proteins, fats, hormones and salts. It contains white cells, mainly lymphocytes, together with waste products that the system is dealing with at any particular time, e.g. dead cells, micro-organisms.

Formation of lymph

Lymph is formed in the tissues of the body and is a derivative of blood plasma which passes out of the capillaries to form what is called intercellular fluid. Excess intercellular fluid drains into the lymphatic capillaries where it is known as lymph.

Lymphatic capillaries

Lymphatic capillaries are fine, hollow, blind-ended, elastic tubes, similar to blood capillaries in structure although they are wider and less regular in shape. They consist of a single layer of epithelial tissue, i.e. their walls are one cell thick, bound together with connective tissue. Because of this they are more permeable than blood capillaries, allowing for larger substances to pass through their walls. Lymph drains into them from the tissue fluids.

Lymphatic vessels

Lymphatic vessels carry lymph from the lymphatic capillaries to the great veins of the neck. They are composed of connective tissue lined with epithelial cells and they also contain valves to prevent back-flow to ensure that lymph flows away from the tissues.

Lymph nodes

Before lymph is discharged into the bloodstream it passes through at least one lymph node. Lymph nodes are situated in clusters around the body and are composed of special cells which include *macrophages* which are phagocytic, i.e. they ingest foreign particles thereby filtering the lymph of toxins. Major groups of lymph nodes are in the head and neck, under the arms (axillae), in the breast area, abdomen and groin (inguinal). When there is localised infection within the body the lymph nodes in that particular area will become swollen as they are engorged with toxins.

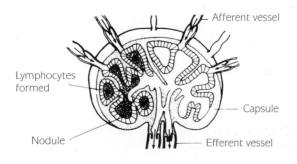

Cross-section of a lymph node

The great veins of the neck

As has been mentioned previously, lymph travels through at least one lymph node before it returns to the blood stream. The vessels which allow lymph to re-enter the blood stream are called:

● The right lymphatic duct. This is a dilated vessel situated at the base of the neck and feeds into the right subclavian vein. It drains lymph from the right half of the head, neck, chest area and right arm.
● The thoracic duct. This vessel begins at the *cisterna chyli*, a specialised lymph sac found in front of the first two lumber vertebrae. It connects into the left subclavian vein at the base of the neck. It drains lymph from the left side of the head and neck, the left arm, left side of the chest area and both legs.

The spleen

The spleen is a large nodule of lymphoid tissue which is a deep purplish-red in colour. It is situated high up at the back of the abdomen on the left side behind the stomach. The functions of the spleen are:

● Formation of lymphocytes.
● A reservoir for blood.
● Formation of antibodies and antitoxins.
● Destruction of worn-out erythrocytes.

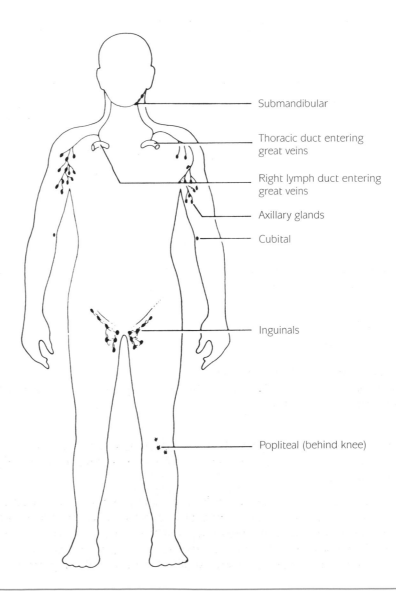

Submandibular

Thoracic duct entering great veins

Right lymph duct entering great veins

Axillary glands

Cubital

Inguinals

Popliteal (behind knee)

Lymph nodes of the body

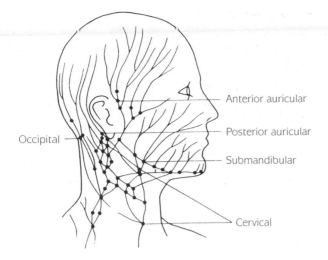

Lymph nodes of the face

Labels on the figure: Anterior auricular, Posterior auricular, Submandibular, Cervical, Occipital

ACTIVITY

Research the ABO system of blood grouping.

SELF-CHECKS

1   Name and describe the principal cells of the circulatory system.

2   Describe the flow of blood through the heart.

3   What is the main function of the lymphatic system?

The neurological system

The neurological system is involved in transmitting messages from the brain to all other parts of the body. It consists of three main divisions:

- The central nervous system.
- The peripheral nervous system.
- The autonomic nervous system.

The central nervous system

The central nervous system consists of the brain and spinal column and is at the centre of the neurological system.

The brain

The brain is the most important part of the entire neurological system. It receives impulses and stores them. It also transmits impulses to all parts of the body to stimulate organs to work.

The adult brain weighs approximately 1.5 kg and contains millions of neurones. Each neurone is composed of a cell body that is similar in composition to other animal cells in that it contains a nucleus and is surrounded by cytoplasm. However, it differs in that it has a long tail known as its axon, the purpose of which is to control impulses away from the cell body. Attached to the cell body are small fibres

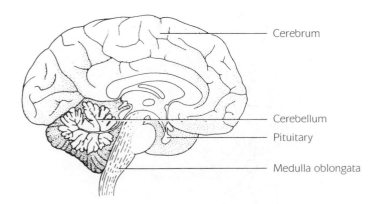

Cross-section through the brain

called dendrites and these carry impulses into the cell. Groups of neurones together form what are termed nerves and in order for impulses to travel along a nerve they must move from the axon of one to the dendrite of the next. Where axons and dendrites meet is called the synapse.

For neurones to remain undamaged in the brain they need to be well protected and this is accomplished first by the skull – a hard outer casing of bone – and secondly by a specialised layer called the *meninges*.

The meninges consist of three distinct layers. These are:

- the *dura mater* – a tough, fibrous outer membrane which cushions the brain against the inside of the cranium
- the *arachnoid mater* – the middle layer, which is much more delicate
- the *pia mater* – the inner layer which folds into the convoluted surface of the brain.

A special fluid is found between the arachnoid and pia mater which acts as a further cushion. It is called *cerebrospinal fluid*.

The brain has three main regions:

- *Cerebrum.* The largest region of the brain, it is a dome-shaped area of nervous tissue split into two halves called cerebral hemispheres. The surface of the cerebrum is made of what is termed grey matter – this is where the main functions of the cerebrum are carried out. These functions include all forms of conscious activity. Sensations such as touch, vision, taste, hearing and smell originate here. Control of voluntary muscular movements and emotion, powers of reasoning and memory are also handled in the cerebrum.
- *Cerebellum.* This region of the brain receives impulses from the semi-circular canals in the ears and from stretch receptors in the muscles. It processes this information to maintain muscle tone and a balanced posture. It also co-ordinates muscles during activities such as walking, running, dancing, etc.
- *Medulla oblongata.* This region is often referred to as the *brain stem* and contains a mass of grey matter known as the *vital centre*. It controls the part of the nervous system not under control of will, e.g. regulation of blood pressure, body temperature, etc. It performs these functions through connections with the autonomic nervous system. The medulla oblongata also contains nerve fibres which connect the brain with the spinal cord.

The spinal cord

As mentioned, the spinal cord is continuous with the medulla oblongata and extends downwards through the vertebral column finishing at the level of the lumbar

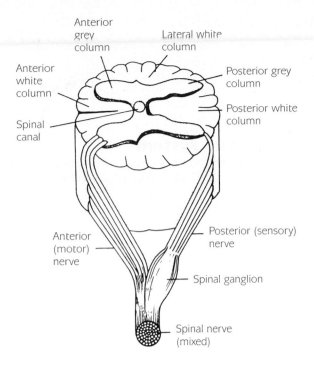

Anterior grey column

Lateral white column

Anterior white column

Posterior grey column

Spinal canal

Posterior white column

Anterior (motor) nerve

Posterior (sensory) nerve

Spinal ganglion

Spinal nerve (mixed)

Cross-section of the spinal cord

vertebrae. It is protected by meninges and cerebrospinal fluid like the brain. Radiating from the spinal column are 12 pairs of cranial nerves and 31 pairs of spinal nerves corresponding to the segments of the vertebral column. The cranial and spinal nerves are part of the peripheral nervous system.

The peripheral nervous system

This part of the neurological system consists of all the nerves situated outside the central nervous system.

There are three types of nerve cell in the peripheral nervous system:

- *Motor (efferent) nerves*. These nerves convey impulses from the brain through the spinal cord to the skeletal muscles, glands and smooth muscular tissue (effector organs).
- *Sensory (afferent) nerves*. This type of nerve conveys impulses from the sensory nerve endings in organs to the brain and spinal cord.
- *Mixed nerves*. These consist of both motor and sensory nerve fibres.

The peripheral nervous system consists of 31 pairs of spinal nerves and 12 pairs of cranial nerves.

The spinal nerves are as follows:

- 8 pairs cervical.
- 12 pairs thoracic.
- 5 pairs lumbar.
- 5 pairs sacral.
- 1 pair coccygeal.

The 12 pairs of cranial nerves are the:

- Olfactory nerves.
- Optic nerves.
- Oculomotor nerves.
- Trochlear nerves.
- Trigeminal nerves.

- Abducent nerves.
- Facial nerves.
- Auditory nerves.
- Glossopharyngeal nerves.
- Vagus nerves.
- Accessory nerves.
- Hypoglossal nerves.

The autonomic nervous system

The autonomic division of the nervous system controls areas of the body over which there is no conscious control. It is divided into two sections:

- the sympathetic system
- the parasympathetic system.

The sympathetic system

The sympathetic system is composed of a gangliated cord which is situated on either side of the anterior surface of the vertebral column.

It is composed of a network of interlaced nerves termed *plexuses*. The main plexuses of the sympathetic division are:

- solar plexus – which supplies the abdominal viscera
- cardiac plexus – which supplies the thoracic viscera
- hypogastric plexus – which supplies the pelvic region.

The parasympathetic system

This division is composed mainly of the vagus nerve which has the largest distribution of all the cranial nerves. It starts from nerve cells in the medulla oblongata and passes through the neck into the thorax and abdomen.

All the internal organs have in effect a double nerve supply, one supply from the sympathetic system and one from the parasympathetic system. The two systems work antagonistically. The sympathetic system increases body activity and the parasympathetic system slows it down.

The other area that the autonomic nervous system is involved with is the *reflex action*. This is an involuntary action designed to protect the body against serious damage. A very good example of this is if you touch a hot surface, before you have had time to register the pain in the normal way the reflex action spontaneously removes the finger.

ACTIVITY

Research the nerve supply for each of the muscles listed in this chapter.

SELF-CHECKS

1 Name and describe briefly the main divisions of the neurological system.
2 List the spinal nerves.

The endocrine system

The endocrine, or hormonal, system is a series of ductless glands that secrete hormones (chemical messengers) which act on parts of the body other than where they were produced. Hormones are carried in the blood stream and influence many activities of the body.

The main endocrine glands of the body are:

- Pituitary hypophysis gland.
- Thyroid gland.
- Prathyroid glands.
- Adrenal glands.
- Pancreas – the islets of Langerhans.
- Ovaries (female only).
- Testes (male only).

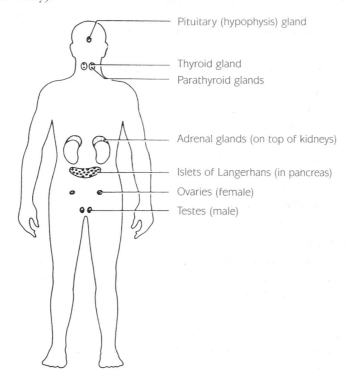

Pituitary (hypophysis) gland

Thyroid gland
Parathyroid glands

Adrenal glands (on top of kidneys)

Islets of Langerhans (in pancreas)

Ovaries (female)

Testes (male)

The endocrine glands

The pituitary hypophysis gland

The pituitary gland is sometimes referred to as the master gland because all the hormones it secretes have a bearing on all the other glands in the system. It is situated in the head in the hypophyseal fossa of the sphenoid bone below the hypothalamus to which it is attached by an isthmus. The gland consists of a posterior and anterior lobe.

Anterior lobe

The anterior lobe of the pituitary gland secretes eight hormones in total, all controlled by what is termed the *negative feedback mechanism*. This means that when the level of any particular hormone is low in the blood supplying the hypothalamus, it stimulates the anterior lobe of the pituitary to produce the appropriate releasing hormone which stimulates the target endocrine gland that produces that hormone to produce more.

The eight hormones secreted by the anterior lobe of the pituitary and their functions are:

- Adrenocorticothrophic hormone (ACTH) – stimulates the adrenal cortex to secrete cortisol.
- Thyroid stimulating hormone (TSH) – stimulates activity and growth of the thyroid gland.
- Prolactin – directly affects the female breast immediately after childbirth to initiate and maintain milk secretion.

- Follicle stimulating hormone (FSH) – controls the maturation of the Graafian follicle in the ovary.
- Luteinising hormone (LH) – controls the activity of the gonads.
- Melanocyte stimulating hormone (MSH) – stimulates the production of melanin with the skin.
- Samatotrophin (HGH) – also known as human growth hormone, it promotes protein synthesis in growth and repair of all tissues.
- Interstitial cell stimulating hormone (ICSH) – controls gonad activity.

Posterior lobe

The posterior lobe of the pituitary gland secretes two hormones: *oxytocin* and *anti-diuretic hormone*.

Oxytocin promotes contraction of the uterine muscle and stimulates cells in the lactating breast to squeeze milk into the large ducts behind the nipple.

Anti-diuretic hormone (ADH) has two main functions:

- The *anti-diuretic effect* prevents water being lost from the kidneys and is influenced by osmotic pressure of the circulating blood.
- In large quantities ADH stimulates contraction of smooth muscle, especially in blood vessel walls, raising the blood pressure. This is called the *pressor effect*.

The thyroid gland

Situated in the lower part of the neck, the thyroid consists of a right and left lobe that lie either side of the trachea connected by an isthmus.

The thyroid secretes two main hormones:

- Thyroxin – necessary for controlling the metabolic rate, growth and differentiation of tissues, mental functioning and skin and hair condition.
- Calcitonin – reduces blood calcium levels by inhibiting the absorption of calcium from bones.

Parathyroid glands

The parathyroid glands are four small glands, two embedded in the posterior surface of each lobe of the thyroid gland. They secrete the hormone called *parathormone* which maintains the blood calcium concentration within its normal limits. It works in conjunction with calcitonin to control blood calcium levels.

Adrenal glands

There are two adrenal glands, one situated on the upper aspect of each kidney enclosed within the renal fascia. The glands are composed of two distinctive layers: the *adrenal cortex* and the *adrenal medulla*.

Adrenal cortex

The adrenal cortex produces three groups of hormones:

- Glucocorticoids – hormones which affect the regulation of carbohydrate metabolism, as well as helping in the formation of liver glycogen and helping *gluconeogenesis* (raising blood sugar levels). They suppress the body's inflammatory and allergic reactions and are connected with sodium and water reabsorption from the renal tubules.
- Mineral corticoids – hormones associated with the maintenance of the electrolyte balance in the body. They stimulate the reabsorption of sodium by the kidneys.
- Gonadocorticoids – sex hormones. The gonadocorticoids are *androgens* (male sex hormones) and the adrenal production is of little importance compared to the production of sex hormones by the ovaries/testes.

Adrenal medulla

The adrenal medulla is completely surrounded by the cortex. It is an extension of tissue from the same source as the nervous system and is closely linked to the sympathetic part of the autonomic nervous system.

The adrenal medulla secretes two hormones:

- Adrenaline (epinephrine) – associated with conditions needed for 'fight or flight'. Readies the body for immediate action. It triggers the constriction of peripheral blood vessels and the dilation of muscle fibres, enabling energy (food and oxygen) to be channelled where it is most needed. It also accelerates the conversion of glycogen to glucose.
- Noradrenaline (norepinephrine) – causes vasoconstriction and raises both systolic and diastolic blood pressure.

The pancreas

Hormones are produced in the pancreas by clusters of cells called *islets of Langerhans* which are distributed irregularly throughout the organ. There are three main types of cell in the islets of Langerhans. One of these cell types, the B cells, secrete the hormone insulin which together with glucagon, affects the level of glucose in the blood. The effect of insulin balances the effect of glucagon. Glucagon raises blood sugar levels while insulin reduces it.

The ovaries

The ovaries are the female gonads or sex glands. They are situated in shallow depressions on the lateral walls of the pelvis. The ovaries consist of a cortex and a medulla.

The ovarian cortex surrounds the medulla and contains ovarian follicles each of which contains an ovum. Throughout the reproductive years, one ovarian follicle matures, ruptures and releases its ovum during each menstrual cycle. The ovarian medulla lies in the centre of the ovary and consists of fibrous tissue, blood vessels and nerves.

The two main hormones produced by the ovaries are:

- Oestrogen – influences the menstrual cycle. It stimulates the uterine lining to thicken to prepare for implantation should fertilisation occur. It is also partly responsible for breast development – the growth of milk ducts in the breast. It also influences health and growth of bones, subcutaneous fat distribution and skin condition.
- Progesterone – connected with the development of the placenta and the maintenance of pregnancy when it occurs. It also prepares the mammary glands for lactation.

The testes

The testes are the male gonads. They consist of 200 to 300 lobules composed of germinal epithelial cells. Between these lobules are interstitial cells that secrete the main male hormone *testosterone*.

Testosterone is responsible for the secondary sexual characteristics that occur at puberty in males. Secondary sexual characteristics in males include:

- Increase in body hair.
- Deepening of the voice.
- Broadening of muscles.

SELF-CHECKS

1 State the importance of the endocrine system.
2 Research the main disorders of the endocrine system.

The respiratory system

The respiratory system is involved in the taking in of oxygen and the removal of carbon dioxide from the body. This process is achieved through a number of specialised organs and tissues.

The respiratory system consists of:

- Nose.
- Pharynx.
- Larynx.
- Trachea.
- Two bronchi.
- Bronchioles.
- Two lungs.
- Intercostal muscles.
- Diaphragm.

Nose

The function of the nose is to warm, filter and moisten air. This function is achieved by tiny, ciliated, columnar epithelium which trap bacteria and dust. They secrete mucous which moistens the air as well as acting as an adhesive medium to prevent bacteria and dust entering the throat. Once air has passed through the nose it moves on to the pharynx.

Pharynx

The pharynx has both a respiratory and a digestive function. The respiratory function of the pharynx is similar to that of the nose – it further warms and moistens air before it travels on to the next air passage, called the larynx.

Larynx

At the top of the larynx there is a flap of tissue called the epiglottis which closes to stop food entering the trachea during swallowing. Air passing over the vocal cords within the larynx produces the voice.

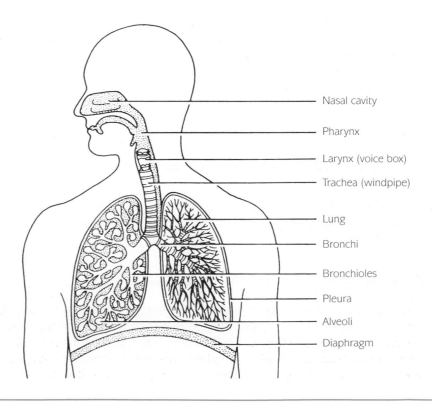

Nasal cavity

Pharynx

Larynx (voice box)

Trachea (windpipe)

Lung

Bronchi

Bronchioles

Pleura

Alveoli

Diaphragm

The respiratory system

Trachea

Also referred to as the windpipe, the trachea consists of a tube surrounded by c-shaped rings of cartilage that act to keep the trachea open even when the neck is bent. It is lined with ciliated epithelium which secrete mucous – a further air-filtration system.

Bronchi

There are two bronchi: the left bronchus and the right bronchus. The bronchi are branches of the trachea that supply the left and right lungs. The right bronchus is wider and more vertical than the left. Both are further divided into a network of narrower passages called bronchioles.

Bronchioles

As mentioned above, bronchioles are narrow passageways which branch from the bronchi. They can branch many times and end in tiny air sacs called alveoli.

Alveoli

Alveoli are extremely tiny, thin-walled, elastic air sacs. They are lined by a flat epithelium and surrounded by pulmonary capillaries. The barrier between the gas in the alveoli and the blood in the vessels is so thin that oxygen and carbon dioxide can pass across it.

Lungs

The lungs are a pair of conical organs each surrounded by a specialised membrane called the *pleura*. The pleura consists of two layers moistened by a special fluid, resembling lymph, which acts as a lubricant enabling the two surfaces to glide smoothly over each other during respiration.

Intercostal muscles

There are both external and internal intercostal muscles. Both sets lie between the ribs. They are responsible for raising and lowering the chest during inspiration (breathing in) and expiration (breathing out).

Diaphragm

The diaphragm is a sheet of muscle that separates the thorax from the abdomen. It is a little unusual in that when it is contracted it becomes flattened and when relaxed it is dome-shaped. The muscle originates from the tip of the sternum, the lower ribs and the cartilages of the lumbar vertebrae and is inserted into the central aponeurosis (a flattened-out tendon). Three openings in the diaphragm allow for the passage of the oesophagus, the aorta and the vena cava. The flattening of the diaphragm increases the volume of the chest cavity, aiding inspiration. Relaxing the diaphragm decreases the volume of the chest cavity, aiding expiration.

How the respiratory system works

The processes of respiration can be summarised in four parts:

- Movement of air in and out of the lungs.
- Free passage of air down the airways.
- Gaseous exchange.
- Control of respiration.

Movement of air in and out of the lungs

During inspiration the intercostal muscles contract, moving the rib-cage upwards and outwards, and the diaphragm contracts downwards to a more flattened position. This causes the thorax to increase in volume, hence decreasing the pressure in the chest cavity. This causes a pressure difference to develop between the inside and outside of the lungs. Air moves from the region of higher pressure (outside the lungs) to the region of lower pressure (inside the lungs) until the pressure difference is removed.

Air is composed of approximately:

- Nitrogen, 78%
- Oxygen, 21%
- Inert gases, 0.07%
- Carbon dioxide, 0.03% (variable)
- Water vapour (variable).

During expiration the diaphragm and intercostal muscles relax and the ribcage returns to the normal position. This has the effect of reducing the volume within the thorax, increasing the air pressure in the lungs, forcing air out of the lungs.

Free passage of air down the airways

As air is breathed in through the nose it passes over hairs and mucous which filter and warm the air. The air passes through the naso-pharynx where it is further filtered and warmed, to the larynx and down the trachea. The trachea also contains mucous secreting ciliated cells which remove any debris from the inhaled air not already dealt with. The air then moves into the bronchial tree, through the bronchi and bronchioles to reach the alveoli.

The air retraces this journey through expiration.

Gaseous exchange

In the lungs, oxygen from the inspired air in the alveolus passes across the alveolar membrane and the capillary walls to combine with haemoglobin in the red blood cells. Simultaneously, carbon dioxide diffuses back from the blood into the alveolar air so that it can be exhaled.

Control of respiration

Control of respiration is achieved through both chemical and neurological means. Respiration is controlled by nerve cells in the medulla oblongata in what is known as the *respiratory centre*. It is further controlled by chemoreceptors in the walls of the aorta and carotid arteries which are sensitive to changes in oxygen and carbon dioxide concentrations in the blood.

SELF-CHECKS

1 State the composition of air.
2 Describe briefly the mechanism of breathing.

The digestive system

The digestive system is concerned with the taking in and breakdown of food. There are two phases to digestion, mechanical and chemical.

The digestive system consists of the alimentary tract or canal and the glands secreting digestive juices which act upon the food matter. The alimentary canal is a passage over 9 metres long leading from the mouth to the rectum. It is lined throughout with a mucous membrane which lubricates the system. Muscular walls act upon the foodstuffs eaten and help their passage along the alimentary canal. The alimentary canal consists of:

- Mouth
- Pharynx
- Oesophagus
- Stomach
- Small intestine
- Large intestine.

The glands are:

- Salivary glands – secreting saliva in the mouth
- Gastric glands – secreting gastric juices in the stomach
- Pancreas – secreting pancreatic juice in the duodenum
- Liver – secreting bile in the duodenum
- Intestinal glands – secreting intestinal juice in the small intestine.

Mouth

Digestion commences mechanically and chemically in the mouth with the action of the teeth and salivary glands respectively. There are 32 permanent teeth of four types in the adult mouth. Each type of tooth has a specific function in the breakdown of food; the *incisors* are adapted to break off food, the *canines* are adapted to tear at meat and the *premolars* and *molars* are adapted to grind and chew.

The tongue also plays a part in mechanical digestion. It consists of striated voluntary muscle attached mainly to the mandible and hyoid bones and helps in the swallowing action by forming the food into a suitably sized ball, or *bolus*, and moving it to the pharynx at the back of the mouth.

The salivary glands in the mouth begin chemical digestion. There are two parotid glands, two mandibular glands and two sublingual glands (the names indicate their positions in the mouth). They secrete a watery substance called *saliva* which contains the digestive enzyme *ptyalin* (amylase) which in involved in the first stage of the digestion of carbohydrates.

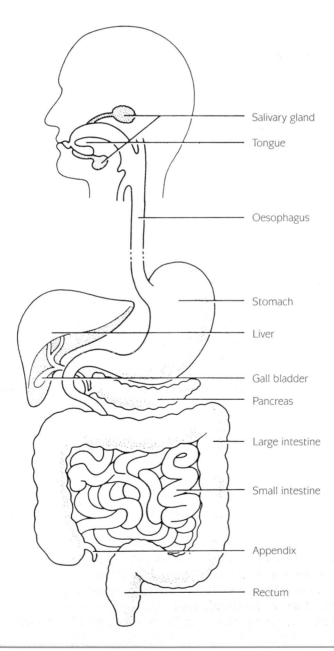

Salivary gland

Tongue

Oesophagus

Stomach

Liver

Gall bladder

Pancreas

Large intestine

Small intestine

Appendix

Rectum

The digestive system

Pharynx

At the back of the mouth lies the pharynx which is about 13 cm long and leads backwards from the mouth. It consists of three areas – the naso pharynx, the oral pharynx and the larygeal pharynx. The oral pharynx is shared by both air and food and the larygeal pharynx merges with the oesophagus. When food is swallowed, the pharynx contracts forcing food downwards into the oesophagus.

Oesophagus

The oesophagus is a muscular tube 25–30 cm long leading from the pharynx to the stomach. It is composed of voluntary and involuntary muscle fibres which work in a wave-like motion called *peristalsis* to propel food into the stomach.

Stomach

The stomach is a muscular sac-like organ placed on the left side of the abdominal cavity beneath the diaphragm. At either end of the stomach are valves, called *sphincters*, which allow or restrict the movement of food into or out of the stomach. The *cardiac sphincter* lies between the oesophagus and the top of the stomach and the *pyloric sphincter* lies between the bottom of the stomach and the duodenum.

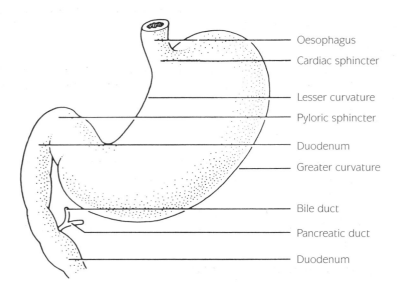

Oesophagus
Cardiac sphincter
Lesser curvature
Pyloric sphincter
Duodenum
Greater curvature
Bile duct
Pancreatic duct
Duodenum

The stomach

The stomach has several distinct layers. The outermost layer is called the peritoneum and its main function is to prevent friction with other organs in the abdominal cavity. The peritoneum is a serous membrane, that is it produces a fluid called serum which acts as a lubricant. Next there is a muscular layer, then a layer which is composed of connective tissue and is rich in blood vessels. Forming the stomach lining is a mucous layer. The layers of the stomach have the ability to expand and contract according to the amount of food consumed. The surface of the inner stomach is convoluted. This provides a greater surface area for the action of secreted acidic gastric juices on the food. Food is held in the stomach until it becomes liquefied and has been partially digested.

Chemical digestion continues in the stomach. Protein digestion commences; proteins are broken down to *peptones*. Gastric juice contains *hydrochloric acid* and the enzymes *pepsin* and *rennin*. The acid is antiseptic in action and provides the correct medium for the digestive juices to work in. Mechanical digestion is also continued in the stomach. The food is churned with strong muscular movements and leaves the stomach in a series of gushes. Some substances ingested are absorbed directly into the body from the stomach; these include water, alcohol and glucose.

information point

Another important function of the stomach is to produce an anti-anaemic factor which controls the formation of blood cells in the bone marrow.

HEALTH AND BEAUTY THERAPY: A PRACTICAL APPROACH

Small intestine

This part of the digestive tract leads from the stomach to the large intestine and is 6–7.4 metres in length. It has three main sections: the *duodenum*, the *jejunum* and the *ileum*.

The duodenum is the first part of the small intestine and is attached to the back of the abdominal wall by peritoneum. It is approximately 24 cm long and curves like the letter C. Lying within the curve is the pancreas.

The jejunum and ileum form most of the total length of the small intestine and lie to the front of the abdominal cavity. The structure of the small intestine is similar to the stomach externally but internally it is puckered and covered with hair-like projections called *villi*. These have the effect of increasing the surface area of the small intestine. Digestion products are absorbed into the villi.

Within the small intestine, the digestion of protein, carbohydrate and fats takes place. Enzymes from three types of digestive juice – *pancreatic juice* from the pancreas, *bile* from the liver, *succus entericus* from the small intestine – affect this digestion. Peptones from the stomach are broken down to polypeptides and finally to amino-acids; carbohydrates are broken down to simple sugars, e.g. glucose; fats and oils are broken down to fatty acids and glycerol. Fatty acids and glycerol after absorption may be used for energy by muscles in activity, or stored.

Large intestine

The large intestine is the last stage of the alimentary tract and begins at the ileum and ends at the rectum. It is about 1.5 metres in length and is divided into three parts:

- the ascending colon
- the transverse colon
- the descending colon.

The first part of the ascending colon consists of a lined pouch called the *caecum* from which extends the *vermiform appendix*. It contains the *ileo-caecal valve* which allows on-flow, but prevents back-flow, of intestinal contents. The remainder of food undigested, plus roughage and unabsorbed digestive juice, pass from the small intestine into the large intestine in a liquid form. Here the water is reabsorbed and the solid faeces are formed.

Glands of the digestive system

The liver

The liver is the largest gland in the body, weighing between 1 and 2.3 kg. It is situated in the upper part of the abdominal cavity and consists of four lobes. Blood rich in nutrients is supplied to the liver via the *hepatic portal vein* which carries blood from the stomach, spleen, pancreas and the intestines. Arterial blood is supplied to the liver via the *hepatic artery*. The right and left *hepatic ducts* carry bile from the liver to the gall bladder. The main digestive functions of the liver are:

- Production of bile, which together with lipase from the pancreas commences the first stage of fat digestion.
- Synthesis of vitamin A from carotene.
- Storage of vitamins, namely B12, A, D, E, K and iron.

The pancreas

The pancreas is a pale grey gland weighing approximately 60 g. It is situated high on the left side of the abdominal cavity behind the stomach. The pancreas consists of a large number of lobules made up of small alveoli and these secrete pancreatic juice which contains the enzymes *lipase*, *trypsin*, *chymotrypsin* and *amylase*. Lipase converts fats into monoglycerides, diglycerides and fatty acids. Trypsin and chymotrypsin convert peptones (protein) into polypeptides. Amylase converts carbohydrates (starch) into maltose.

> **information point**
>
> The pancreas is both an endocrine and an exocrine gland as it secretes hormones (see p. 353) and also has a digestive function.

The urinary system

The urinary system consists of:

- The kidneys.
- Ureters.
- Bladder.
- Urethra.

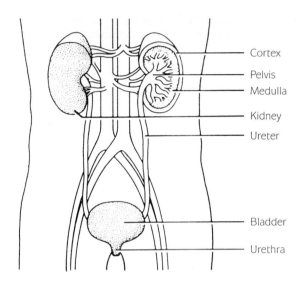

The urinary system

The kidneys

There are two kidneys, each approximately 11 cm in length by 6 cm in width. They lie high on the posterior wall of the abdomen. Each kidney consists of an outer layer called a fibrous capsule, a *cortex*, an inner *medulla* which contains *renal pyramids* and the pelvis. Each kidney receives blood at very high pressure through a renal artery. Once inside the kidney, the artery divides into smaller capillaries which carry the blood to tiny cup-shaped structures called *glomerular capsules*.

The glomerular capsules are the beginning of lengths of narrow tubes, approximately 3 cm long called *nephrons*. Urine is produced in the nephrons.

Formation of urine

The capillary inside each glomerular capsule divides into a tiny bundle of intertwined blood vessels called a *glomerulus*. Blood pressure is so high in this area that liquid is forced out through the capillary walls into the space inside the glomerular capsule. This liquid is known as *glomerular filtrate*. It contains urea to be excreted together with many useful substances (e.g. glucose, amino acids, mineral salts, vitamins and large amounts of water) which the body cannot afford to lose. These substances are reabsorbed in the nephron.

Reabsorption

Glomerular filtrate flows out of the glomerular capsules into the tubular part of each nephron; it is here that reabsorption occurs. The walls of the nephron extract useful substances from the filtrate and these pass into blood flowing through capillaries surrounding the nephron. What is left now is urine, which consists of waste products such as urea, uric acid and small amounts of mineral salts.

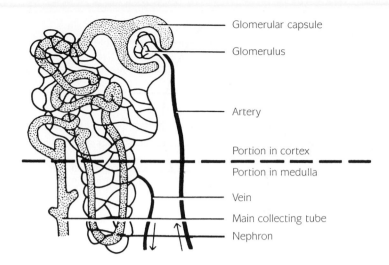

Glomerular capsule

Glomerulus

Artery

Portion in cortex

Portion in medulla

Vein

Main collecting tube

Nephron

The internal structure of a kidney

The ureters, bladder and urethra

A thin tube called a *ureter* which is attached to the concave side of each kidney conveys the urine to a single large bag called the *bladder*. The bladder has only one exit, a tube called the *urethra*, which leads to the body's surface. The bladder end of the urethra is closed by means of a sphincter. Urine drains continuously out of the kidneys into the ureters, where it is forced downwards into the bladder by wave-like contractions. The bladder stretches and expands as it fills with urine. When the bladder is full, the stretching stimulates sensory nerve endings in its walls which convey nerve impulses to the brain letting you know when your bladder must be emptied. The sphincter muscles around the urethra are then voluntarily relaxed allowing urine to drain from the bladder through the urethra and out of the body.

SELF-CHECKS

1   Explain briefly how urine is produced.

2   Describe the appearance of a kidney.

Anatomy of the female breast

The breasts are the accessory glands of the female reproductive system and are composed of fatty, fibrous and glandular tissues. Breasts mature in the female at puberty under the influence of the female hormones oestrogen and progesterone.

The breasts are structured for breast feeding with each consisting of about 15–20 lobes of glandular tissue. These are formed from lobules and are connected by areolar tissue, blood vessels and ducts. Each lobule is made up from tiny little sacs called alveoli which collectively form lactiferous ducts. These converge towards the nipple (or areolar) where they form a lactiferous sinus whose function is to act as a reservoir for milk in the event of lactation.

Fatty tissue covers the entire surface of the breast whilst fibrous tissue, in conjunction with the pectoral muscle group lying directly underneath on the chest wall, provides support for the breast.

information point

Suspensory ligaments in the form of fibrous tissue give the breasts their firm contour. The firm contour decreases as we age. It is therefore extremely important to wear a good, properly fitted, supporting bra at all times.

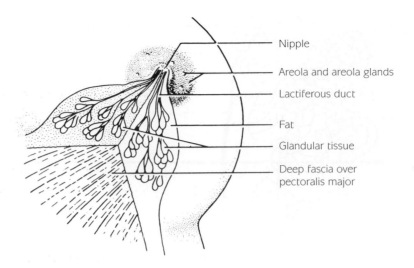

Section through the breast

SELF-CHECKS

1   What is the main function of the female breast?

2   Explain the importance of the pectoralis muscle group.

Anatomy relevant to massage

The bones

When carrying out a facial massage you will feel below your hands the underlying bones. Bone is the hardest structure in the body: it protects the underlying structures, gives shape to the body, and provides an attachment point for our muscles, thereby allowing movement. Bones have different shapes, according to their function. Some have surfaces so that one can move against another. The point where two or more bones meet is known as a joint.

Bones of the head

The bones that form the head are collectively known as the skull. The skull can be divided into two parts, the face and the cranium, which together are made up of 22 bones:

- The 14 facial bones form the face.
- The 8 cranial bones form the rest of the head.

As well as forming our facial features, the facial bones support other structures such as the eyes and the teeth. Some of these bones, such as the nasal bone, are made from cartilage, a softer tissue than bone.

The cranium surrounds and protects the brain. The bones are thin and slightly curved, and are held together by connective tissue. After childhood, the joints become immovable, and are called *sutures*.

The arm

The arm is made up of three bones. The upper arm bone is the *humerus*. This bone is connected at the top to the shoulder by a ball and socket joint. The lower end of the humerus is connected to the two lower arm bones – *ulna* and *radius* at the elbow – a hinge joint.

Bone	Number	Location	Function
Facial bones			
Nasal	2	The nose	Form the bridge of the nose
Vomer	1	The nose	Forms the dividing bony wall of the nose
Palatine	2	The nose	Form the floor and wall of the nose and the roof of the mouth
Turbinate	2	The nose	Form the outer walls of the nose
Lacrimal	2	The eye sockets	Form the inner walls of the eye sockets; contain a small groove for the tear duct
Malar (zygomatic)	2	The cheek	Form the cheekbones
Maxillae	2	The upper jaw	Fused together, to form the upper jaw, which holds the upper teeth
Mandible	1	The lower jaw	The largest and strongest of the facial bones; holds the lower teeth
Cranial bones			
Occipital	1	The lower back of the cranium	Contains a large hole called the foramen magnum: through this pass the spinal cord, the nerves and blood vessels
Parietal	2	The sides of the cranium	Fused together to form the sides and top of the head (the 'crown')
Frontal	1	The forehead	Forms the forehead and the upper walls of the eye sockets
Temporal	2	The sides of the head	Provides two muscle attachment points: the mastoid process and the zygomatic process
Ethmoid	1	Between the eye sockets	Forms part of the nasal cavities
Sphenoid	1	The base of the cranium the back of eye sockets	A bat-shaped bone which joins together all the bones of the cranium
Bones of the neck and arms			
Cervical	7	The neck vertebra	These vertebrae form the top of the spinal column: the atlas is the first vertebra, which supports the skull; the axis is the second vertebra, which allows rotation of the head
Hyoid	1	A U-shaped bone at the front of the neck	Supports the tongue
Clavicle	2	Slender long bones at the base of the shoulder	Commonly called the collar bone: these form a joint with the sternum and the scapula bones, allowing movement at neck
Scapula	2	Triangular bones in the upper back	Commonly called the shoulder blade: scapulae provide attachment for muscles which move the arm. The shoulder girdle, which allows movement at the shoulder, is composed of the clavicles and the scapulae
Humerus	2	The upper bones of the arms	Form ball-and-socket joints with the scapulae: these joints arms allow movement in any direction

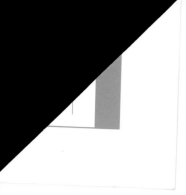

The wrist and the hand

The wrist is connected to the ulna and radius. These bones allow the forearm and hand to rotate. The carpals are a group of eight bones that make up the wrist, they are located between the ulna and radius bones of the arm and the metacarpals. This area is known as the *carpus*. The following bones make up the group of bones in this area:

- Hamate
- Capitate
- Multangular (trapezoid)
- Greater Multangular (trapezoid)
- Navicular (scaphoid)
- Lunate
- Triquetrum
- Pisiform.

The palm contains five bones called metacarpals, four of the fingers have three phalanges, and the thumb has only two. Flexible ligaments connect all these bones.

- *Metacarpals* – bones between the wrist and the fingers.
- *Phalanges* – bones of the fingers.

The leg

The leg is constructed much like the arm and contains the strongest bones and muscles of the body. The upper bone is called the *femur*. It joins the hip at the top by a ball joint and at the bottom it is connected to the larger of the two lower leg bones, the *tibia* (shin) at the knee joint. The other bone of the lower leg, the *fibula*, connects to the tibia just below the knee.

The knee

The knee joint is the most complex joint in the human body. Unlike the elbow, it is more than a simple hinge joint. A series of outer ligaments and internal crossing ligaments provided the structural strength to allow weight bearing at the same time as complex rotational and bending movements. The *patella*, or kneecap, protects the interior parts of the knee joint.

The ankle

The ankle joint is formed at a hinge joint between the lower ends of the tibia and fibula, and with a bone in the upper foot called the *talus*. Below the talus is the heel bone, or *calcaneous*, which actually carries most of the body's weight. The talus, calcaneous and the other bones of the upper foot are called *tarsals*.

The *tarsals* are made up of seven bones which form the compact arrangement of the ankle, or *tarsus*, and the heel. These tarsal bones include the navicular, the three cuneiform, the cuboid, the talus, and the calcaneous (which also forms the heel) bones. These tarsal bones are arranged generally in two rows, the proximal (nearer the body) and distal (nearer the toes). The distal tarsals articulate with the five metatarsals.

The foot

The foot is constructed much like the hand, however it is much stronger to bear the weight and impact of the body. The bones and joints of the foot are held closely together by strong tendons and ligament. The seven bones that make up the ankle are called the *tarsus structure*. These include the heel bone and bones that make up the upper portion of the foot arch.

Five *metatarsals* are the longest bones in the foot and connect the toes to the ankle. These bones make up the remainder of the arch structure. The phalanges or toe bones are similar to those of the fingers. There are fourteen bones, three on four of the toes and two on the large toe. Prolonged or persistent use of improperly sized footwear can cause deformities of the foot structure.

The muscles

Muscles are responsible for the movement of body parts. Each is made up of a bundle of elastic fibres bound together in a sheath, the fascia. Movement occurs when these fibres contract. Most muscles are usually anchored by strong tendons to the bones. The point of attachment is known as the muscle's origin. The muscle is likewise joined to a second bone: this attachment in this case is called the muscle's insertion. It is this second bone that is moved: the muscle contracts, pulling the two bones towards each other. A different muscle, on the other side of the bone, has the contrary effect. Not all muscles are connected to the bones, some insert into adjacent muscles, or into the skin itself.

Facial muscles

Many of the muscles located in the face are very small and are attached to ('inserted into') another small muscle or the facial skin. When the muscles contract, they pull the facial skin in a particular way: it is this that creates the facial expression. With age, the facial expressions that we make every day produce lines on the skin – frown lines. The amount of tension, or tone, also decreases with age. When performing facial massage, the aim is to improve the general tone of the facial muscles.

MUSCLES OF FACIAL EXPRESSION

Muscle	Expression	Location	Action
Frontalis	Surprise	The forehead	Raises the eyebrows
Corrugator	Frown	Between the eyebrows	Draws the eyebrows together
Orbicularis occuli	Winking	Surrounds the eyes	Closes the eyelid
Risorius	Smiling	Extends diagonally, from the corners of the mouth	Draws mouth corners outwards
Buccinator	Blowing	Inside the cheeks	Compresses the cheeks
Zygomaticus	Smiling, laughing	Extends diagonally from corners of the mouth	Lifts the mouth's corners upwards and outwards
Orbicularis oris	Pout, kiss, doubt	Surrounds the mouth	Purses the lip, closes the mouth
Triangularis	Sadness	The corner of the lower lip extends over the chin	Draws down the mouth's corner
Mentalis	Doubt	Chin	Raises the lower lip, causing the chin to wrinkle
Depressor labii	Sulking	The lower lip extends over the chin	Draws down the mouth's corners
Platysma	Fear, horror	The sides of the neck and chin	Draws the mouth's corners downwards and backwards
Labii superioris	Smiling, laughing	The upper lip extends towards the eye	Draws the mouth's corners to lift upper lip

The muscles responsible for the movement of the lower jawbone (the mandible) when chewing are called the muscles of mastication.

MUSCLES OF MASTICATION

Muscle	Location	Action
Masseter	The cheek area: extends from the zygomatic bone to the mandible	Clenches the teeth; closes and raises the lower jaw
Temporalis	Extends from the temple region at the side of the head to the mandible	Raises the jaw and draws it backwards, as in chewing

MUSCLES THAT MOVE THE HEAD

Muscle	Location	Action
Sternocleidomastoid	Runs from the sternum to the clavical bone and the temporal bone	Flexes the neck; rotates and bows the head
Trapezius	A large triangular muscle, covering the back of the neck and the upper back	Draws the head backwards and allows movement at the shoulder

Upper arm

All the muscles on the upper arm are superficial to some degree; the entire arm is covered by a fascia which smoothes muscles into deep segments that attach to the bone. The fascia divides the flexors from the extensors and impacts the surface form only in a couple of places. Flexors are on the front of the arm (supine position) and extensors are on the back. For the entire arm the origins are above, the insertions below.

Descriptions of form and function are based on the arm in supination.

Coracobrachialis – smallest muscle
- Origin: coracoid process.
- Insertion: approximately halfway down the medial side of the humerus.
- Function: helps raise the arm forward; helps pull arm to the side (adducts it) and to turn the arm inward.
- Form: mostly covered by other muscles when arm at the side – becomes evident when the arm is raised ('crucifixion muscle').

Brachialis anticus
- Origin: right below insertion of coracobrachialis – covers entire lower half of upper arm and front of arm.
- Insertion: into coronoid process of ulna.
- Function: flexor – in contraction pulls ulna towards humerous.
- Form: does not quite cover the epicondyles – responsible for outline on lower outside of the upper arm.

Biceps – two heads: long and short
- Long head origin: above glenoid fossa of scapula.
- Long head insertion: tendon passes over head of humerus down through bicipital groove and becomes part of the muscle.

- Short head origin: coracoid process.
- Short head insertion: joins main muscle by single tendon to radial tuberosity.
- Function of biceps:
  Flexor. Flexes elbow: since it has its origin on the scapula it can also function as a flexor of the shoulder; it aids in supination. When fully flexed as in supination the biceps are fullest. The flexor is pulled down when the bones rotate in pronation and is in an elongated form. The flexor forms the entire front profile of upper arm. It creates the entire anterior thickness of arm.

Triceps

The triceps is a large muscle that is located in the back of the upper. The main movement of the arm is controlled by the triceps. The triceps have three heads and one point of insertion.

Lateral and medial heads

- Origin: on humerus:
  Lateral is located just below head of humerus on the outside.
  Medial is located just below head of humerus on inside.
- Insertion: into common tendon with a broad flat strap attached to olecranon process: this tendon is the characteristic flattened area on the back of the upper arm above the elbow.

Long head

- Origin: on scapula right beneath glenoid fossa: thicker than medial head and gives characteristic bulge high on the arm.
- Insertion: olecranon process.
- Function: long head adducts the arm, draws it backward; the three heads together extend forearm. The muscles of the back of the arm create most of the outline of the front of the arm just as the muscles of the back create the outline of the front of the torso.

Anconeus extensor of the elbow (forearm)

- Origin: back of lateral epicondyle of humerus.
- Insertion: olecranon process and partly on ulnar ridge.
- Form: It helps to create the characteristic V shape on back of elbow.

Muscles of the forearm

The muscles of the forearm are numerous and complex they operate not only supination and pronation but also create flexion and extension of wrists and fingers. Flexors of the fingers are deep muscles. Flexors and extensors of wrist are more superficial.

Two major groups designated according to function and position

Anatomically the division of hand and arm is based on the palm forward position when the arm is supinated.

- **Interior-anterior/flexor-pronator group**. These all arise from the inner or medial epicondyle of the humerus. Four muscles in the anterior-interior group are responsible for flexing the wrist/hand. One of the muscles in the group crosses from the inner epicondyle to the radius; when it contracts it pronates the arm (the *pronator teres*). These four muscles create the interior-anterior-flexor-pronator group which are thick above and thin below.
- **External-posterior/extensor-supinator group**. They start in the back of the arm at the external epicondyle of the humerus and for the most part pass over the wrist to the fingers and the tendons on the back of the hand.

  These muscles extend the hand (extensors).

  One of these muscles starts on the lateral epicondylar ridge of the humerus and inserts on the radius when flexed the arm is fully supinated (the *brachioradialis*).

Flexor-pronator group of forearm

Flexor muscles have short bodies with tendons going the rest of the way.

Pronatorteres
- Origin: inner epicondyle of humerus.
- Insertion: halfway down radius on the lateral side.
- Function: pronates and flexes forearm.

Flexor carpi radialis
- Origin: inner epicondyle of humerus.
- Insertion: base of metacarpal of first and second finger.
- Function: pronates arm; flexes and abducts hand.

Palmaris longus
- Origin: inner epicondyle of humerus.
- Insertion: tendon spreads out into fascia of palm (palmar aponeurosis).
- Function: pronates forearm, flexes hand.

Flexor carpi ulnaris

The largest muscle of the group.

- Origin: inner epicondyle of humerus.
- Insertion: wraps around to back of the arm and follows ulnar crest down to the carpal mass on the little finger side.
- Function: flexes and adducts hand.

Extensor-supinator group of the forearm – extensors longer, thinner

Extensor carpi ulnaris
- Origin: lateral epicondyle, passes over the anconeous slightly.
- Insertion: base of metacarpal 5 (little finger).
- Function: adducts hand, extends it somewhat.

Extensor digitorium (communis)
- Origin: lateral epicondyle.
- Insertion: phalanges of fingers (dorsal surface).
- Function: extends hand and fingers, spreads fingers apart.

Extensor carpi radialis brevis
- Origin: lateral epicondyle of humerus.
- Insertion: base of metacarpal of middle finger.
- Function: extends and abducts hand.

The next two muscles create a strong visual and physical link between the upper and lower arm; both originate on the condyloid ridge of the humerus.

Extensor carpi radialis longus
- Origin: condyloid ridge of humerus.
- Insertion: base of the metacarpal of the index (second) finger.
- Function: flexes forearm; supinates forearm in extension; pronates arm in flexion; abducts and extends the hand.
- Form: along with the brachioradialis, creates a visual link between the upper arm and the forearm.

Brachioradialis (supinator longus)
- Origin: lateral epicondylar ridge of humerus, between triceps and brachialis.
- Insertion: styloid process of the radius.
- Function: flexes forearm; supinates forearm in extension; pronates it in flexion.
- Form: along with the extensor carpi radialis longus creates a visual link between the upper arm and the forearm.

The hand

There are two groups of interosseus muscles between the metacarpals and the outside of the little finger; one set is on the dorsal side, one on the palmar side. The biggest muscles are between the metacarpal of the thumb and finger; these are triangular in shape and they bulge when the thumb is adducted. The other group is on the little finger side and they partly account for the padding in that location. They do not cover the carpal mass but rather leave the carpal mass subcutaneous.

There are no muscles on the back of the hand (only tendons) – on the palm side there is padding and muscle.

The extensors of the thumb

These continue the spiral effect of the posterior forearm.

- Origin: about halfway up the radius and the ulna.
- Insertion: base of the thumb.
- Function: extend and abduct thumb.
- Form: some softening effect on harsh line of the radius (two muscles): one muscle has the tendon which creates a depression when the thumb is flexed.

Thenar eminence

The largest of the two.

- Origin: carpals of the thumb and metacarpal 3 (covers about half of the palm).
- Insertion: base of the first phalanx of the thumb.
- Function: pulls thumb in across palm.
- Form: very rounded on inside of palm.

Hypothenar eminence

Located on little finger side, this muscle is longer and flatter; it rises from a little higher on the carpal mass than the thenar eminence; blends with the interosseus muscle on the little finger to create padding on the medial edge of the hand.

The webbing between the fingers, on the palm side, extends about halfway down the first phalanx. Hence fingers look longer when viewed on the dorsal side of hand.

The blood supply

A healthy muscle is activated by a nerve supply, which effects movement; the necessary oxygen and nutrients are brought by the blood. Blood transports various substances around the body:

- It carries oxygen from our lungs, and nutrients from our digested food to supply energy – these allow the cells to develop and divide, and the muscles to function.
- It carries waste products and carbon dioxide away for elimination from the body.
- It carries various cells and substances which allow the body to prevent or fight disease.

The main constituents of blood

- Plasma. A straw-coloured liquid, mainly water, with foods and carbon dioxide.
- Red blood cells (erythrocytes). These cells appear red because they contain haemoglobin; it is this that carries oxygen from the lungs to the body cells.
- White blood cells (leucocytes). There are several types of white blood cells; their main role is to protect the body, destroying foreign bodies and dead cells, and carrying away the debris (a process known as *phagocytosis*).
- Plateletes (thrombocytes). When blood is exposed to air, as happens when the skin is injured, these cells bind together to form a clot.
- Other chemicals. Hormones also are transported in the blood.

Functions of blood

The blood is a liquid tissue that has three major functions:

- Transportation – Blood transports materials to and from all the cells of the body. Wastes produced by the cells are carried away in the blood to organs which remove the wastes.

- Regulation – Blood acts as a regulator. Blood can absorb heat from warm areas of the body and releases the heat in cooler areas. The blood usually maintains a constant pH and water balance.
- Protection – Blood protects the body. It holds specialised cells and chemicals that defend the body against diseases. Blood has the ability to clot, preventing the body from losing large amounts of blood due to an injury.

The circulation

Blood helps to maintain the body temperature at 36.8 °C; varying blood flow near to the skin surface increases or decreases heat loss. The circulation of blood is under the control of the heart, a muscular organ that pumps the blood around the body. The pumping of the blood under pressure through the carotid arteries can be felt as a pulse the neck. Press gently on the neck just inside the position of the sternomastoid muscle. Blood leaving the heart is carried in large, elastic tubes called arteries. The blood to the head arrives via the carotid arteries, which are connected via other main arteries to the heart. There are two main carotid arteries, one on each side of the neck. These arteries divide into smaller branches, the internal carotid and the external carotid. The internal carotid artery passes the temporal bone and enters the head, taking blood to the brain. The external carotid artery stays outside the skull, and divides into branches:

- The occipital branch supplies the back of the head and the scalp.
- The temporal branch supplies the sides of the face, the head, the scalp and the skin.
- The facial branch supplies the muscles and tissues of the face.

Pulmonary circulation

The pulmonary circulation circuit describes the process whereby oxygen and carbon dioxide are delivered to and from the lungs. Oxygen-poor blood travels to the right atrium via the inferior and superior vena cavae, then to the right ventricle. The right ventricle subsequently pumps the blood into the pulmonary artery, which branches to the right and left lungs. The pulmonary arteries subdivide until reaching the arteriole, then capillary levels. After gas exchange, the capillaries recombine to form venules and veins. Ultimately two right and two left pulmonary veins carry oxygen-rich blood to the heart for distribution, via the aorta/systemic circuit, to the rest of the body.

Capillaries

The strength of capillary walls can be damaged, for example by a blow to the tissues. These arteries also divide repeatedly, successive vessels becoming smaller and smaller until they form tiny blood capillaries. These vessels are just one cell thick, allowing substances carried in the blood to pass through them into the tissue fluid that bathes and nourishes the cells of the various body tissues. The blood capillaries begin to join up again, forming first small vessels called venules, and then larger vessels called veins. These return the blood to the heart. Veins are less elastic than arteries, and are closer to the skin's surface. Along their course are valves which prevent the backflow of blood.

The main veins are the external and internal jugular veins. The internal jugular vein and its main branch, the facial vein, carry blood from the face and head. The external jugular vein carries blood from the scalp and has two branches: the occipital branch and the temporal branch. The jugular veins join to enter the subclavian vein, which lies above the clavicle.

Blood returns to the heart, which pumps it to the lungs, where the red blood cells take on fresh oxygen, and where carbon dioxide is expelled from the blood. The blood returns to the heart, and begins its next journey round the body.

Blood supply to the head and neck

Most arteries in the anterior cervical triangle arise from the common carotid artery or one of the branches of the external carotid artery, for blood supply to the brain.

Most veins in the anterior cervical triangle are tributaries of the large internal jugular vein, for the venous sinuses of the dura mater.

The common carotid arteries
- The right common carotid artery begins at the bifurcation of the brachiocephalic trunk, posterior to the right sternoclavicular joint.
- The left common carotid artery arises from the arch of the aorta and ascends into the neck, posterior to the left sternoclavicular joint.
- Each common carotid artery ascends into the neck within the carotid sheath to the level of the superior border of the thyroid cartilage.
- Here it terminates by dividing into the internal and external carotid arteries.

The internal carotid artery
- This is the direct continuation of the common carotid artery and it has no branches in the neck.
- It supplies structures inside the skull.
- The internal carotid arteries are two of the four main arteries that supply blood to the brain.
- Each artery arises from the common carotid at the level of the superior border of the thyroid cartilage.
- A plexus of sympathetic fibres accompany it.

The external carotid arteries
- This vessel begins at the bifurcation of the common carotid, at the level of the superior border of the thyroid cartilage.
- It supplies structures external to the skull.
- It terminates by dividing into two branches, the maxillary and superficial temporal arteries.
- The stems of most of the six branches of the external carotid artery are in the carotid triangle.

The superior thyroid artery
- This is the most inferior of the three anterior branches of the external carotid.
- It arises close to the origin of the vessel, just inferior to the greater horn of the hyoid.

The lingual artery
- This arises from the external carotid artery as it lies on the middle constrictor muscle of the pharynx.
- At the anterior border of this muscle, it turns superiorly and ends by becoming the deep lingual artery.

The facial artery
- This arises from the carotid artery either in common with the lingual artery, or immediately superior to it.
- In the neck the facial artery gives off its important tonsillar branch and branches to the palate and submandibular gland.
- It loops anteriorly and enters a deep groove in the submandibular gland.
- The facial artery hooks around the inferior border of the mandible and enters the face. Here the pulsation of this artery can be felt (anterior to the masseter muscle).

The ascending pharyngeal artery
- This is the first or second branch of the external carotid artery.
- This small vessel ascends on the pharynx, deep to the internal carotid artery.

The occipital artery
- This arises from the posterior surface of the external carotid near the level of the facial artery.

- It ends in the posterior part of the scalp.
- During its course, it is superficial to the internal carotid artery and three cranial nerves.

The posterior auricular artery
This is a small posterior branch of the external carotid artery.

The internal jugular vein
- This is usually the largest vein in the neck.
- The internal jugular vein drains blood from the brain and superficial parts of the face and neck.
- Its course corresponds to a line drawn from a point immediately inferior to the external acoustic meatus to the medial end of the clavicle.
- This large vein commences at the jugular foramen in the posterior cranial fossa, as the direct continuation of the sigmoid sinus.
- Near its termination is the inferior bulb of the jugular vein which contains a bicuspid valve similar to that of the subclavian vein.
- The deep cervical lymph nodes lie along the course of the internal jugular vein, mostly lateral and posterior.

Tributaries of the internal jugular vein
This large vein is joined at its origin by the inferior petrosal sinus, the facial, lingual, pharyngeal, superior and middle thyroid veins, and often the occipital vein.

The nerve supply
All muscles are made to work by electrical stimulation via the nerves. These, together with the brain and the spinal cord, form the nervous system. Nerve cells do not reproduce; when damaged, only a limited repair occurs.

Kinds of nerve
There are two types of nerve: sensory nerves and motor nerves. Both are composed of white fibres enclosed in a sheath.

- Sensory nerves. These receive information and relay it to the brain. They are found near to the skin's surface and respond to touch, pressure, temperature and pain.
- Motor nerves. These are situated in muscle tissue and act on information received from the brain, causing a particular response, typically muscle movement.

Appropriate massage manipulations, though applied to the skin, produce a stimulating or relaxing effect on nerves.

Nerves of the face and neck
These nerves link the brain with the muscles of the head, face and neck. There are 12 pairs of cranial nerves. Those of concern to the beauty therapist when performing a facial massage are as follows:

- The fifth cranial nerve, or trigeminal.
- The seventh cranial nerve, or facial.
- The eleventh cranial nerve, or accessory.

Fifth cranial nerve
This nerve carries messages to the brain from the sensory nerves of the skin, the teeth, the nose and the mouth. It also stimulates the motor nerve to create the chewing action when eating. The fifth cranial nerve has three branches:

- The ophthalmic nerve serves the tear glands, the skin of the forehead, and the upper cheeks.
- The maxillary nerve serves the upper jaw and the mouth.

- The mandibular nerve serves the lower jaw muscle, the teeth and the muscle involved with chewing.

Seventh cranial nerve

This nerve passes through the temporal bone and behind the ear, and then divides. It serves the ear muscle and the muscles of facial expression, the tongue and the palate.

The seventh cranial nerve has five branches:

- The temporal nerve serves the orbicularis occuli and the frontalis muscles.
- The zygomatic nerve serves the eye muscles.
- The buccal nerve serves the upper lip and the sides of the nose.
- The mandibular nerve serves the lower lip and the mentalis muscle of the chin.
- The cervical nerve serves the platysma muscle of the neck.

Eleventh cranial nerve

This nerve serves the sternomastoid and trapezius muscles of the neck.

The lymphatic system

The lymphatic system is closely connected to the blood system, and can be considered as supplementing it. Its primary function is defensive: to remove bacteria and foreign materials, thereby preventing infection. It also drains away excess fluids for elimination from the body.

The lymphatic system consists of the fluid lymph, the lymph vessels, and the lymph nodes (or glands). You may have experienced swelling of the lymph nodes in the neck when you have been ill. Unlike the blood circulation, the lymphatic system has no muscular pump equivalent to the heart. Instead, the lymph moves through the vessels and around the body because of movements such as contractions of large muscles. Facial massage can play an important part in assisting this flow of lymph fluid, thereby encouraging the improved removal of the waste products transported in the lymph.

Lymph

Lymph is a straw-coloured fluid, derived from blood plasma, which has filtered through the walls of the capillaries. The composition of lymph is similar to that of blood, though less oxygen and fewer nutrients are available. In the spaces between the cells where there are no blood capillaries, lymph provides nourishment. It also carries lymphocytes (a type of white blood cell). Lymph travels only in one direction: from body tissues back towards the heart.

The functions of the lymphatic system

The lymphatic system has three primary functions:

- It returns excess interstitial fluid to the blood. Of the fluid that leaves the capillary, about 90% is returned. The 10% that does not return becomes part of the interstitial fluid that surrounds the tissue cells. Small protein molecules may 'leak' through the capillary wall and increase the osmotic pressure of the interstitial fluid. This further inhibits the return of fluid into the capillaries, and fluid tends to accumulate in the tissue spaces. If this continues, blood volume and blood pressure decrease significantly and the volume of tissue fluid increases, which results in oedema (swelling). Lymph capillaries pick up the excess interstitial fluid and proteins and return them to the venous blood. After the fluid enters the lymph capillaries, it is called lymph.
- It absorbs fats and fat-soluble vitamins from the digestive system and transports these substances to the venous circulation. The mucosa that lines the small intestine is covered with fingerlike projections called villi. There are blood capillaries and special lymph capillaries, called lacteals, in the centre of each villus. The blood capillaries absorb most nutrients, but the fats and fat-soluble

vitamins are absorbed by the lacteals. The lymph in the lacteals has a milky appearance due to its high fat content and is called *chyle*.

- It defends against invading micro-organisms and disease. Lymph nodes and other lymphatic organs filter the lymph to remove micro-organisms and other foreign particles. Lymphatic organs contain lymphocytes that destroy invading organisms.

Lymph vessels

Lymph vessels often run very close to veins, forming an extensive network throughout the body. The lymph moves quite slowly and there are valves along the lymph vessels to prevent backflow of the lymph.

The lymph vessels join to form larger lymph vessels, which eventually flow into one or other of two large lymphatic vessels: the thoracic duct (or left lymphatic duct) and the right lymphatic duct. The thoracic duct receives lymph from the left side of the head, neck, chest, abdomen and lower body; the right lymphatic duct receives lymph from the right side of the head and upper body.

These principal lymphatic vessels then empty their contents into a vein at the base of the neck, which in turn empties into the vena cava. The lymph is mixed into the venous blood as it is returned to the heart.

Lymph nodes

Lymph nodes or glands are tiny oval structures that filter the lymph, extracting poisons, pus and bacteria, and thus defending the body against infection by destroying harmful organisms. Lymphocytes, found in the lymph glands, are special cells which produce antibodies which enable us to resist invasion by micro-organisms.

When performing massage, the hands should be used to apply pressure to direct the lymph towards the nearest lymph node: this encourages the speedy removal of waste products. Various groups of lymph nodes drain the lymph of the head and neck.

Lymph nodes of the head

- The buccal group drain the eyelids, the nose and the skin of the face.
- The mandibular group drain the chin, the lips, the nose and the cheeks.
- The mastoid group drain the skin of the ear and the temple area.
- The occipital group drain the back of the scalp and the upper neck.
- The submental group drain the chin and the lower lip.

Lymph nodes of the neck

- The external cervical group drain the neck below the ear.
- The upper deep cervical group drain the back of the head and the neck.
- The lower deep cervical group drain the back area of the scalp and the neck.

Lymph nodes of the chest and arms

- The nodes of the armpit area drain various regions of the arms and chest.

Chapter 13 Elementary science

After working through this chapter you will be able to:

● list the different states of matter

● state the difference between compounds and elements

● outline the differences between mains and battery electricity

● describe the effects of an electric current

● give examples of different electric currents used in therapy treatments.

It is beneficial for the therapist to have an understanding of elementary science, particularly before studying electrical treatments. A whole book could be dedicated to this subject, which many therapists find fascinating and may wish to study at greater depth. There is a variety of books and articles available for further research to assist in performing effective electrical treatment programmes.

Forms of matter

Matter is anything that occupies space and possesses mass. All substances can exist in three different physical states:

● Solid.

● Liquid.

● Gas.

Solids have a definite shape and distinct boundaries, e.g. ice, hair. The particles in a solid are packed closely together and remain in a definite position.

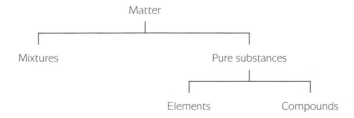

Forms of matter

Liquids have a definite volume and take up the shape of their container. The particles in a liquid are closely packed but have a certain freedom to move around.

Gases take up both the shape and volume of their container. The particles in a gas have large spaces between them and move freely (this is why we can smell perfume vapour from a bottle across a room).

All matter is composed of minute particles. In solids these particles are in definite positions, they vibrate in position but do not move from one part of the solid to another. The state of a substance depends on the energy that the substance contains. The solid state has a minimum energy content. When a solid is heated the internal energy is increased and particles vibrate more vigorously until it melts to form a liquid.

The state of matter is affected by temperature and pressure, e.g. if a solid such as ice is placed in a hot temperature, it heats beyond its melting point and becomes a liquid. Water, when heated beyond its boiling point becomes steam, a gas. This *change of state* from liquid water to gaseous steam is utilised in the salon environment when the therapist uses a steam cabinet.

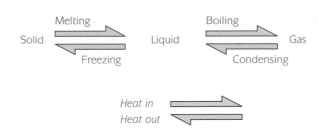

Changing states

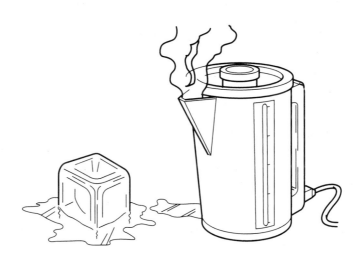

The three states of water: ice, water, steam

Atoms

Matter is made up of small indivisible particles called *atoms*, which cannot be created or destroyed. For a variety of reasons, atoms can be attracted to each other to form *molecules*. A molecule is defined as the smallest part of an element or compound that can exist alone. Under normal conditions, elements which are gases rarely exist as single atoms, the atoms join together in pairs to form molecules, e.g. nitrogen:

Nitrogen atom + Nitrogen atom = Nitrogen molecule

Atomic structure

An atom is a particle of matter with clouds of *electrons* (which can be considered as concentric rings or shells) revolving around a small, dense mass of *protons* and *neutrons*, which form the *nucleus* of the atom.

- Electrons have a negative electrical charge.
- Protons have a positive electrical charge.
- Neutrons have no electrical charge.

In atoms the positive and negative charges are equal, as they contain equal amounts of electrons and protons, therefore making them neutral.

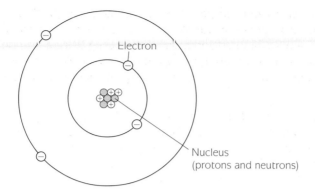

Electrons fill the shells around the nucleus in a systematic manner. The first shell holds two electrons, the second shell holds eight electrons and the third holds 18. Elements are held together by forces called bonds. The ease of making or breaking these bonds is referred to as *chemical reactivity*. The ionic bond is formed by the complete transfer of one or more electrons from one atom to another resulting in the formation of charged particles called *ions*.

An ion is an atom or molecule which has gained or lost electrical charge. The addition of an electron makes the atom or molecule negatively charged, i.e. it has gained the negative charge of one electron, and is known as an *anion*. The atom or molecule losing an electron will become positively charged, i.e. it loses the negative charge of one electron, and is known as a *cation*.

When therapists apply electrical galvanic treatments and products, they need to know the relevant electrical charge of the ion in the product in order to perform an effective treatment. (See Chapter 5.)

Elements and compounds

An element may be defined as a substance which cannot, by any known chemical means, be split into two or more simpler substances. Elements are made up of one type of atom which cannot be broken down any further, e.g. atoms of carbon make an element, atoms of oxygen are also an element. When elements combine chemically together, i.e. *react* with each other, they form a substance. This substance is known as a *compound*, e.g. sodium chloride (table salt) is a compound composed of sodium ions and chlorine ions.

A compound is a pure substance containing two or more elements chemically combined together. Sodium chloride, hydrogen peroxide, keratin, etc. are compounds. Compounds have a fixed composition and their appearance and properties are usually quite different from those of the elements composing them.

When heated, copper nitrate gives off a brown gas and oxygen and leaves a black, solid residue. This indicates that copper nitrate is composed of at least three simple substances. The black solid and the brown gas can be split further. The brown gas (nitrogen dioxide) can be made to yield nitrogen and oxygen. The black solid (copper oxide) can be made to yield copper and oxygen. Copper nitrate is made of copper, nitrogen and oxygen. Copper, oxygen and nitrogen are all elements. There are over a hundred elements, most of which are present in the Earth's crust either in a free state or combined with other elements in compounds.

Mixtures

Mixtures contain two or more substances which may be elements or compounds mechanically combined. The constituents of a mixture do not react chemically with each other. A large number of preparations used on the skin are mixtures, e.g. calamine lotion, mascara and cosmetic creams are mixtures of fatty materials and water. A mixture can be separated into its constituents by physical means.

1   List the three states of matter.

2   What two factors can affect states of matter?

3   Describe the atomic structure.

4   State what is meant by the following:

   a element

   b compound

   c mixture.

Electricity

We use the phenomenon and power of electricity every day for heating, lighting, washing, ironing, cooking, etc. We use it to look after our appearance (shavers, hairdryers, etc.) and for entertainment (television, video, radio, etc.), but how much do we know about it? Electricity can be defined as the movement of electrons from atom to atom. The moving electrons create an electrical charge which can be classed as either *dynamic* or *static*.

information point

- *Dynamic electricity* is created by either chemical reactions or magnetic fields.
- *Static electricity* is created by friction. A common example is the rubbing of hair with a plastic comb or brush. The friction between the comb and the hair can cause electrons to move from the hair to the comb. The comb becomes negatively charged as it gains electrons and the hair becomes positively charged as it loses electrons. As the hair and comb have opposite electrical charges they are attracted to each other making the hair stand out from the head and reach towards the comb.
- *Electric current* is the term used to describe the movement of electrons flowing freely in the same direction through a conductor to an area deficient in electrons.
- *Conductors* allow electrons to move freely through them, e.g. metals.
- *Insulators* prevent the flow of electrons, e.g. plastic, wood, rubber.

Electric circuits

An electric circuit can be defined as the path of an electric current linking the electrical appliance to the electricity supply. To create a circuit two ingredients are required:

- a device capable of supplying electricity, e.g. a battery or a generator (mains)
- a complete path of conducting materials in which electricity can flow.

A circuit is made mostly of metals, but sometimes water containing dissolved acids, alkalis or salts can form part of a circuit.

Electric current

Electric current is the name given to a flow of electricity; it tells us the number of electrons passing a fixed spot in the circuit each second. Electric current is measured in amps (A).

Electrical pressure

This is a measure of the ability of a battery or generator to drive the current around a circuit. Electrical pressure is measured in volts (V).

REMEMBER

- It is important that electrical equipment be kept away from water.
- Moist skin is a better conductor of electricity than dry skin. Ensure that your hands are dry when you use electrical equipment.

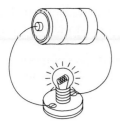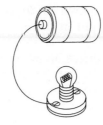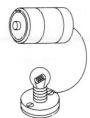

(a) An electrical circuit must be made from a complete path of conducting material

When the switch is open the circuit is *broken*. No current flows and the bulb does not light

When the switch is closed the circuit is *made*. Current flows and the bulb lights.

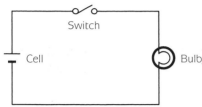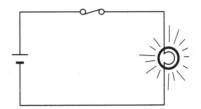

Switch

Cell   Bulb

(b) Switches – 'making' and 'breaking' a circuit

Electric circuits

Electric power

This is a measurement of the power used to run a piece of electrical equipment. Electrical power is measured in watts (W).

Electric cells and batteries

An electrical cell consists of:

- a plate of a reactive metal, e.g. zinc
- a plate made of an unreactive conductor, e.g. graphite, carbon
- a solution or paste, called the electrolyte, containing acid, alkali or salt.

A chemical reaction between the metal plates and the electrolyte produces electricity. A battery consists of several cells joined together.

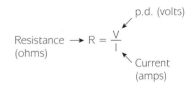

$$\text{Resistance (ohms)} \rightarrow R = \frac{V}{I}$$

p.d. (volts)

Current (amps)

Ohm's law

The differences between mains and battery electricity

- Batteries need replacing or recharging.
- Mains pressure, or voltage, is much higher than most batteries. In the United Kingdom the mains voltage is 240 volts.
- Battery equipment is usually portable.
- Battery circuits conventionally have the current flowing from the positive terminal to the negative terminal all the time. This flow of current is in one

direction only and is known as *direct current* or DC. An example of the application of DC current in therapy treatments is galvanic treatment (see Chapter 5).

- The mains circuit produces an *alternating current* or AC (sometimes referred to as sinusoidal current) by continually reversing the polarity (direction of flow) of the current. An example of the application of AC in therapy treatments is high frequency treatment (see Chapter 5).

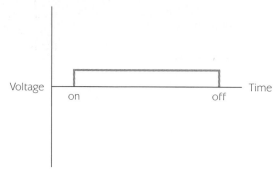

(a) Direct current

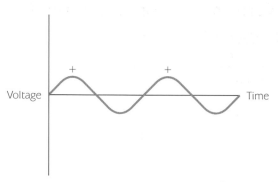

(b) Alternating current

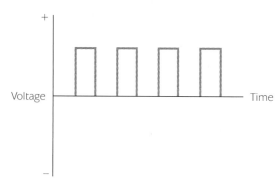

(c) Interrupted direct current (as used in NMES)

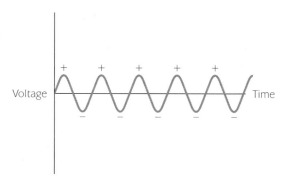

(d) High frequency alternating current

Electrical graphs

Earthing electrical appliances

Electrical appliances are earthed to protect the user from possible shock or electrocution.

Note: Appliances need not be earthed if:

- they have an all plastic body
- they are double insulated.

Fuses

There are two types of fuse:

- Cartridge fuses. These are placed in plugs to protect the cable of the appliance from overheating.
- Wire fuse/circuit breaker. These protect the wiring of the building from overheating.

In order to ensure the correct size of fuse and electrical cable diameter are selected for an electrical appliance, the current (measured in amps) must be calculated using the following equation:

$$\text{Watts} = \text{Amps} \times \text{Volts}$$

or

$$\frac{\text{Watts}}{\text{Volts}} = \text{Amps}$$

If an appliance is rated at 1000 W (1 kW) and the supply is 240 V, what current is drawn by the appliance?

The effects of an electric current

Heating effect

Heat is produced if you use:

- large currents
- thin wires
- resistance wires.

The heating effect can be used to good purpose in therapy, for example in the sauna stove and infrared lamp element.

The chemical effect

The addition of salts, acids and alkalis (*electrolytes*) makes water a good conductor of electricity. An application of this effect in therapy treatments is the use of saline solution on the skin to enable conduction of an electric current, e.g. in neuro-muscular electrical stimulation. If direct current supplies are used, chemical effects occur at the electrodes. An example of the application of this effect in therapy treatments is galvanic iontophoresis, which describes the absorption of ions into the skin.

Magnetic effect

A current passing through a coil of wire (*solenoid*) causes the coil to behave as if it were a magnet, i.e. one end behaves like a north pole, the other end like a south pole. If such a coil has a central iron core, the coil behaves as a much stronger magnet. The arrangement is called an *electromagnet*. This is a magnet which can be switched on or off as it only acts as a magnet when current is flowing in the coil.

An electromagnet supplied with alternating current will keep reversing its polarity. This is the basis on which an AC motor operates. An example of the application of electromagnets in therapy treatments are mechanical massagers.

Electromagnetic waves

Wave motion

A wave motion is a disturbance travelling through a medium. Two sets of waves using the same medium can either reinforce or cancel each other out. This is known as *interference* and it can be used to prove that any type of electromagnetic radiation (i.e. heat, light, ultraviolet) consists of waves.

Wavelength and frequency

The *wavelength* is the distance between corresponding points on successive waves. It can be measured in metres (m), centimetres (cm), millimetres (mm), micrometers (μm) or nanometres (nm).

The *frequency* is the number of waves that pass any fixed point in a second. It is measured in hertz (Hz), kilohertz (kHz) or megahertz (MHz). The higher the frequency, the shorter the wavelength.

- The frequency of the mains electricity supply (AC) is 50 Hz.
- A transformer alters the voltage of an AC electricity supply but not the frequency.
- A capacitor charges with electricity and stores it until it is discharged. (A capacitor can be considered as acting as a spring, collecting power as it is compressed and then slowly releasing it as required.)
- Rectifiers change AC to DC as they allow the current to flow through them in one direction only. If a rectifier is used, then a capacitor is needed in the same circuit to smooth the current out.
- The inductance of a coil will oppose the flow of AC current. This type of coil is known as a choke.
- A potentiometer (often referred to as a 'pot') is used to control the intensity of currents. (The control knob on many beauty therapy appliances, e.g. galvanic or NMES, is a potentiometer.)
- The frequency of a high frequency machine will depend on the values of the capacitor and the coil.

Costing of electricity

Electrical costs are based on the number of *units* used. The scientific name for a unit is a kilowatt-hour. To calculate the number of units the following equation is used:

$$\text{Units} = \frac{\text{Watts} \times \text{Hours}}{1000}$$

To calculate hours we transpose the formula thus:

$$\text{Hours} = \frac{1000 \times \text{Units}}{\text{Watts}}$$

Examples

1 How long will a 750 watt appliance operate for on 1 unit of electricity?

$$\text{Hours} = 1000 \times \frac{\text{Units}}{\text{Watts}}$$

$$= 1000 \times \frac{1}{750}$$

$$= 1\tfrac{1}{3} \text{ hours} = 1 \text{ hour } 20 \text{ minutes}$$

2 Calculate the cost of using a 3000 watt convection heater for 5 hours at a cost of 7.18p per unit.

$$\text{Units used} = \text{Watts} \times \frac{\text{Hours}}{1000}$$

$$= 3000 \times \frac{5}{1000}$$

$$= 15 \text{ units}$$

$$\text{Cost} = \text{Number of units used} \times \text{Cost per unit}$$
$$= 15 \times 7.18$$
$$= 107.7\text{p}$$

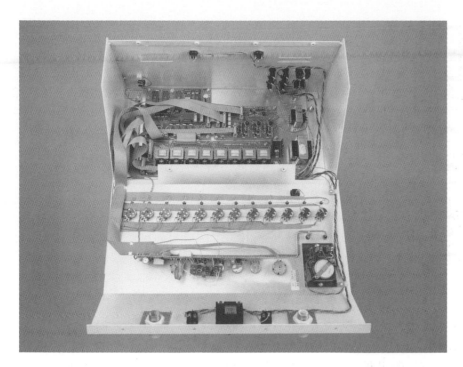

Inside of a dynatone machine

Research and compare the differences in the manufacturing of galvanic and high frequency machines.

SELF-CHECKS

1 Give a definition of electricity.

2 Give an example of:
   a a conductor
   b an insulator.

3 What is:
   a an anion
   b a cation?

4 State the two components required for the flow of electricity.

5 Explain what is meant by the following terms:
   a alternating current
   b direct current
   c volts
   d ohms.

6 What effect do the following have on an electric current:
   a a capacitor
   b a rectifier
   c a transformer?

KEY TERMS

You need to know what these words and phrases mean. Go back through the chapter to find out.

Atoms

Compounds

Earthing

Effects of an electric current

Electric cell

Electric current

Electric pressure

Electrical circuits

Electricity

Electromagnetic waves

Elements

Fuses

Gases

Liquids

Mixtures

Solids

Chapter 14

Elementary diet and exercise

After working through this chapter you will be able to:

- list the different nutrients required for a balanced diet
- identify the different food sources for the different nutrients
- list the reasons why people may wish to gain or lose weight
- list different types of diet
- recognise the different body types
- identify a number of postural problems
- list the components of fitness
- understand the factors that should be considered when offering corrective exercise home-care advice.

As many clients attend health spas and clinics to support them in a weight loss programme, it is important that the therapist has an understanding of basic nutrition. It must be stressed, however, that the role of the therapist is not that of a dietician who undertakes specialist training in this field. Health spas employ medical staff to carry out a client's initial consultation and will refer them to the dietician if a special diet is needed due to medical conditions such as diabetes or if the client wishes to lose weight. Many therapists in salons work in close liaison with doctors, particularly if offering specialised treatments such as alpha hydroxy acids or collagen injections, and some salons extend their range of treatments to include dietary advice under medical supervision. It is strongly recommended that the therapist should only supplement their clients' weight loss programmes with information on healthy eating.

The therapist must refer the client to their doctor if they have any underlying medical problems or a serious weight condition.

Basic nutrition

In order for our body to operate efficiently it requires a well-balanced diet. In general a normal varied diet will provide all the nutrients required for health, though during illness or pregnancy the diet will require additional supplements, e.g. iron is often needed to supplement the diet of expectant mothers. During the latter half of the twentieth century there was a greater tendency for mothers to take up employment and this trend, along with the advancements in convenience foods, has been responsible for a move away from the traditional diet. However, more recently, people have become health conscious and realise that trends in lifestyle may lead to an unbalanced diet. Many people now pay more care and attention to their diet.

Nutrition, in conjunction with digestion, is the process by which the body absorbs foodstuffs and converts them to substances that it requires for life. Food is made up of differing amounts of substances and these can either be used directly by our bodies or converted into other substances our bodies need. The types of food required by a healthy individual are: proteins, carbohydrates, fats, water, fibre, mineral elements and vitamins.

Proteins

Proteins are used by the body for the growth and repair of body tissues. They also act as a secondary source of energy. Proteins are broken down during digestion into amino acids. Proteins are made up of varying amounts of different amino acids and can be subdivided into two categories: first class proteins and second class proteins.

First class proteins

First class proteins are those that contain all the essential amino acids required by the body. Sources of first class proteins are meat, milk, eggs, fish and soya beans.

Second class proteins

Second class proteins are those that do not contain all the essential amino acids. Sources of second class proteins are pulses and nuts.

Carbohydrates

Carbohydrates provide the body with energy. If an excess of carbohydrates is eaten the body converts them and stores them as fat. Sources of carbohydrates are starchy and sugary foods such as cereals, bread, potatoes, sugar, vegetables and fruits.

Carbohydrates are digested in the alimentary canal and are absorbed into the body in the form of monosaccharides, the simplest chemical form in which carbohydrates can exist. Examples of monosaccharides are glucose, fructose and galactose.

Disaccharides consist of two monosaccharide molecules which chemically combine. Sucrose, maltose and lactose are disaccharides.

Polysaccharides are complex molecules consisting of large numbers of monosaccharide molecules chemically combined. Starches, glycogen, cellulose and dextrin are polysaccharides. The body cannot digest all polysaccharides. For example, cellulose, present in vegetables and fruit and some cereals, passes through the alimentary canal almost unchanged.

> **information point**
>
> Amino acids not needed by the body are broken down in the liver. The nitrogeneous part is converted into urea and excreted in urine and the rest, if needed, is used for energy or stored as fat.

> **information point**
>
> - Proteins are made up of carbon, hydrogen, oxygen and nitrogen. Some also contain phosphorous and sulphur.
> - Most sources of first class protein are of animal origin. Vegetarian diets, particularly vegan diets, can be deficient in certain essential amino acids.

> **information point**
>
> - Carbohydrates are made up of carbon, hydrogen and oxygen.
> - Starch forms the larger proportion of the carbohydrates we eat in our food. It must be broken down by the body into simple sugars before it can be used as an energy source.
> - The body breaks down complex sugars and starch into glucose which is the form in which fuel is transported to the different organs of the body.

Fats

The body needs a certain quantity of fat to protect organs, provide insulation, transport fat-soluble vitamins and provide energy. Excess fat in the diet is converted into fatty acids and stored until it is needed. Fats come from either animal or vegetable sources. Examples of foods containing animal fats are meat, cheese, butter, milk and eggs. Vegetable oils and margarine contain vegetable fats.

Cholesterol is a fat-like substance which is produced naturally in the bodies of all animals. A high level of cholesterol in the blood encourages the build up of deposits of fat on the inside walls of arteries, which can lead to heart problems.

Water

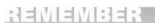

REMEMBER

Approximately two-thirds of body weight is made up of water.

A large proportion of body weight is made up of water. Water is found in the blood and tissue fluids and aids in digestion, maintaining the body temperature and health of cells. It also dilutes waste products and assists in their elimination. It is found throughout the body in varying quantities and is essential to life. The body excretes around two litres of water per day in the form of urine and perspiration. The body rebalances its fluid loss by absorbing water from drinks and food.

The majority of foods we eat contain some water.

Fibre

Fibre is a nutrient that is not digestible but is required by the body to assist in the digestion process, in particular excretion. It provides the diet with bulk, helping to satisfy the appetite and provides a medium on which peristalsis can work, hence aiding the movement of food through the alimentary canal.

Mineral elements

Minerals are needed by the body to maintain health. They are not required in large quantities in the diet.

Calcium

Calcium is needed for the formation and maintenance of healthy teeth and bones and for muscular activity. It can be found in foods such as milk, cheese and eggs.

Iodine

Iodine is essential for the formation of the hormone thyroxine from the thyroid gland. It is only needed in very small quantities and can be found in foods such as watercress, seafood and iodised salt.

Iron

Iron is used by the body to manufacture haemoglobin. Women generally require more iron in their diet than men as they lose blood, and therefore iron, during menstruation. During pregnancy expectant mothers often need to supplement their diet with additional iron to maintain their own health and that of the foetus. Iron can be found in foods such as liver and green vegetables, e.g. spinach.

Magnesium

Magnesium is needed by the body for metabolism and the composition of bones, nerves and muscles. It can be found in foods such as green vegetables, wholegrain cereals and lentils.

Manganese

Manganese is necessary for metabolism and can be found in foods such as kidneys, lentils, almonds, apricots, wheatgerm and watercress.

Phosphorous

Phosphorous is needed for the formation of teeth and bones. It is a constituent of cells and plays a part in the maintenance of body fluid balance and aids in the utilisation of energy from foods. It can be found in foods such as cheese, eggs, meat, fish, yeast, wheatgerm and green vegetables.

Potassium

Potassium is needed to maintain the body's fluid balance and is also involved in the functioning of nerves and muscles. It can be found in the majority of foods, especially milk, cheese, seafood, bananas, spinach, butter and baked potatoes.

Sodium

Sodium is required to maintain the fluid balance of the body. It also plays an important role in the transmission of impulses from the nerves and in muscular contraction. It can be found in the majority of foods, in particular salt.

Sulphur

Sulphur helps with the formation of body tissues and can be found in foods such as eggs, fish, cheese, meat and beans.

information point

- Mineral elements are often called mineral salts.
- Deficiency in iron leads to anaemia.
- Calcium absorption diminishes in females over 50.
- Anti-oxidants are nutrients that help to protect the body from damage caused by preventing and treating disease. The main anti-oxidants are considered to be Vitamins A, C, E and beta-carotene (the precursor of vitamin A found in fruit and vegetables).

Trace elements

Trace elements are found in extremely small quantities within the body and are needed for a variety of body processes such as digestion. Examples of trace elements are copper, cobalt, fluorine and zinc.

Zinc

Zinc is found in foods such as fish and nuts and is important for a healthy skin. It protects and repairs DNA and can be found in high levels in animals and fish. Oysters contain the highest dietary sources of zinc. Zinc is essential for male and female fertility and it must be noted that stress, smoking and alcohol deplete zinc.

information point

Some vegan diets can be deficient in zinc.

Vitamins

Vitamins have no energy value but are essential organic substances required in small quantities for health and certain chemical activities of the body.

They can be categorised into two groups:

- Water-soluble vitamins such as B complex and C.
- Fat-soluble vitamins such as A, D, E and K.

Vitamin A (retinol)

Vitamin A is needed for growth of the majority of body cells and is particularly important for healthy eyesight. Deficiency in vitamin A can lead to poor night vision and dry skin. Good sources of vitamin A are milk, butter, cream, eggs, cheese, carrots, green vegetables and oily fish, e.g. sardines.

information point

The liver can convert carotene, which is found in foods such as carrots and spinach, into vitamin A.

Vitamin B complex

Vitamin B includes a complex of vitamins:

- Vitamin B1 (thiamine) helps the nervous system to function and controls the release of energy from carbohydrates. Examples of food sources are wheatgerm, offal, yeast, eggs and nuts.
- Vitamin B2 (riboflavin) is needed for energy and health of the mouth and skin. It can be found in foods such as eggs, cheese, kidneys and liver. It is resistant to heat but can be destroyed by sunlight.
- Pantothenic acid is essential for the body's nervous system and in the burning of fat for energy. Examples of food containing pantothenic acid are liver, egg yolk and vegetables. It is present in most types of food.
- Vitamin B6 (pyridoxine) helps with many of the body's functions and is obtained from foods such as brewer's yeast, bread, wholegrain cereal, milk, eggs and liver.
- Niacin or nicotinic acid is crucial for the utilisation of energy and healthy skin. It plays a part in both the digestive and nervous systems. It can be found in food such as liver, eggs, cheese, brewer's yeast and bread.
- Folic acid is important for the formation of red blood cells and can be found in foods such as liver, kidneys and fresh green vegetables.
- Vitamin B12 is needed in the body for the production of red blood cells. Examples of food sources are meat and dairy products.
- Biotin is required for healthy skin and hair. It is produced naturally by the body and can be obtained from such food stuffs as liver, yeast, kidneys and egg yolk.

Vitamin C (ascorbic acid)

Vitamin C assists in the formation of connective tissue, the absorption of iron and the development and maintenance of healthy bones. It can be found in foods such as vegetables and citrus fruits, e.g. oranges.

Vitamin D (calciferol)

Vitamin D assists in depositing phosphorous and calcium in the bones and is therefore required for the formation of healthy, strong bones and teeth. Examples of foods with a rich supply of vitamin D are cheese, eggs, margarine, butter and fatty fish. The body can produce vitamin D when exposed to sunlight and is able to store it in the liver.

Vitamin E (tocopherol)

The function of vitamin E is not known, however it is thought that a deficiency prevents growth. It can be found in foods such as peanuts, milk, vegetable oils, eggs, fish, wholemeal bread and cereals. Deep-frying destroys a lot of this vitamin.

Vitamin K

Vitamin K is needed for the clotting mechanism of blood. It can be obtained from green vegetables, fruit and liver.

Vitamin P (rutin)

Vitamin P strengthens capillary walls. A rich source can be found in green buckwheat tea.

ACTIVITY

Compile lists of a child's and an adult's daily food intake and note the different nutrients that will have been absorbed by their bodies.

Metabolism

Metabolism is the process by which the body makes use of the food it takes in and utilises it for energy, growth and general health. The body metabolises basic food elements in two general ways:

- Catabolism is the way in which the body releases energy by breaking down food.
- Anabolism is the way in which the body builds up or utilises cell structures from digested food materials.

Calorific requirements

The body needs a well-balanced diet to meet its individual daily requirements. The calorific requirement of an individual is the amount of energy the body needs to stay warm and do any work required of it. Fats have a higher calorific value than carbohydrates, i.e. they contain more energy per unit weight, and carbohydrates have a higher calorific value than proteins. As people vary in size, age, gender and way of life, each individual will have different nutritional needs. It is therefore impossible to state a general energy requirement to suit everybody. Women generally require less energy than men; manual workers require more energy than sedentary office workers; older people require less energy than younger people.

Basal metabolism

The basal metabolism is the minimum energy output required by the body for vital functioning, e.g. respiration, heart beat, peristalsis, etc. The basal metabolic rate varies according to gender, age, lifestyle and body size. It also tends to decrease with age. If the body absorbs more energy from foods than it needs for basal metabolism and the work it does (e.g. exercise), it will store the excess as fat around the body.

Diets

Social and peer-group pressures regarding the way individuals look can create a great deal of stress in people's lives. One of the major influencing factors in how people feel about themselves often relates to how they truly feel about their body shape and size. It cannot be stated that obese people are more unhappy with their appearance than extremely thin people as feelings are individual and other factors in people's lives often alter their emotions, e.g. the excitement of a new job or home, or a

information point

Different nutrients provide different quantities of calories, e.g. 1 g of fat contains 9 calories, whereas 1 g of carbohydrate contains 4 calories.

information point

- As the body ages the basal metabolic rate will fall by an average of 5% every 10 years.
- Regular exercise increases the metabolic rate as muscle cells burn up more calories than fat cells even when at rest.

A general indicator to assess a client's frame size is the circumference of their wrist:

- 14 cm (5½ inches) = Small
- 15.25 cm (6 inches) = Medium
- 16.5 cm (6½ inches) = Large

loving relationship can all detract from past insecurities and can bring about weight loss or gain! There are a variety of reasons why a person may be over- or underweight, e.g. a lack of, or excessive exercise, poor diet. Some people suffer with weight problems due to medical conditions such as an over- or under-active thyroid gland.

GOOD PRACTICE

For figure assessment, when measuring a client:

- Remember to consider their modesty – only expose the areas you need to measure.
- Do not pull the tape measure tight.
- Always record the measurements accurately.

There are a variety of reasons why people may wish to lose or gain weight including:

- To feel healthy and fit.
- To feel happy with their appearance.
- To restore their figure after childbirth.
- To prevent coronary conditions.

It is a common misconception that it is only women who worry about weight problems. In today's society men take a lot more time and effort over their appearance and although some may not show it they often suffer in the same way as women if they are not happy with the way they look. People may wish to diet to improve their total shape whilst others may feel that they have problems with particular areas such as the abdomen, thighs and hips. For whatever reason a person wishes to lose or gain weight they must be sensible in adjusting their diet to ensure it meets the body's nutritional requirements and suits their lifestyle.

There are many books available on different types of diet and fact sheets available through doctors, hospitals and slimming organisations. The important thing to remember if wishing to lose weight is that the body stores excess energy obtained from fats, carbohydrates and proteins in the form of fat around the body. As a person continually takes in surplus energy requirements, the fat cells will increase in size and thus they will gain more and more weight. Therefore the diet will need to be balanced and they will need to increase their energy output to burn up the excess fat. For those wishing to gain weight it is often quite difficult to increase the intake of foods with a high calorific value and the process of weight gain for many people is a slow and arduous task.

REMEMBER

- Weight loss should be slow and controlled, as often people who lose weight rapidly find it returns fairly quickly.
- Individuals develop different eating habits, e.g. some people like to nibble whilst others like full meals and others need to satisfy a sweet tooth.

Body mass index (BMI) can be calculated by dividing the client's weight (in kilograms) by the square of the client's height (in metres). This can be used as a guide to five BMI groups:

- Underweight: BMI 19.9 and below
- Normal: BMI 20–24.9
- Grade 1 obesity: BMI 25–29.9
- Grade 2 obesity: BMI 30–39.9
- Grade 3 obesity: BMI 40 and above.

REMEMBER

If food intake is reduced drastically the dieter will often feel hungry and tired, whereas a slow reduction allows the stomach time to adjust.

Women

ft in	cm	Small lb	Small kg	Medium lb	Medium kg	Large lb	Large kg
4 10	147	102–111	46–50	109–121	49–55	118–131	54–59
4 11	150	103–113	47–51	111–123	50–56	120–134	55–61
5 0	152	104–115	47–52	113–126	51–57	122–137	56–62
5 1	155	106–118	48–54	115–129	52–59	125–140	57–61
5 2	158	108–121	49–55	118–132	54–60	128–143	58–65
5 3	160	111–124	50–56	121–135	55–61	131–147	59–67
5 4	163	114–127	52–58	124–138	56–63	134–151	61–69
5 5	165	117–130	53–59	127–141	58–64	137–155	62–70
5 6	168	120–133	55–60	130–144	59–65	140–159	63–72
5 7	170	123–136	56–62	133–147	60–67	143–163	65–74
5 8	173	126–139	57–63	136–150	62–68	146–167	66–76
5 9	175	129–142	59–64	139–153	63–69	149–170	68–77
5 10	178	132–145	60–66	142–156	64–71	152–173	69–79
5 11	180	135–148	61–67	145–159	66–72	155–176	70–80
6 0	183	138–151	63–69	148–162	67–74	158–179	72–81

Men

ft in	cm	Small lb	Small kg	Medium lb	Medium kg	Large lb	Large kg
5 2	158	128–134	58–61	131–141	59–64	138–150	63–68
5 3	160	130–136	59–62	133–144	60–65	140–153	61–69
5 4	163	132–138	60–63	135–145	61–66	142–156	64–71
5 5	165	134–140	61–63	137–148	62–67	144–160	65–72
5 6	168	136–142	62–64	139–151	63–69	146–164	66–75
5 7	170	138–145	63–66	142–154	64–70	149–168	68–76
5 8	173	140–148	61–67	145–157	66–71	152–172	69–78
5 9	175	142–151	64–69	148–160	67–72	155–176	70–80
5 10	178	144–154	65–70	151–163	69–74	158–180	72–82
5 11	180	146–157	66–71	154–166	70–75	161–184	73–84
6 0	183	149–160	68–72	157–170	71–77	164–188	75–85
6 1	185	152–164	69–75	160–174	72–79	168–192	76–87
6 2	188	155–168	70–76	164–178	75–81	172–197	78–90
6 3	190	158–172	72–78	167–182	76–83	176–202	80–92
6 4	193	162–176	74–80	171–187	78–85	181–207	82–94

Charts to show an example of accepted weight norms of gender, height and frame size

Types of diet

There are many types of diet available to suit individual requirements. Some of these are outlined below.

Calorie-controlled diet

This type of diet limits the quantity of calories the individual takes in per day, but enables them to select the types of food they eat. It is also a useful diet for those who eat out socially as it allows them to save calories for that special meal without everyone they eat with focusing on the fact that they are on a diet. It can also assist those who have a sweet tooth by enabling them to save calories for a treat.

High protein diet

A high protein diet is suitable for people who want to build muscles. However, a diet high in protein can still produce excess energy requirements as protein is a secondary source of energy. Also, protein type foods often contain saturated fats which can increase the body's cholesterol level.

Low fat diet

A low fat diet will obviously reduce the main energy source from outside the body. Some of the fat which was laid down and stored when the body was consuming an excess to the body's requirements is utilised instead.

Low carbohydrate diet

A low carbohydrate diet means reducing the quantity of sugars and starch in the diet. Some people find this hard to do particularly if they have a sweet tooth. As the body obtains most of its daily energy requirements from carbohydrates, it works by reducing the readily available energy. The body calls on its reserve of energy, the stock-pile of fat!

High fibre diet

A high fibre diet provides a lot of bulk to the diet which generally makes the dieter feel full. High fibre diets also improve bowel conditions such as constipation.

Vegetarian diets

Over the years many people have opted to become vegetarians. There are two types of vegetarian:

- Lacto-vegetarians, who do eat some animal products such as milk, cheese and eggs.
- Vegans, who do not eat any form of animal produce.

Health diets

Health diets are prescribed by doctors or nutritionists for the benefit of their patients' health. Examples of people who require health diets are coronary sufferers and diabetics.

Acid and alkaline diet

A balanced body chemistry is of utmost importance for the maintenance of health and correction of disease. Acidosis, or over-acidity in the body tissues, is one of the basic causes of many diseases, especially the arthritic and rheumatic diseases.

All foods are 'burned' in the body, more commonly known as 'digested', leaving an ash as the result of the 'burning', or the digestion. This food ash can be neutral, acid or alkaline, depending largely on the mineral composition of the foods. Some foods leave an acid residue or ash, some alkaline. The acid ash (*acidosis*) results when there is a depletion of the alkali reserve or the diminution in the reserve supply of fixed bases in the blood and the tissues of the body.

It is vitally important, therefore, that there is a proper ratio between acid and alkaline foods in the diet. The natural ratio in a normal healthy body is approximately 4:1 (four parts alkaline to one part acid), or 80%:20%. When such an ideal ratio is maintained, the body has a strong resistance against disease.

In the healing of disease, when the patient usually has acidosis, the higher the ratio of alkaline elements in the diet, the faster will be the recovery. Alkalis neutralise the acids. Therefore in the treatment of most diseases it is important that the patient's diet includes plenty of alkaline-ash foods to offset the effects of acid-forming foods and leave a safe margin of alkalinity.

A healthy body usually keeps large alkaline reserves which are used to meet the emergency demands if too many acid-producing foods are consumed. But these normal reserves can be depleted. When the alkaline:acid ratio drops to 3:1, health can be seriously affected. Your body can function normally and sustain health only in the presence of adequate alkaline reserves and the proper alkaline:acid ratio in all the body tissues and the blood.

The chart on pp. 394–5 is only a general guide to alkalising and acidifying type foods.

Commercial diet products

There is a large variety of products which can be purchased over the counter in many shops. They include solid food substances, e.g. diet bars, and powders which are mixed with water to produce liquid meals. The main problem with commercial diet products is that people tend to totally replace their diet with them and do not balance their diet nutritionally. Often these products' calorific values are way below the body's daily needs.

Slimming clubs

Over recent years the number of slimming and similar clubs has increased rapidly. Many people gain support and comfort from other dieters.

Alternative weight control

There is a variety of alternative ways in which weight can be controlled:

- Acupuncture. This can prove to be quite a costly method depending how quickly the dieter responds to treatment. However, many people find it helps to suppress their appetite.
- Hypnosis. Depending on an individual's response to hypnotherapy this method may encourage weight loss.
- Cosmetic surgery. This is a fairly drastic and expensive method to remove surplus fat.
- Tablets. There is a variety of slimming tablets that can be purchased over the counter. These are taken a number of hours before eating to suppress the appetite.
- Drugs. Doctors sometimes prescribe drugs to people whose life is threatened by their weight to help suppress their appetite.

Eating problems

There is a variety of different types of eating problems, some of which can prove to be fatal.

Stress-induced eating

Stress affects everyone differently, but it can be noted that weight is either lost or gained according to how it affects an individual's eating patterns. Some people eat more under stress as they often take comfort from eating, whilst others eat a great deal less as they find their appetite reduced. Quite often when the anxieties disappear the normal eating pattern will gradually re-emerge. It is important to note that help in some form should be sought to cope with the problem creating the stress, particularly if rapid weight loss is noted. There are many self-help groups for people suffering with stress depending on the cause, e.g. living with cancer, losing a child. However, it may be just the support of family or friends that is needed to reduce anxiety and bring comfort or a relaxing massage.

Bulimia nervosa

Bulimia nervosa is a disease where sufferers will 'binge' and afterwards make themselves sick. It is sometimes very difficult to realise that a person close to you is suffering with this disease, particularly in the early stages, as they mainly eat in front of people. It is important that medical help is sought as soon as possible.

Anorexia nervosa

Anorexia nervosa is a slimmer's disease where sufferers slowly starve themselves of food. This disease is often brought on by social pressure to be slim. The sufferer starts by dieting, quite often drastically, to lose weight. Once the weight is lost the sufferer still perceives him/herself as 'too fat' and comes to believe that any food he/she eats will increase his/her weight. This can be a life-threatening disease and medical help should be sought as soon as possible.

ALKALISING VEGETABLES

Alfalfa
Barley grass
Beet greens
Beets
Broccoli
Cabbage
Carrot
Cauliflower
Celery
Chard greens
Chlorella
Collard greens
Cucumber
Dandelions
Dulce
Edible flowers
Eggplant
Fermented veggies
Garlic
Green beans
Green peas
Kale
Kohlrabi
Lettuce
Mushrooms
Mustard greens
Nightshade veggies
Onions
Parsnips (high glycemic)
Peas
Peppers
Pumpkin
Radishes
Rutabaga
Sea veggies
Spinach, green
Spirulina
Sprouts
Sweet potatoes
Tomatoes
Watercress
Wheat grass
Wild greens

ALKALISING ORIENTAL VEGETABLES

Daikon
Dandelion root
Kombu
Maitake
Nori
Reishi
Shitake
Umeboshi
Wakame

ALKALISING FRUITS

Apple
Apricot
Avocado
Banana (high glycemic)
Berries
Blackberries
Cantaloupe
Cherries, sour
Coconut, fresh
Currants
Dates, dried
Figs, dried
Grapes
Grapefruit
Honeydew melon
Lemon
Lime
Muskmelons
Nectarine
Orange
Peach
Pear
Pineapple
Raisins
Raspberries
Rhubarb
Strawberries
Tangerine
Tomato
Tropical fruits
Umeboshi plums
Watermelon

ALKALISING PROTEIN

Almonds
Chestnuts
Millet
Tempeh (fermented)
Tofu (fermented)
Whey protein powder

ALKALISING SWEETENERS

Stevia

ALKALISING SPICES AND SEASONINGS

Chilli pepper
Cinnamon
Curry
Ginger
Herbs (all)
Miso
Mustard
Sea salt
Tamari

ALKALISING OTHER

Alkaline antioxidant water
Apple cider vinegar
Bee pollen
Fresh fruit juice
Green juices
Lecithin granules
Mineral water
Molasses, blackstrap
Probiotic cultures
Soured dairy products
Veggie juices

ALKALISING MINERALS

Calcium: pH 12
Cesium: pH 14
Magnesium: pH 9
Potassium: pH 14
Sodium: pH 14

Although it might seem that citrus fruits would have an acidifying effect on the body, the citric acid they contain actually has an alkalinising effect in the system.

ACIDIFYING VEGETABLES

Corn
Lentils
Olives
Winter squash

ACIDIFYING FRUITS

Blueberries
Canned or glazed fruits
Cranberries
Currants
Plums
Prunes

ACIDIFYING GRAINS, GRAIN PRODUCTS

Amaranth
Barley
Bran, oat
Bran, wheat
Bread
Corn
Cornstarch
Crackers, soda
Flour, wheat
Flour, white
Hemp seed flour
Kamut
Macaroni
Noodles
Oatmeal
Oats (rolled)
Quinoa
Rice (all)
Rice cakes
Rye
Spaghetti
Spelt
Wheat germ
Wheat

ACIDIFYING BEANS AND LEGUMES

Almond milk
Black beans
Chick peas
Green peas
Kidney beans
Lentils
Pinto beans
Red beans
Rice milk
Soy beans
Soy milk
White beans

ACIDIFYING DAIRY

Butter
Cheese
Cheese, processed
Ice cream
Ice milk

ACIDIFYING NUTS AND BUTTERS

Cashews
Legumes
Peanut butter
Peanuts
Pecans
Tahini
Walnuts

ACIDIFYING ANIMAL PROTEIN

Bacon
Beef
Carp
Clams
Cod
Corned beef
Fish
Haddock
Lamb
Lobster
Mussels
Organ meats
Oyster
Pike
Pork
Rabbit
Salmon
Sardines
Sausage
Scallops
Shellfish
Shrimp
Tuna
Turkey
Veal
Venison

ACIDIFYING FATS AND OILS

Avocado oil
Butter
Canola oil
Corn oil
Flax oil
Hemp Seed oil
Lard
Olive oil
Safflower oil
Sesame oil
Sunflower oil

ACIDIFYING SWEETENERS

Carob
Corn syrup
Sugar

ACIDIFYING ALCOHOL

Beer
Hard liquor
Spirits
Wine

ACIDIFYING OTHER FOODS

Catsup
Cocoa
Coffee
Mustard
Pepper
Soft drinks
Vinegar

ACIDIFYING DRUGS AND CHEMICALS

Aspirin
Chemicals
Drugs, medicinal
Drugs, psychedelic
Herbicides
Pesticides
Tobacco

ACIDIFYING JUNK FOOD

Beer: pH 2.5
Coca-Cola: pH 2
Coffee: pH 4

Figure and postural analysis

In order to perform an effective body-treatment consultation, the therapist must have an understanding of the figure and postural problems that a client may have.

Body types

Body types are generally categorised into three types: *ectomorph*, *mesomorph* and *endomorph*. However, it should be noted that the majority of people tend to be a combination of these types.

The ectomorph

Ectomorphs tend to be recognised by:

- Narrow shoulders and hips.
- Long bones.
- Not much muscle bulk.
- Low percentage of fat.
- General lack of curves.

The mesomorph

Mesomorphs tend to be recognised by:

- Athletic build.
- Well-developed shoulders.
- Slim, 'boyish' hips.
- Well-toned muscles.
- Low percentage of fat.

The endomorph

Endomorphs tend to be recognised by:

- Rounded shoulders.
- Heavy build.
- Higher percentage of fat to muscle bulk.
- Inclination to be overweight.

REMEMBER

Although the appearance of the body can be altered through diet and exercise, the actual body type remains constant through life.

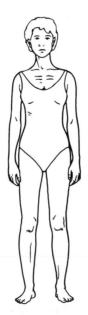

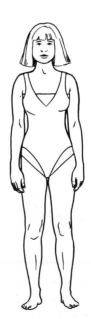

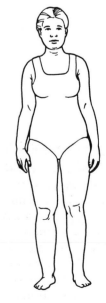

Ectomorph   *Mesomorph*   *Endomorph*

HEALTH AND BEAUTY THERAPY: A PRACTICAL APPROACH

Good posture

It is rare to find perfect posture. This is mainly due to the lifestyles that we lead: company representatives who spend a great deal of their day driving often suffer with tense, round shoulders; busy mothers who carry young children around on their hips or carry heavy shopping bags on one side whilst holding their child's hand for example often suffer with scoliosis.

We naturally take notice of the person who holds him/herself well. A person with good posture often creates a good first impression compared to the person who slouches. Watch men and women when they are attracted by a member of the opposite sex – they automatically react by stretching their bodies upright! Besides enhancing the body's appearance, good posture also maximises the lung capacity which obviously has a beneficial effect on the body.

Recent studies around the world show a relationship of blood types to diet and lifestyle and there is increased attention to the body shape according to the effects on metabolism and main areas of fat storage (and cellulite) of the endocrine glands. Body shapes/types, identified according to the predominant endocrine influence are described as four main types: gonad (G), thyroid (T), super-adrenal (S), and hypophysis/pituitary (H).

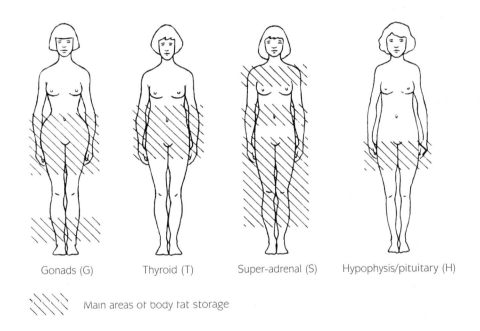

| Gonads (G) | Thyroid (T) | Super-adrenal (S) | Hypophysis/pituitary (H) |

Main areas of body fat storage

Fat storage

Points to look for in good posture

- The head should not abnormally extend or retract beyond the mid line.
- The arms, when relaxed, should lie evenly.
- The spinal column should be straight.
- The distances from the right and left scapulae to the spine should be even.
- The abdomen should appear flat.
- The waist curves should be level.
- The buttocks should not protrude abnormally.
- The legs and knees should be straight and facing forwards.
- The feet should face forwards and should be either together or slightly apart.
- The body weight should be evenly distributed.

If an imaginary, lateral line is drawn down the side of the body it should pass in a straight line through the ear, shoulder, elbow, waist, hip, knee and ankle. Trainee therapists often use a plumbline to assist in postural analysis.

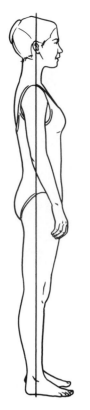

Correct postural stance (lateral view)

SELF-CHECKS

1 State four reasons why clients may wish to gain or lose weight.

2 Explain briefly four different types of diet.

3 Describe three different eating problems.

4 Name the three main body types and for each give a brief description of how you would recognise them.

5 What points would you look for to establish good posture in a client?

Distribution and type of body fat

Many clients are concerned about the distribution of their body fat which influences their shape. The most common problem in women is the rounded, heavy thighs, buttocks and hips commonly referred to as a 'pear-shape'. The therapist needs to assess the client fully and analyse whether the body fat is evenly distributed. They should also note any stretch marks and their cause, e.g. rapid weight loss or pregnancy, and the type of fat, e.g. cellulite, soft or hard. It is also important to build up a picture of the client's lifestyle, eating habits and dietary intake.

Soft fat

Soft fat is the easiest type of fat condition to mobilise. It is not firm and moves easily when touched. It is easy to manipulate and generally responds well to diet and exercise.

Hard fat

This type of fat is difficult to disperse and is firm to touch.

Cellulite

Cellulite is not a term that is recognised by the medical profession but it clearly exists and is not identifiable as any other fat type. Cellulite affects mainly women and causes unsightly dimpling and puckering of the skin. It is normally found in the thigh and buttock areas. It gives a characteristic 'cool feel' to the skin as the blood circulation is diminished in the area. The formation of cellulite is linked to the female hormones, namely oestrogen and progesterone, which play a part in subcutaneous fat distribution. A person does not have to be overweight to be affected by cellulite. As well as being unattractive, cellulite can be painful as it can compress nerve endings. For these reasons, many women resort to the therapist for treatment. There are varying degrees of cellulite, namely hard and soft.

The stages of hard and soft cellulite development are described as Stage 1, 2, 3 or 4 according to the degree of change to the circulation pattern and aesthetic appearance.

Stretch marks

Stretch marks, or *striations* as they are technically known, are caused by thinning and loss of elasticity in the dermis. On fair skins they first appear as red, raised lines becoming purple later on, whereas on darker skins they initially appear as dark raised lines and eventually flatten to form shiny streaks usually between 6 and 12 mm long. They often occur on the hips and thighs during adolescent growth spurts and occur on approximately 75% of all pregnant women, especially on the abdomen and breast areas. It is for the latter reason that most women seek the advice of the therapist and provided they are caught in the early stages treatment can

---

information point

Contact thermography (using special heat active material) is sometimes used to illustrate these stages prior to and during treatment.

HEALTH AND BEAUTY THERAPY: A PRACTICAL APPROACH

be effective. (See Chapter 6.) The two main reasons why stretch marks can occur are due to *endocrine cause* or *mechanical cause*.

It is known that corticosteroid hormones suppress fibre formation in the skin which in turn causes collagen found within the dermis to waste away. Consequently the organisation and texture of tissues is seriously affected and this can lead to a state of well-defined marking of the skin. This is the endocrine cause of stretch marks.

It is thought that sudden and excessive weight increase does not allow the skin time to stretch gently, therefore 'ripping' of the collagen and elastin fibres occurs and leads to the appearance of stretch marks. This is a mechanical cause.

Figure and postural conditions

Deviation in body alignment can lead to a variety of figure and postural conditions, the main ones being outlined below.

Dowager's hump

This is a condition associated with old age. Fatty deposits build up at the back of the neck over a period of time as the client holds his/her head forward of the normal postural alignment.

Protruding abdomen

This often relates to the postural condition of lordosis. However, it may also be the result of fatty deposits around the area or as a result of weak abdominal muscles, a condition often found in postnatal mothers.

Midriff bulge

This is a fairly common condition, often associated with the over 35 age group, where, as a result of the ageing process, fatty deposits accumulate in this area. It tends to be more apparent in women than men.

Flat feet

Flat feet is a condition due to the absence or sinking of the medial longitudinal arch of the foot, caused by weakness of the ligaments and tendons.

Hallux valgus

Hallux valgus is a condition recognised by a deviation of the big toe from the mid-line. It is commonly referred to as a bunion.

Tibial torsion

Commonly referred to as 'knock knees', tibial torsion is generally due to a slack tendon supporting the knee. This results in the knees rotating inwards towards the mid-line.

Winged scapulae

The shoulder blades protrude as they are adducted towards the mid-line. This is a fairly common condition in backpackers who carry heavy weights on their backs.

Round shoulders

Round shoulders are generally a result of the postural condition kyphosis. The pectoral muscles shorten creating a 'barrel chest'. Round shoulders are often associated with tall people who round their shoulders to appear smaller, ladies with large chests who try to conceal the size of their breasts and people suffering with severe asthma.

Kyphosis

Kyphosis may be recognised by the client's rounded shoulders. This shortens the pectoral muscles and curves the thoracic area of the vertebral column outwards. In women it can lead to sagging breasts as the suspensory ligaments and pectoral muscles normally hold the breasts upright. This condition is quite common in young

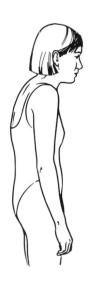

Kyphosis

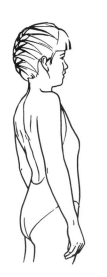

Lordosis

girls with large breasts who through embarrassment curve their shoulders round to conceal themselves. It is also common in office workers, drivers and therapists whose everyday bodily posture involves rounding their shoulders.

Lordosis

Lordosis is recognised by the hollow back created by the inward curvature of the lumbar area of the spinal column. The muscles of the back tighten and this often leads to back ache. In severe cases the pelvis tends to tilt forward, the abdomen and gluteals appear to protrude. The knees will hyper-extend, shortening the hamstrings in order to counter-balance the body weight. This condition is common in small people who often, through trying to appear taller, hollow out their backs. Gymnasts and ballet dancers can also suffer with this condition.

Scoliosis

Scoliosis is recognised by a lateral deviation of the vertebral column. The shortening of muscles on one side of the body can lead to dropped shoulders, uneven waist and scapulae and a tilting pelvis. Busy mothers who tend to hold their children on one side of their waist can suffer with scoliosis. Carrying heavy bags or standing with the body weight to one side can also lead to this condition.

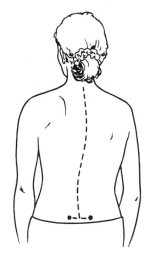

Scoliosis

information point

- Postural spinal curvatures can appear as an S or concave or convex C shape.
- Stiletto heeled shoes distort the natural body alignment and can lead to postural conditions such as lordosis.
- Some spinal curvatures are structural and cannot be altered by the therapist.

Postural assessment of the client

1   The therapist first assesses the client by observing their postural stance from a side view and notes any deviations to the points listed on p. 397.

Note: Whilst training it is common practice to use a weighted string (plumb line) as a guide to check that the body is in alignment or whether the client's head, shoulders, abdomen, pelvis, buttocks or knees are protruding forwards or behind the plumb line.

2   The therapist assesses the anterior then posterior view of the client.

Note: It is common practice whilst training for the trainee to:

- mark the individual vertebrae to see if there is any curvature of the spine
- mark the scapulae and measure the distance between them and the spine
- place their hands on either side of the waist to see if they are even
- place their hands on both shoulders to see if they are even.

3   The therapist observes the client's normal seating position noting the position of the head, shoulders, arms, waist, pelvis, legs, knees and feet.

4   The therapist notes the client's normal walking pattern, observing the gait of movement, the positioning of the skeleton and the distribution of body weight.

REMEMBER

The majority of postural conditions can be assisted by gentle corrective exercise undertaken by the client at home.

ACTIVITY

Perform a postural analysis on three different colleagues. Note your findings and research suitable corrective exercises for postural improvement.

Corrective exercise as home-care advice

In order for the therapist to assist the client in gaining the maximum benefit from some salon treatments, e.g. neuro-muscular electrical stimulation, they need to have a basic understanding of the use of corrective exercise. A number of therapists develop an interest in exercise and take up specialist exercise courses which enable them to teach and fully advise on exercise programmes. There are also a great many books on types of exercises, mobility, muscle strength and fitness testing that would be useful further study.

Before advising any corrective exercises it is important to consider the:

- Age and mobility of the client.
- Muscle strength of the client.
- General health of the client.
- Past history of exercise of the client.
- Environment in which the exercises will be carried out.

information point

- Youth does not always indicate that the fitness and mobility of a client are good.
- Mobility often deteriorates with age as people tend not to use their full range of movement. The therapist can test a client's mobility by checking the extent of their range of movement through the joints.
- Muscle strength can be determined by testing through resistance-type exercises the strength of the client's muscles in different areas of the body.
- The strength and tone of a muscle increase with regular exercise.

Isotonic exercise

Isotonic exercise is a form of exercise that produces lengthening and shortening of the muscle fibres by movement of the joints, e.g. active exercise (exercise with movement).

Concentric and *eccentric* muscle work relates to isotonic exercise. Concentric is where the fibres, through shortening, become thicker, e.g. the biceps when the arm is bent. Eccentric is where the muscle fibres, through movement, lengthen, e.g. the triceps when the arm is bent.

Isometric exercise

Isometric exercise causes the muscle fibres to contract without an overall change of length in the muscle, e.g. passive exercise (exercise without movement).

Corrective exercise

Corrective exercises may be recommended to supplement salon treatments providing the therapist is happy that there are no underlying medical conditions. The normal pattern of exercise sequences would include warm-up exercises, aerobic exercises, strengthening and stretching exercises and a cool-down/relaxation period.

Warm-up exercises

Warm-up exercises prepare the body's physiology for action and so reduce the risk of injury. They should include:

- Mobility exercises (within the normal range of movement).
- General activity to gradually increase the heart and respiration rates and to stimulate circulation.
- Static stretches of the muscles to be exercised, held for 6–8 seconds.

Aerobic exercises

Aerobic exercises provide a sustained period of exercise at the correct level of intensity to increase the heart rate into the training zone. They should include:

- Build-up aerobics.
- Peak aerobics.
- Cool-down aerobics.

Strengthening and stretching exercises

Strengthening and stretching exercises are used to build up muscle strength and improve mobility. They can be used to correct postural conditions. Examples of exercises follow.

1 Arm lift – a strength exercise for kyphosis

Purpose – To strengthen scapular adductors and help prevent or correct round shoulders and kyphosis.

Position – **a** Least difficult: lie prone with arms in reverse 'T'; forehead resting on floor.

      – **b** More advanced: same as before except arms are extended overhead and held against the ears.

Movement – Maintain the arm position and contract the muscles between the shoulder blades, lifting the arms as high as possible without raising head and trunk. Hold, relax and repeat.

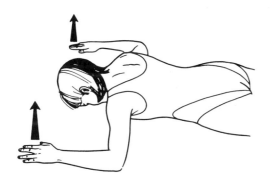

Arm lift

2 Wand exercise – a stretch exercise for kyphosis

Purpose – To help prevent and correct round shoulders and kyphosis by stretching the muscles on the anterior side of the shoulder joint.

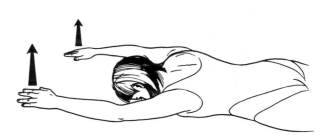

Position – Sit with wand grasped at ends. Raise wand overhead. Be certain that the head does not slide forward into a 'poke neck' position. Keep the chin tucked and neck straight.

Movement – Bring the wand down behind the shoulder blades. Keep spine erect. Hold.

Hands may be moved closer together to increase stretch on chest muscles.

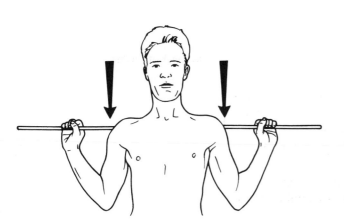

Wand exercise

HEALTH AND BEAUTY THERAPY: A PRACTICAL APPROACH

3 Pelvic tilt – a strength exercise for lordosis

Purpose – To strengthen the abdominals and help prevent or correct lumbar lordosis and backache.

Position – Supine with knees bent.

Movement – Tighten the abdominal muscles and tilt the pelvis backward; try to flatten the lower back against the floor. At the same time, tighten the hip and thigh muscles. Hold then relax. Breathe normally during the contraction, do not hold the breath.

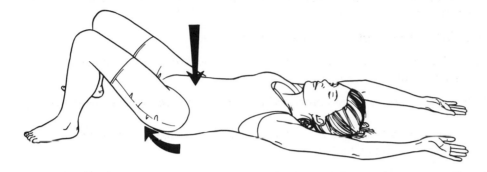

Pelvic tilt

4 Low back stretcher – a stretch exercise for lordosis

Purpose – To stretch hip flexors and lumbar muscles, and help prevent or correct lumbar lordosis and backache.

Position – Supine position.

Movement – Draw one knee up to the chest and pull it down tightly with the hands, then slowly return it to the original position. Repeat with other knee. Do not grasp knee, but the thigh. If a partner or a weight stabilises the extended leg, the hip flexor muscles of that leg will also be stretched.

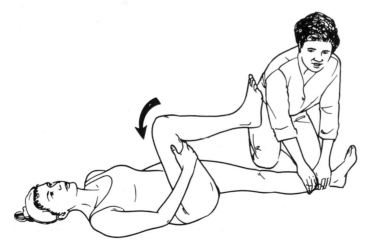

Low back stretcher

The therapist needs to advise on suitable exercises to stretch the shortened muscles and strengthen the lengthened muscles, ensuring the starting position is appropriate to the client's mobility, muscle strength, balance and age range, e.g. an older client with unsteady balance would be more suited to exercises performed in a sitting position on a steady chair.

Isotonic and isometric exercises can be used and gradually, as muscle strength improves, resistance exercises using available home weights, e.g. jars of coffee, can be used to strengthen the arm muscles.

Cool-down/relaxation period

Cool down/relaxation exercises allow the body to cool down gradually and control breathing.

SELF-CHECKS

1 Describe how you would recognise the following conditions:
   a soft fat
   b hard fat
   c cellulite
   d stretch marks
   e dowager's hump
   f midriff bulge.

2 Explain what is meant by the following terms:
   a kyphosis
   b lordosis
   c scoliosis.

3 Before recommending corrective exercise home-care advice, what factors would you take into consideration?

4 Define the following terms:
   a isotonic exercise
   b isometric exercise
   c concentric muscle work
   d eccentric muscle work.

Physical fitness

Every physical activity undertaken needs the body to produce energy from food digested and absorbed by the body. There are two systems which release energy from food: the aerobic system and the anaerobic system.

The aerobic system provides energy for prolonged activity, i.e. for most activity. The anaerobic system provides energy for short periods of activity (up to 10 seconds) and can be thought of as an 'emergency' system. The aerobic system utilises carbohydrates and fats to obtain energy whereas the anaerobic system utilises only carbohydrates. The body switches to the anaerobic system when the aerobic system cannot produce enough energy for the body's needs. Once the anaerobic system cannot produce enough energy, the body tires and needs to rest until waste products produced by the anaerobic system are removed. How well the aerobic and anaerobic systems work is one measure of physical fitness and is important for health.

Components of physical fitness may be classified as either health-related components or skill-related components.

Health-related components of physical fitness are:

- Cardiovascular fitness.
- Muscular endurance.
- Muscular strength.
- Flexibility.
- Body composition.

Skill-related components of physical fitness are:

- Agility.
- Balance.
- Co-ordination.
- Speed.
- Power.
- Reaction time.

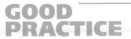

Cardiovascular fitness

Cardiovascular fitness is a measure of the efficiency of the respiratory and circulatory systems. It is a term used to indicate how effectively oxygen is taken into the body and transported to the working muscles for energy and how effectively the waste produced is removed by the body.

A person who is considered to have a high cardio-respiratory endurance, i.e. they can exercise for a fair period of time at increased heart rate and recover reasonably fast, can be assumed to be 'aerobically fit'.

Exercise to test for cardiovascular fitness – running in place
Run in place for 1½ minutes (at a rate of 120 steps per minute). Rest for 1 minute and count the heart rate for 30 seconds. A heart rate of 60 or lower passes.

Examples of aerobic activity, i.e. activity that improves cardiovascular fitness, are jogging, swimming, brisk walking and aerobics.

Muscular endurance

This refers to the individual's ability to repeatedly use the same muscle or muscles without getting tired. Many athletes display high muscular endurance, e.g. swimmers and long distance runners.

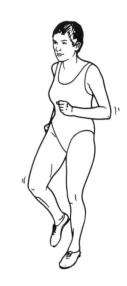

Running in place

Exercise to test for muscular endurance – side leg raise
Lie on the floor on your side. Lift your leg up and to the side of the body until your feet are 24–36 inches apart. Hold for as long as possible. Perform ten repetitions with each leg.

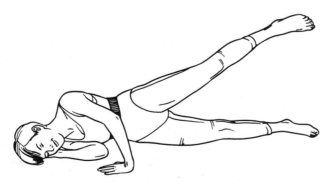

Side leg raise

Isometric examples of muscular endurance exercises are: gluteal squeeze, pelvic tilt, arm press.

Isotonic examples of muscular endurance exercises are: squats, curl ups, back extensions.

Muscular strength

Muscular strength describes the amount of force an individual muscle or group of muscles can produce in overcoming a resistance in one maximum voluntary contraction, e.g. lifting a heavy weight.

Muscular strength can be tested by using dynamometers or manual tests for different parts of the body, e.g. press ups for the arms and chest.

Exercise to test muscular strength – press ups

Lie face down on the floor. Place the hands under the shoulders. Keeping the legs and body straight, press off the floor until the arms are fully extended. Women repeat once, men three times.

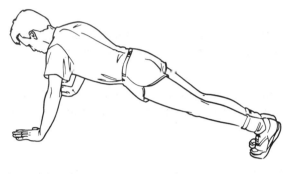

Press ups

Examples of muscular strength exercises are press ups and exercises done with variable resistance machines and free weights.

Flexibility

Flexibility can be measured by a person's range of movement. Flexibility will actually determine how an athlete can perform, because if muscles are tight and joints are inflexible, agility, range of movement, balance and speed are all restricted.

Exercise for testing flexibility of the hamstrings and lower back – toe touch

Sit on the floor with your feet against a wall. Keep the feet together and the knees straight. Bend forward at the hips. Reach forward and touch your closed fists to the wall. Bend forward slowly, do not bounce.

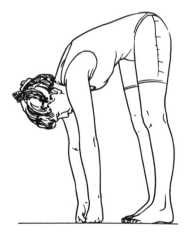

Toe touch

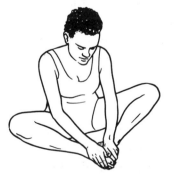

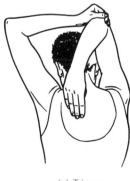

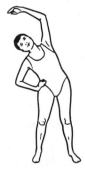

(a) Triceps	(b) Adductors	(c) Obliques

Examples of flexibility exercises

Body composition

The composition of a person's body refers to the relative percentages of muscle, fat, bone and other tissues that make up the body. It can be thought of as a measure of whether a person is under- or overweight, i.e. has a low or high percentage of body fat.

Body composition can be measured by using calibrated skin callipers. Four measurements are taken from different parts of the body. These measurements are then compared with a chart of accepted norms and an estimate of the percentage of body fat read off. This test can also be performed manually.

Manual measurement of body composition – the pinch

Have a partner pinch a fold of skin on the back of your upper arm halfway between the tip of the elbow and the tip of the shoulder. Measurements of 2.5 cm (1 inch) for men and 4 cm (1½ inches) for women are acceptable.

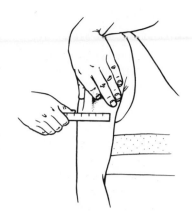

Measuring body composition

Agility

Agility is the ability to rapidly and accurately change the direction of the entire body in space. Examples of sports that require agility are skiing and wrestling.

Balance

Balance is the maintenance of equilibrium whilst stationary or moving. Balance is very important in gymnastic beam exercises and water skiing.

Co-ordination

Co-ordination is a person's ability to use the senses, e.g. sight and hearing, in conjunction with the body parts to perform motor tasks smoothly and accurately. Good co-ordination is needed for golf.

Speed

Speed is the ability to perform a movement in a short period of time, e.g. running.

Power

Power is a person's ability to transfer energy into force at a fast rate. Discus throwing requires power.

Reaction time

A person's reaction time is the time elapsed between stimulation and the beginning of reaction to that stimulation, e.g. from starting block to sprint take-off.

Fitness testing

Before anyone undertakes an exercise regime in a professionally supervised leisure club or gym it is usual, after their initial consultation, that they be given a test to establish their level of fitness. A fitness test is used to assess where an individual's strengths and weaknesses lie, to meet the perceived needs of the client and to prevent injury.

Tests vary in their degree of sophistication depending upon the requirement of the client. Such tests should include measurements of:

- Height and weight.
- Peak flow.
- Cardiovascular fitness.
- Body composition, i.e. percentage body fat.

Conclusions are reached on an individual's fitness by comparing test results against accepted norms related to age, sex and body type.

information point

- Research indicates that a person's weight at the age of 21 could indicate how long their life expectancy will be. Those that achieve their ideal weight (based on BMI) at a youthful age are more likely to remain healthy and have a long life.
- A healthy BMI range is gauged between 18.5–25; 25–30 is overweight; 30+ is obese.
- To calculate your BMI: write down your height in metres; multiply your height by itself (which gives you your height squared); write down your weight in kilograms; divide your weight by your height squared.

ACTIVITY

Perform tests to identify a client's level of cardiovascular fitness, muscular strength and endurance and flexibility.

Considerations for safe exercise

All the following should be taken into consideration when assessing whether exercise at a particular level is safe for a client:

- Heart conditions; high blood pressure; dizziness.
- Severe respiratory conditions; asthma.
- Fever.
- Recent operations.
- Broken bones.
- Other medical conditions such as diabetes, epilepsy and pregnancy.
- Whether the client has eaten a heavy meal or consumed alcohol.

Always remember that every exercise if not performed correctly is potentially dangerous!

ACTIVITY

Devise a suitable exercise plan for:

a a 50-year-old female client with lordosis
b a 30-year-old female office worker with kyphosis
c a 40-year-old postman with scoliosis.

Name   Date

Address

Tel. no.

Date of birth

Medical history

High blood pressre   Medication

Asthma   Number of pregnancies

Dizziness/fainting   Ages of children

Anaemia

Weight   Frame size

Height   % Body fat

Reason for exercise:

Lose fat ( )   Change appearance ( )   Gain strength ( )   Feel fitter ( )

Sports performance ( )   Doctor's advice ( )   Social ( )   Other

---

Example of an exercise consultation card

1. Explain the difference between the aerobic and anaerobic systems.
2. Describe the following components of health-related fitness:
   a cardiovascular fitness
   b muscular strength
   c muscular endurance
   d flexibility
   e body composition.
3. Explain the different components of skill-related fitness.
4. State the considerations for safe exercise.
5. List the points that should be noted on an exercise consultation card.

You need to know what these words and phrases mean. Go back through the chapter to find out.

Basal metabolism

Body types

Carbohydrates

Components of fitness

Eating problems

Fats

Fibre

Good posture

Isotonic and isometric exercise

Metabolism

Mineral elements

Nutrition

Proteins

Types of diets

Vitamins

Bibliography and further reading

Arnould-Taylor, William, *A Textbook of Anatomy and Physiology*, 3rd edition, Stanley Thornes (Publishers) Ltd, 1998.

Brown, Denise, *Aromatherapy*, Headway Lifeguides Series, 1993.

Burns, E. and Blamey, C., 'Soothing Scents in Childbirth' in *International Journal of Aromatherapy*, 1994 vol. 4 no. 1.

Cartwright, Elizabeth, Morris, Gill and Severn, Michelle, *Electro-epilation: A Practical Approach*, 2nd edition, Nelson Thornes, 2001.

Corney, J., *Anthropology for Designers*, Batsford Academic and Educational Ltd, 1980.

Cowmeadow, O., *The Art of Shiatsu*, Element Books Ltd, 1992.

Cullum, Rodney and Mowbray, Leslie, *YMCA Guide to Exercise Music*, YMCA.

Davis, P., *Aromatherapy, an A–Z*, C. W. Daniel Company Ltd, 1990.

Fire, M., 'Providing Massage Therapy in a Psychiatric Hospital' in *International Journal of Alternative and Complementary Medicine*, June 1994.

Franks, B. Don and Howley, Edward T., *Fitness Leader's Handbook*, Human Kinetics Europe Ltd, 1989.

Goldberg, Lyn, *Massage and Aromatherapy: A Practical Approach*, 2nd edition, Nelson Thornes, 2001.

Gray FRS, Henry, *Gray's Anatomy*, Courage Books, 1999.

Henry, J. *et al.*, 'Lavender for Night Sedation of People with Dementia' in *International Journal of Aromatherapy*, 1994 vol. 6 no. 2.

International School of Aromatherapy, *A Safety Guide on the Use of Essential Oils*, Nature by Nature Oils Ltd, London, 1993.

Kasner, K. and Tindall, D. H., *Ballière's Nurses Dictionary*, Ballière Tindall, 1984.

Lavabre, M., *Aromatherapy Workbook*, Healing Arts Press, USA, 1990.

Lawless, Julia, *The Encyclopaedia of Essential Oils*, Element Books Ltd, 1992.

Lewis, Roger and Trevitt, Roger, *Business for Advanced GNVQ*, 2nd edition, Nelson Thornes, 2001.

Mernagh-Ward, Dawn and Cartwright, Jennifer, *Good Practice in Salon Management*, Stanley Thornes (Publishers) Ltd, 1997.

Pitman, V. and MacKenzie, K., *Reflexology: A Practical Approach*, Stanley Thornes (Publishers) Ltd, 1997.

Price, S., *Practical Aromatherapy*, Thorsons Publishing Group, 1987.

Sanderson, H. and Ruddle, J., 'Aromatherapy and Occupational Therapy' in *British Journal of Occupational Therapy*, 1992, 55(8).

Simmons, John V., *Science and the Beauty Business: The Beauty Salon and its Equipment*, Vol. 2, Thomson Learning, 1995.

Simms, Janet, *A Practical Guide to Beauty Therapy*, 3rd edition, Nelson Thornes (Publishers) Ltd, 2003.

Simpkins, J. and Williams, J. I., *Advanced Human Biology*, Collins Educational, 1992.

Tisserand, R., 'Aromatherapy Today' in *International Journal of Aromatherapy*, 1993 vol. 5 no. 4.

Winwood, R. S. and Smith, J. L., *Sear's Anatomy and Physiology for Nurses*, Edward Arnold, 1985.

Woolfson, A. and Hewitt, D., 'Intensive Aroma Care' in *International Journal of Aromatherapy*, 1992 vol. 4 no. 2.

Index

Page references in *italics* indicate figures or tables

HEALTH AND BEAUTY THERAPY: A PRACTICAL APPROACH